Quality of life : the
new medical dilemma /

QUALITY OF LIFE

THE NEW
MEDICAL
DILEMMA

EDITED BY
JAMES J. WALTER
THOMAS A. SHANNON

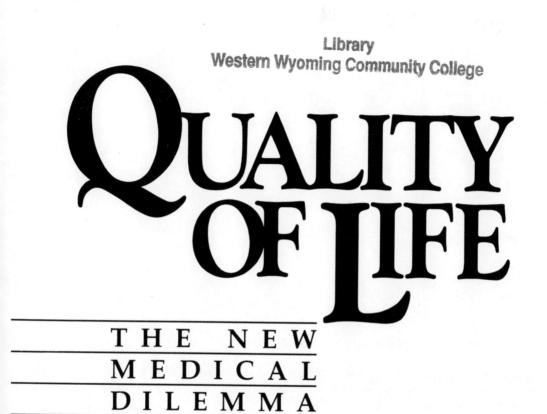

PAULIST PRESS
New York and Mahwah, N.J.

Library of Congress Cataloging-in-Publication Data

Quality of life: the new medical dilemma/by James J. Walter and
    Thomas A. Shannon, eds.
        p.   cm.
    Includes bibliographical references.
    ISBN 0-8091-3191-9
    1. Medical ethics.   2. Quality of life.   I. Walter, James J.
II. Shannon, Thomas A. (Thomas Anthony), 1940–
R724.Q35   1990
174′.24—dc20   90-41235
                                                                                                 CIP

Published by Paulist Press
997 Macarthur Boulevard
Mahwah, New Jersey 07430

Printed and bound in the United States of America

Contents

Medical Issues

Part 2
APPLICATIONS

Prenatal Diagnosis and Abortion

Imperiled Newborns

The Permanently Unconscious Patient

Care of the Elderly

Euthanasia and Assisted Suicide

Part 3
PUBLIC POLICY

Precedents

Guidelines

TO
MARYANNE WALTER
CATHERINE HAENN SHANNON

Who, through their constancy, patience, and good humor
have graciously increased the quality of our lives.

Foreword: An Overview of "Quality of Life"

We live in a society that is increasingly concerned with quality. Automobile manufacturers appeal to us to buy their cars by trying to convince us that for them "Quality is Job 1," and the motels in which we stay are even called "Quality Inns." The ecology movement has made us patently aware that the quality of the air we breathe is being compromised, if not poisoned, by the burning of fossil fuels. It should not be surprising, then, that our concerns about the quality of the products we buy and with the quality of the environment we inhabit have led to discussions about the very quality of life itself. When the term "quality of life" is used in a medical setting, some think that it is a code to justify the disposal of all the people whom individuals or society find problematic in one way or another. In this case, the term conjures up pejorative connotations and sinister overtones. For others, quality of life is a term which captures the very essence of how we evaluate the benefit-burden ratio involved in various medical treatments that are offered to us.

"Quality of life" obviously has a variety of meanings and connotations. Its use ranges from judgments about whether one should live at all, to the conditions under which one will live, to evaluations of life-style, and to considered judgments by patients about how medicine corresponds to their beliefs and aspirations. None of these usages is synonymous, of course, and frequently they are contradictory.

Consider, for example, quality of life in relation to the question of whether one should be allowed to live. Here we can think of the Nazi era and the term *lebenunwertes Leben*—life unworthy of life. What made such a life unworthy, of course, was primarily the fact of being Jewish, but it also included the conditions of mental illness and insanity. The critical issue here is that certain lives were considered unworthy of being lived. Today quality of life is often used in a neonatal context, and its application initiates a process of decision making when there is, for example, a genetic abnormality or a major physiological defect. In this situation the child's life is not considered unworthy, but perhaps it is so burdened or compromised that continued existence itself may be too onerous.

Quality of life has also been used in reference to the conditions under which one lives. In many ways this term refers to the traditional concepts of "burdensomeness" or "extraordinary means" that are found in traditional moral analysis. The insight here is that the conditions under which one lives or is forced to live may be so burdensome that there is no obligation to pursue medical treatment in order to preserve life. Yet this concept, too, has been extended in ways that are quite controversial, e.g., abortion for sex selection. While this practice does not appear to be common, it is nevertheless a reality. Morally less abhorrent but equally problematic are technologies that assist in the conception of a child. When quality of life is applied in this context it can refer to the intellectual powers, artistic capabilities, athletic abilities, or physical attributes that are desired by parents for their children. What is interesting in such lists is the universal absence of qualities such as kindness, gentleness, honesty, and generosity. Thus quality of life frequently reflects the social biases and prejudices that are used to evaluate the conditions under which we live. Similar to several other interpretations of quality, this concept equates the value of life with the presence or absence of various characteristics or attributes.

Quality of life can also refer to our expectations and aspirations, and the only boundaries of its application in these instances may be our imagination or the limit of our credit card. The connotation here is distinctively consumerist, and the intent is to get the best deal one can. The bumper-sticker slogan "Whoever Dies With The Most Toys Wins" and the television program "Life Styles of the Rich and Famous" quickly come to mind. Quality of life is interpreted in terms of the quantity of material goods that can be amassed during one's life, and conspicuous consumption is used as a minimal standard of well-being. Those who are on the margins of society or those who refuse to take part in such a life-style are simply dismissed or defined as insignificant.

Finally, one can also think of quality of life as referring to how a person chooses to live under the constraints imposed by biological and social conditions and the limits (technical or ethical) of modern medicine. In other words, the term can refer to personal choices about one's own life, how it is to be lived and the extent to which medicine will or will not be utilized in achieving one's own goals. This individualist perspective, which is also open to the problems of the consumerist model, can effectively blunt any social evaluation of the conditions under which people should live or of the personal qualities that they should possess.

The purpose of this book is to present an overview of many aspects of the quality of life debate vis-à-vis medical decision making. That the question is significant is attested to by the sheer quantity of articles available on the topic. Thus we were faced with the typical editorial difficulty of choosing criteria for the inclusion or exclusion of various articles. We resolved this issue by focusing on three broad areas: definitional, applications, and public policy. In this way we hope to indicate the range of the discussion and yet make the topic manageable by thematically arranging the articles.

In the definitional section we focus on the various ways of defining quality of life: philosophical, theological and medical. While each of these disciplines approaches the topic differently, common issues and concepts do, in fact, emerge.

Part 2 presents a variety of applications of quality of life to specific medical situations. Here we examine issues surrounding prenatal diagnosis and abortion, imperiled newborns, the permanently unconscious patient and the use of fluids and nutrition, the care of the elderly, and finally the questions of euthanasia and assisted suicide of the critically ill. These are all areas in which quality of life has been frequently and often problematically applied. Because it is in the area of application that most of the controversies about the term have occurred, we wish to offer a representative sample of perspectives.

Finally, in Part 3 we turn to the discussion of public policy, because it is at this level that the social implications of quality of life will be debated and, perhaps, implemented. We present two areas for examination: precedents and guidelines. The intent of this section is to concentrate clearly on how quality of life has recently been discussed or implemented through legislative, professional and ecclesiastical bodies. This section will show the present state of the question and will also suggest ways for shaping future debates.

We would like to thank Loyola University of Chicago for the support that it has given to this project.

James J. Walter
Loyola University of Chicago

Thomas A. Shannon
Worcester Polytechnic Institute

Part 1

DEFINITIONAL ISSUES

part 1

Introduction

The purpose of this first section of the volume is to present a variety of definitions of quality of life from different points of view. Because there is no one definition of the concept, the use of quality of life considerations in the clinical setting becomes somewhat problematic. If these considerations are to play any role in our decisions to forgo or withdraw medical treatment, then it is important at the start to establish a proper definition of quality of life itself.

A range of issues is involved in attempting to define what is meant by quality of life. Are all quality of life judgments necessarily subjective and thus, implicitly at least, involve social and personal biases, or are there any objective criteria to which one can appeal in making these judgments? In other words, can we locate any objective medical indicators that can truly measure quality of life, or do all these indicators themselves reflect prior human evaluations or value judgments? If we cannot escape value judgments in establishing and formulating criteria, then whose value judgments should be included in the criteria?

Some argue that quality of life refers to a specific characteristic or attribute that must be present before we can consider a patient worthy of moral respect and therefore a candidate for medical treatment. Others believe that the concept should not focus on the conditions which allow patients to act comfortably, well or without burden, but rather it should focus on the conditions which allow patients to act at all. Yet others argue that we should never permit the use of quality of life judgments in medical decision making because inevitably these judgments involve a comparison of the social worth of patients' lives.

One of the major tenets of the Judeo-Christian tradition has been that each person is created in the image of God, and consequently this tradition has considered every human life to be inherently valuable. The moral principle of "sanctity of life" has often been derived from this religious tenet. Is it the case that the use of quality of life considerations in the clinical setting will ultimately undermine this moral principle, or do these considerations in fact further specify the very meaning of sanctity of life? The Judeo-Christian tradition has historically sought to avoid any form of medical vitalism, which is a view that requires patients to be treated in all circumstances and under any condition because life is considered an absolute value. Consequently, one might ask if some form of the quality of life principle is not already implicit in the sanctity of life position adopted by this religious tradition? Answers to these questions necessarily involve not only a theological judgment about what is worthy of being an absolute value, but also entail normative moral judgments about what is valuable about human life itself. Such theological and moral issues are at least implicit in each of the essays that follow in this section.

Further Readings

Baier, Kurt. "Towards a Definition of 'Quality of Life.' " In *Environmental Spectrum,* eds. Ronald
    O. Clarke and Peter C. List (New York: D. Van Nostrand Co., 1974), pp. 58–81.

Callahan, Daniel. "The Quality of Life: What Does It Mean?." In *That They May Live: Theological
    Reflections on the Quality of Life,* ed. George Devine. Proceedings of the College Theology
    Society. (New York: Alba House/Society of St. Paul, 1972), pp. 3–16.

Cohen, Carl. "On the Quality of Life: Some Philosophical Reflections," *Circulation* 66(1982):
    29–33.

Connery, John R., S.J. "Prolonging Life: The Duty and Its Limits," *Linacre Quarterly* 47(May 1980):
    151–165.

Diamond, Eugene F. "Quality vs. Sanctity of Life in the Nursery," *America* 135(December 4, 1976):
    396–398.

Edlund, Matthew and Tancredi, Laurence R. "Quality of Life: An Ideological Critique," *Perspec-
    tives in Biology and Medicine* 28(Summer 1985): 591–607.

Jonsen, Albert, Ph.D.; Siegler, Mark, M.D.; and Winslade, William J., Ph.D., J.D., eds. "Quality of
    Life." In *Clinical Ethics: A Practical Approach to Ethical Decisions in Clinical Medicine,* 2nd
    ed. (New York: Macmillan, 1986), pp. 101–116.

McCormick, Richard A., S.J. "A Proposal for 'Quality of Life' Criteria for Sustaining Life," *Hospi-
    tal Progress* 56(September, 1975): 76–79.

——— "The Quality of Life, The Sanctity of Life," *Hastings Center Report* 8(February, 1978):
    30–36.

Pellegrino, Edmund D. and Thomasma, David C. "Quality-of-Life Judgments and Medical Indica-
    tions." In *For the Patient's Good: The Restoration of Beneficence in Health Care* (New York:
    Oxford University Press, 1988), pp. 92–98.

Reich, Warren T. "Quality of Life." In *Encyclopedia of Bioethics,* Vol 2, ed. Warren T. Reich (New
    York: The Free Press, 1978), pp. 829–840.

PHILOSOPHICAL AND
THEOLOGICAL ISSUES

1

Four Indicators of Humanhood—
The Enquiry Matures

Joseph F. Fletcher

Jean Rostand describes a meeting of French
Catholic intellectuals; they spoke of a prosecution for infanticide following the thalidomide
disaster of the Sixties.[1] Morvan Lebesque:
"After centuries of morality, we still cannot
answer questions like those raised by the trial
in Liege. Should malformed babies be killed?
Where does man begin?" Father Jolif: "No one
knows what man is any longer."

That is the situation, exactly. Whether or
not we ever knew in the past what man is, in
the sense of having a consensus about it, we do
not know now. To realize this, make only a
quick scan of the wild confusion and variety
on the subject gathered together by Erich
Fromm and Ramon Xirau in their historical
compendium.[2]

First There Was One

Yet it is this question, how we are to define
the *humanum*, which lies at the base of all serious talk about the quality of life. We cannot
appraise quality or enumerate human values if
we cannot first say what a human being is. The
Hastings Center Report (November, 1972)
published a shortened version of an essay of
mine in which I made a stab at this problem,
under the title "Indicators of Humanhood: A
Tentative Profile of Man."[3]

In substance I contended that the acute
question is what is a *person;* that rights (such as
survival) attach only to persons; that out of
some twenty criteria one (neocortical function) is the cardinal or hominizing trait upon
which all the other human traits hinge; and
then I invited those concerned to add or sub-
tract, agree or disagree as they may. This was
intended to keep the investigation going forward, and it worked; the issue has been vigorously discussed pro and con.

What crystals have precipitated? Without
trying to explore them in any detail, as each of
them deserves to be, four different traits have
been nominated to date as the singular *esse* of

---

*"Four Indicators of Humanhood—The Enquiry Matures" by Joseph Fletcher. Reprinted with
permission of Joseph Fletcher and* The Hastings Center Report 4*(December, 1975):4–7.*

The original

INDICATORS OF HUMANHOOD: A TENTATIVE PROFILE OF MAN

by Joseph F. Fletcher

Positive Human Criteria

1. Minimal intelligence
2. Self-awareness
3. Self-control
4. A sense of time
5. A sense of futurity
6. A sense of the past
7. The capability to relate to others
8. Concern for others
9. Communication
10. Control of existence
11. Curiosity
12. Change and changeability
13. Balance of rationality and feeling
14. Idiosyncrasy
15. Neo-cortical function

Negative Human Criteria

1. Man is not non- or anti-artificial
2. Man is not essentially parental
3. Man is not essentially sexual
4. Man is not a bundle of rights
5. Man is not a worshiper

---

humanness: neocortical function, self-consciousness, relational ability, and happiness—the last being included more in a light than a heavy vein. Various additional criteria of the optimal or *bene esse* kind are mentioned in a growing correspondence, but no argument *against* any one of them has been offered; e.g., one correspondent (Robert Morison) wants concern for the meek and dependent stipulated under my eighth trait, "concern for others."

But on the question which one of the optimal traits and capabilities is the *sine qua non*, the essential one without which no combination of the others can add up to humanhood, there are now four contenders in the running. It should be noted at the outset that of the four discrete cardinal criteria thus far entered, none of them is mutually exclusive of any of the others, any more than the optimal indicators are (sense of time, curiosity, ideomorphous identity, obligation, reason-feeling balance, self-control, changeability, etc.). The decisive question therefore appears to be about precondition. Which one of these traits, if any, is required for the presence of the others? To answer this is to find *the* criterion among the criteria.

Now There Are Four

I. Michael Tooley of Stanford contends that the real precondition to "having a serious right to life" or to being the kind of moral entity we call a person, as in the Sixteenth Amendment sense, is subjectivity or self-awareness (no. 2 in my original list). He called it "the self-consciousness requirement."[4] As he points out, fetuses and infants lack that requirement. Machines have no consciousness at all, and therefore may be sacrificed in a competing values situation. Animals are probably not self-conscious, although a few pet lovers claim they are. Once a growing baby's neurological "switchboard" gets hooked up, allowing consciousness of self to emerge, he or she is a person. (Mind is, as Dubos points out, a verb—not a noun; it is not something given but acquired, a process rather than an event.[5] It is what the mind does, not what it is.) So runs Tooley's thesis.

II. Richard McCormick of the Kennedy Center for Bioethics at Georgetown University, on another tack, says "the meaning, substance, and consummation of life is found in human relationships," so that when we try to make quality of life judgments ("and we must"), as in cases of diseased or defective newborns, "life is a value to be preserved only insofar as it contains some potentiality for human relationships."[6] On this basis anencephalics certainly, and idiots probably, lack personal status, with a consequent lack of claim upon rights. If you lack what he calls "the relational potential" (what I call "the capability to relate to others," no. 7) you cannot be human. "If that potential is simply nonexistent or would be utterly submerged and undeveloped in the mere struggle to survive, that life has achieved its potential" and we need not save it from death's approach.

III. When a pediatrician at the Texas Medical Center (Houston), whose work takes her daily into a service for retarded children, heard me at a grand rounds expound my suggestion that minimal intelligence or cerebral function is the essential factor in being human, she rejected it: "I know a little four-year-old boy, certainly 20 minus or an idiot on any measurement scale and untrainable, but just the same he is a human being and nobody is going to tell me different. He is happy and that makes him human, as human as you or I." By "human" she meant morally, not only biologically. She described the child's affectionate responses to caresses and his constant euphoria. I thought of my neighbor's kitten and recalled the euphoria symptom as happiness without any reason for it, and I remembered Huxley's *Brave New World* where everybody was happy on drugs—except the rebellious intellectuals. I asked her if she really meant to say that euphoria qualifies us for humanhood. I took her silence to be an affirmative answer.

IV. As far as I can yet see, I will stand by my own thesis or hypothesis that neocortical function is the key to humanness, the essential trait, the human *sine qua non*. The point is that without the synthesizing function of the cerebral cortex (without thought or mind), whether before it is present or with its end, the person is nonexistent no matter how much the individual's brain stem and mid-brain may continue to provide feelings and regulate autonomic physical functions. To be truly Homo sapiens we must be sapient, however minimally. Only this trait or capability is necessary to *all* of the other traits which go into the fullness of humanness. Therefore this indicator, neocortical function, is the first-order requirement and the key to the definition of a human being. As Robert Williams of the University Medical Center (Seattle) puts it, "Without mentation the body is of no significant use."[7]

Discussion Goes On

This search for a *shared* view of humanness, a consensus, may not find a happy ending. James Gustafson's (University of Chicago Divinity School) skepticism about reaching agreement has now been graduated into skepticism also about applying whatever criterion we might agree to.[8] He thinks now that "intuitive elements, grounded on beliefs and profound feelings," would color our judgments seriously. More sharply, Rostand warns us (p. 66) that looking for a single trait is "a temptation for the fanatics—and there are always fanatics everywhere—to think that his adversary is less human than himself because he lacks some mental or spiritual quality." In scientific and medical circles I find that a *biological* definition is thought to be feasible, but not a list of moral or psychological traits—to say nothing of picking out only one cardinal trait subsumed in all the rest.

One slant on the problem is to deny the problem itself, not as insoluble but as specious (no pun intended). For example, William May of Catholic University, trying to justify the pro-

hibition of abortion, objects to "the thought of Fletcher, Tooley, and those who would agree with them" that membership in a *species* is of no moral significance.[9] He argues that we are human by virtue of what we are (our species), not what we achieve or do. A member of the biological species is, as such, a human being. Thus, we would be human if we have opposable thumbs, are capable of face-to-face coitus and have a brain weighing 1400 grams, whether a particular brain functions cerebrally or not. (I put in the thumbs and coitus to exclude elephants, whales and dolphins, the only other species having brains as big or bigger than man's.) In this reasoning the term "human" slides back and forth between meaning sometimes the biological, sometimes the moral or personal, thus combining fallacy of ambiguity with the fallacy of ostensive definition. ("He has opposable thumbs, therefore he is a person.")

Tristram Engelhardt of the Texas Medical Branch (Galveston) takes a different path; he renounces not the need to define humanhood but the attempt to single out any one crucial or essential indicator.[10] Instead, he is synoptic in the same manner that René Dubos has so superbly shown us in *Man Adapting* and *So Human an Animal*. Engelhardt distinguishes the biological from personal life but follows a multifactorial, non-univocal line. Indeed, he points precisely to the traits elected in all three of the major univocal definitions discussed here; together they compose his own—cerebral function, self-consciousness, and relationship or the societal dimension. Yet it is difficult, studying his language, not to believe that he gives cerebral function the determinative place, as when he says that "for a person to be embodied and present in the world he must be conscious in it," but follows that up by adding, "The brain is the singular focus of the embodiment of the mind, and in its absence man as a person is absent" (p. 21).

Being careful in all this is supremely important. Leonard Weber of Detroit urges "caution in adopting a neocortical definition of death" because this is tantamount to a definition of personhood, although he doesn't throw it out of court. He further asks us to make sure "the biological is not being under-valued as a component of human life."[11] On both scores I agree. I take "caution" to mean carefulness, which is always in order, and I certainly want to affirm our physical side, since why even talk of cerebral function apart from a cerebrum? "Mind is meat" may be too crass, but I agree that it contains a vital truth.

Rapprochement?

To Tooley and McCormick I would want to say, "You are on sound ground, so far." Of all the optimal traits of a full and authentic human life, I am inclined with you to give top importance to awareness of self (Tooley's cardinal and my optimal trait no. 2) and to the capacity for interpersonal and social relations (McCormick's cardinal and my optimal traits no. 7 and no. 8). But I still want to reason that *their* key indicators are only factors at all because of *my* key criterion—cerebral function. Is this not an issue to be carefully weighed?

Rizzo and Yonder of Canisius College, Buffalo, have argued the case for the neocortical definition.[12] Their conclusion is that "when there is incontrovertible evidence of neocortical death, the human life has ceased." To Professor Tooley and Father McCormick I would say, "Neocortical death means that both self-consciousness and other-orientedness are gone, whereas neither non-self-consciousness nor inability to relate to others means the end

of neocortical activity." Just remember amnesia victims when self-consciousness is proposed as the key; just remember radically autistic and schizophrenic patients when the relational key is proposed. The amnesiac has lost his identity, his selfhood, and the psychotic is still *thinking*, no matter how falsely and in what disorder. On these grounds we cannot declare that such individuals are no longer persons, just as we cannot do so at some levels of mental retardation. Only irreversible coma or a decerebrate state is ground for such a serious determination. It seems that possibly the neocortical key is more conservative than some observers of the ethical debate suppose.

The importance of self-awareness is obvious. Abraham Maslow has taught this generation that much. Being able to recognize and respond to others is of the greatest importance to being truly human, as Gordon Allport's interpersonalism made plain. But as Julius Korein, the New York University neurologist, tells us, "Basic to the definition of the death of an individual is identification of the irreversible destruction of that critical component of the system which represents the essence of the person," and that essence, he says, is "cerebral death."[13] The "vegetable" patient, no matter how many spontaneous vital functions may be continuing, is dead, a nonperson, but not at the point he appears to be incapable of self-perception or of relational affect—only when neurologic diagnosis determines that cerebral function has ended permanently.

The non-neocortical theories (or paraneocortical) fall because they do not account for all cases. "Neocortical death," on the other hand, *necessarily* covers all other criteria, because they are by definition impossible criteria when neocortical function is gone. The key trait must be one that covers all cases, no matter how infrequently they are seen clinically.

Incidentally but not unimportantly, the neo-cortical indicator is *medically* determinable, whereas Tooley's and McCormick's are not.

If it proves that very many ethicists feel these issues about a sound hypothesis for the *humanum* are crucial, those whose training has been in the humanities will need the help and advice of psychiatrists, psychologists, neurologists and brain specialists, to teach us the limiting principles involved and expedite our discussion.

Notes

1. J. Rostand, *Humanly Possible: A Biologist's Notes on the Future of Mankind,* trans. by L. Blair (New York: Saturday Review Press, 1973), p. 8.
2. E. Fromm and R. Xirau, *The Nature of Man* (New York: Macmillan, 1968).
3. The full text is "Medicine and the Nature of Man," in *The Teaching of Medical Ethics,* ed. by R. M. Veatch, W. Gaylin and C. Morgan (Hastings-on-Hudson, N.Y.: Institute of Society, Ethics and the Life Sciences, 1973), pp. 47–58. It appeared also in *Science, Medicine and Man* 1 (1973), 93–102.
4. M. Tooley, "Abortion and Infanticide," *Philosophy and Public Affairs* 2 (Fall, 1972), 37–65.
5. R. Dubos, *Man Adapting* (New Haven: Yale University Press, 1965), p. 7n.
6. R. A. McCormick, "To Save or Let Die: The Dilemma of Modern Medicine," *Journal of the American Medical Association* 229 (July 8, 1974), 172–76.
7. R. H. Williams, *To Live and To Die* (New York: Springer-Verlag, 1974), p. 18.
8. J. M. Gustafson, "Basic Ethical Issues in the Bio-Medical Fields," Soundings 53 (1970), 177; and "Mongolism, Parental Desires, and the Right to Live," *Perspectives in Biology and Medicine* 16 (Summer, 1973), 529–57.
9. W. May, "The Morality of Abortion," *Catholic Medical Quarterly* 26 (July, 1974), 116–28.
10. H. T. Engelhardt, Jr., "The Beginnings of Personhood: Philosophical Considerations," *Perkins (School of Theology) Journal* 27 (1973), 20–27.
11. L. J. Weber, "Human Death or Neocortical Death: The Ethical Context," *Linacre Quarterly* 41 (May, 1974), 106–13.
12. R. F. Rizzo and J. M. Yonder, "Definition and Criteria of Clinical Death," *Linacre Quarterly* 40 (November, 1973), 223–33.
13. J. Korein, "On Cerebral, Brain, and Systemic Death," *Current Concepts of Cerebrovascular Disease (Stroke)* 8 (May-June, 1973), 9.

2

The Quality of Life

William Aiken

1. "We should set the highest value, not on living, but on living well," Socrates exclaimed.[1] And with Crito we are still puzzling over what it means to "live well," though today we would be more likely to talk about the "quality of life."

This phrase, "the quality of life," has become unusually popular in contemporary normative debates in such diverse areas as medical ethics (for instance, euthanasia, abortion), environmental ethics (resource use and allocation), moral issues in law (punishment), and social justice (welfare rights, future generations). But it is not used univocally throughout these debates. Consequently an analysis of the concept "quality of life" would be helpful in attaining a clear understanding of the various ways it can be used in practical ethics. But mere sterile analysis is insufficient for we need to know which uses are morally acceptable and which are morally deficient.

To accomplish this task the following steps will be taken: the moral philosopher's use is distinguished from the social scientist's use.

Two traditional moral uses of "quality of life," the "eudaimonistic" use and the "equalitarian" use, are described and advanced as paradigmatic uses. The priority of the latter is advocated. Then two popular contemporary uses of "quality of life," the "exclusionary" use and the "protectionary" use, are briefly analyzed and shown to be morally indefensible.

2. The "quality of life" is a normative concept but it has both a descriptive use and a prescriptive use. In the former, it is seen as an evaluative property admitting of degrees—thus it can serve as a means of comparison, or if appropriately specified by measurable criteria, as a tool of measurement. In this regard it is like the concepts, "efficiency" and "usefulness." I say this is a descriptive use for what is attempted is an "objective" comparison of the measurable degree of quality in two different lives or societies. This is the use frequently adopted by social scientists. They are striving to find indicators of *social* well-being analogous to the economic indices of economic well-being and to produce (eventually) a Qual-

"The Quality of Life" by William Aiken. Reprinted with permission of Applied Philosophy *1(1982):26–36.*

ity of Life measure equivalent to the Gross National Product measure with which to make inter-societal or inter-group comparisons.

As a moralist I am not particularly interested in this "comparative" use of "quality of life" with its debates over appropriate procedures of measurement (do we include preference and subjective satisfaction data or not?) and over the correct procedures for deriving interval scale rankings. Like Mill in his reaction to Bentham's incessant quantification of satisfactions, I resist the complete reduction of quality properties to statistically measurable quantities.

3. The moralist's prescriptive use of the phrase "quality of life" is philosophically more interesting. Here it is used as a value designator such that appeal to the enhancement or preservation of one's "quality of life" provides a good moral reason for acting or refraining from acting. In this prescriptive use we are not particularly interested in comparing differing degrees of quality—rather the task is to discover the means of attainment and maintenance of some desirable level of quality of life. Of course, this will involve determining what *is* the desirable level of quality.

Traditionally, this desirable "level of quality" was analyzed in terms of happiness, beatitude or eudaimonia. It was derived by ontological considerations of the nature of human beings. Having determined human essence, one could know what is required to obtain happiness or fulfillment and thus the desirable "quality of life" for human beings. If to fulfill one's essence meant being rational, or self-sufficient, or just, or pious, then the appropriate "quality of life" (or good life) was a life of activity in accordance with that virtue. Any life which did not obtain or maintain this level of quality was not a life lived well.

I shall call this use of "quality of life" the

"eudaimonistic" use. It is concerned with the "upper limits" of quality of a human life. It seeks to define the "good life" and to provide knowledge of both the necessary *and* sufficient conditions for its attainment. It is concerned with the social environment (be it Polis, Monastery, State, or Class) as an enabler of individuals in reaching this fulfillment level. It has a noble tradition (from Plato and Aristotle through Hegel and Marx) and is alive today in much of the literature of the holistic humanists.

4. However, the focus has changed in the Anglo-American tradition in the last two-hundred years away from the goal of the "good life," that is, the upper level of quality possible to humans. It has shifted to a concern with a much "lower level" of quality, the lower limits of quality necessary to live a minimally "human," that is, moral existence. This shift from maximal level to minimal level was influenced by the Liberal tradition's tolerance of diversity, its equalitarian doctrine of liberty, and its reluctance to *prescribe* the "good life." The protection of liberty was seen as a necessary condition for the pursuit of happiness—but it was left up to the individual to determine the nature of this goal. With concern for liberty as a prerequisite for maintaining a human quality of life came the recognition of the universal equality of human beings and thus universal entitlement to liberty. Slavery was, after many centuries, finally abolished.

Yet, liberty alone is insufficient to insure an equal minimal human quality of life. Liberty is one very important social good necessary for the attainment of a human quality of life but mere free choice and non-interference, no matter how equally distributed, are inadequate. Choice without opportunities, freedom without alternatives, non-interference without some interests to protect are vacuous. During the era circumscribed by Adam Smith and Herbert Spencer—the era of Liberty, *laissez faire,* competition, and social Darwinism—there was a revival, and rightly I think, of concern for what Aristotle called "external goods"—material and social goods. The 19th-century reformers—both radical utilitarians and socialists—stressed the need for basic material amenities to satisfy physical needs. Contra Malthus, the plight of the masses was not doomed to subhuman levels of existence. Social practices and institutions could be changed, reforms could be enacted—by revolution if necessary. The ideal of fundamental human equality had caught on. Not only were all humans entitled to liberty but they were also entitled to a minimal level of physical well-being and the institutions which could guarantee this. The movement continued to expand so as to not only include basic material goods (food, clothing, shelter, health resources) but also social goods: land reform, employment mobility, political participation and franchise, free public education and today it is being extended to recreational and cultural opportunities. In effect, the method of inquiry has been a form of transcendental deduction—asking what are the necessary material and social goods which persons must have if they are to achieve that minimal level of well-being which enables them to live a human quality of life as moral entities and thus to pursue the "good life." The emphasis is upon the minimal necessary conditions and the concern is inherently equalitarian—that is, it stresses the insurance of these minimal goods for all human beings. When the "quality of life" is used in normative argumentation to refer to this equal lower limit of quality, I shall call this the "equalitarian" use.

This use is dominant in social-political theory today. Even those who vehemently disagree with the ever-increasing expansion of entitlements, do not, I believe, fundamentally differ as to what the minimal level should be—rather they disagree on the effectiveness of various means to implement distribution of material goods. The intense concern with distributive justice reawakened by Rawls,[2] the emergence of claims to positive human rights to well-being launched by Vlastos[3] and Wasserstrom,[4] and the examination of equitable international resource allocation prompted by Singer[5] and O'Neill[6] all attest to the dominance of this use today.

And this is as it should be. Once the equal entitlement of all humans to liberty was acknowledged, the equal entitlement of all humans to a minimal level of well-being was inevitable. Short of the somewhat question begging appeal to an exclusive natural right to Liberty, the sole justification for granting Liberty universally is that it is a necessary condition for human beings to live the type of life befitting a moral entity. But then, other social goods and material goods are equally required to achieve this level of quality and so they, too, should be granted universally.

5. But what happens when the values designated by these two uses of "quality of life" come into conflict? Should the attainment of the "good life" by some take precedence over the attainment of a minimal human quality of life by all? I think not. I could argue for the priority of the equalitarian use either by a deontological appeal to universal positive rights or by an "essentialist" type of argument. Since I have done the former elsewhere,[7] and since I think it was the latter type of argument which such eudaimonists as Plato and Marx used to argue a similar point, I will provide an "essentialist" argument. Contra the radical individualist, I start with the premise that we are indeed social creatures by nature and thus that

the fulfillment of our nature is intricately involved with the construction and preservation
of community. But we are not merely social
creatures; we are social creatures capable of
moral action and thus of agency—which is to
say we are potentially moral entities. The type
of community then, which we must foster, to
fulfill our nature, must be a moral community
—that is, a community composed of and conducive to the creation of moral entities. We
could, with Kant, call such a community—a
kingdom of ends. But then the conditions necessary to construct and preserve such a community of moral entities is entailed, for "to will
the end is to will the means." Since these conditions involve the satisfaction of both the
physical and social needs of all individuals
within the community (otherwise they could
not become moral entities), then equal access
to the minimal goods necessary to satisfy these
needs is a prerequisite to the construction of a
moral community. Because my fulfillment is
derivative upon there being such a moral community, a condition for my eudaimonia is the
satisfaction of the needs of others so as to ensure their status as moral entities. Thus the
fulfillment of the equalitarian quality of life is
prior to the fulfillment of the eudaimonistic
quality of life. For Plato, a just man arises only
within a just society. For Marx the attainment
of species-being occurs only in a socialist society. And for me, the equalitarian use is similarly temporally prior to the eudaimonistic—
though not necessarily prior in value. This
priority will become important later in our assessment of the contemporary uses of quality
of life in practical ethics.

It is evident that there is a common prescriptive use of "Quality of Life" concepts em-
bedded in tradition. A distinctive pattern persists throughout both the eudaimonistic use
and the equalitarian use—that is, the unques-

tioned assumptions that humans *should* obtain
the desired level of quality; that actions which
enhance, insure, or protect this level are *prima
facie* right actions; and that we have a good
moral reason to enhance this value whenever
possible.

6. The remainder of this paper is a brief survey of the variety of applications of the phrase
"quality of life" in contemporary debates in
practical ethics. It will be shown that because
these applications ignore the preferred prescriptive use they are rife with confusions and
moral errors. These applications will be divided into two major types of uses of the
phrase "quality of life"—the exclusionary use
and the protectionary use which will be discussed separately.

Unlike the traditional prescriptive uses of
"quality of life" which *promote* this value, the
"exclusionary" use cites "quality of life" as
providing a criterion for exclusion of some
from the moral community and concomitantly
from normal standards of moral treatment.
The judgment is made that because a person's
"quality of life" is below the desirable level,
that person's life is not worth living and we are
justified in treating them accordingly. This use
is similar to the equalitarian use in that it attempts to specify what goods are required to
live a life of minimal human quality. The
equalitarian argument distinguished two types
of goods—social goods and material goods.
Each type has been used in exclusionary
arguments.

The social good of freedom has been used in
an exclusionary way in a rather bizarre defense
of capital punishment.[8] It is argued that since
living under the conditions of life-imprison-
ment is living without the social good of freedom (a necessary good for a human quality of
life), then we should, for humanitarian reasons, execute criminals (if they concur with

our assessment) rather than imprison them for life. That is, we are excused from normal moral treatment when dealing with those who fail to obtain the desired level of quality due to lack of a necessary social good.

In a similar manner some people have been excluded from receiving normal moral treatment on grounds of insufficient material goods. In some societies the material well-being of great numbers of people is below an acceptable quality (due to overpopulation and limited resources). For these people a fully human quality of life is impossible since any increase in their material well-being will exacerbate the population density problem. So rather than being subject to the benefit of others' benevolence, these people should be excluded from all assistance designed to prevent their death by starvation and want. Or, put more crudely, they are too poor to live *human* lives and aiding them would be a waste of money.[9]

In both of these exclusionary uses, the equalitarian argument is being turned on its head. The lack of necessary social or material goods is used not to prescribe alleviation of the deficiency but to justify exclusion of those who lack the goods, from normal moral treatment. In a way this is a bit laughable—like the zealous knights of the Inquisition who felt justified in killing infidels on grounds that these unfortunates were not saved. What they ought to have done, if salvation was so important to living a human life, was to try to convert them —not kill them. So too here, if some are deprived of the social or material goods necessary to live a human quality of life—don't kill them or neglect them to death; rather give them the minimal goods necessary to obtain this level. There are alternative forms of punishment which do not strip a person of *all* liberty and there are forms of assistance which save lives *and* alleviate the pressure on the

carrying capacity of an environment. These examples of the exclusionary argument seem to me to be confused in their judgment of a *moral* outcome.

But there is a more serious exclusionary application of the quality of life criterion in current practical ethics. Rather than focus on the lack of attainment of social or material goods, this application focuses upon the very *capability* of the excluded person to ever achieve the desired level of quality. There are two versions of this use. The first of these confuses the "upper" level of quality with the "lower" level of quality as necessary for a life worth living. The second confuses the distributive decision to override or defeat legitimate claims, with the decision to disregard altogether the moral legitimacy of those claims.

The first of these uses is illustrated by a very popular but poor argument to justify abortion. Since the potential for happiness for a fetus whose mother does not want it is insufficient to ever achieve this quality the mother is justified in aborting the fetus. That is, the fetus, if born, will be unloved, unwanted and inadequately cared for. But without these a child is incapable of achieving a happy adult life. So rather than a life below the desired quality (happiness) better to have no life—better not to be born.[10] This argument confuses the upper and lower levels of quality of life. That parental love is necessary to happiness is not disputed—but it is not clear that a life without this is a life below the minimal quality necessary to be a moral entity. The fetus may be quite capable of attaining the latter, albeit not the former quality. If we bought this argument then it would seem that we could extend it to justify terminating those with mental or physical deficiencies or even those who are ugly since at least the Greeks thought that physical beauty was a prerequisite to eudaimonia. Yet this is absurd. The argument does not make the more common mistake of placing the eudaimonistic use above the equalitarian—it actually fails to differentiate between an adequate moral life and a completely fulfilled one. The lack of capability to achieve complete eudaimonia is not a grounds for termination or exclusion from the moral community.

The second application which focuses upon capability of attaining the desired quality is illustrated by a common argument for euthanasia. Since severely defective newborns and the irreversibly comatose are not capable of attaining even a minimal "lower level" quality of life in spite of all requisite material and social goods, then their lives are not worth living. They can be excluded from the moral community, and treated accordingly (killed or neglected to death).[11] With the advancement of medical technology and the ability to keep people alive, this argument will increase in popularity. And it would appear that if any exclusionary use of quality of life is justified, this one is. But is it a good argument? I think not.

If in fact there were no significant costs involved in keeping these people alive there would be no good reason to kill or neglect them to death even though they could not obtain the minimal level of quality of life. But this seldom happens. It is the excessive cost (financial, resource allocational, and emotional) of maintaining these individuals which makes their death desirable. Valuable resources which could better be used to enhance the quality of the lives of others are being consumed by them. The real argument used here to justify killing them is a utilitarian one involving the equitable distribution of scarce resources so as to maximize derivative benefits. But if this is so, then it is not necessary to exclude these people from the moral community in order to judge that they should be termi-

nated because there are separate reasons for deciding to use the resources elsewhere. This is somewhat complicated but the point of principle is important to make. To override the interest of X without denying the moral validity of those interests is different from denying that X has such interests. In the language of rights we would say that X remains a right-holder even though, for the sake of honoring the rights of others, we must defeat or override, in this circumstance, X's exercise of those rights. X remains a right-holder and member of the moral community though X's claims are defeated. The exclusion model denies that X is a member of the community; it excludes X from the category of right-holder and thus the category of person. This virtually opens the door for unscrupulous experimentation on X, of disregard for X's comfort or X's legal status as an entity worthy of respect and protected against abusive negligence. Though perhaps easier on our conscience to exclude these people from moral personhood, it is better, I believe, to face up to the fact that we choose to intentionally sacrifice them for the sake of others—though this sacrifice is carefully limited by moral constraints on permissible treatment so as not to deny their personhood. The exclusion of these people by a quality of life criterion is undesirable. We need not exclude anyone from the moral community on grounds of deficient capability.

Our analysis of the exclusionary uses of quality of life in contemporary practical ethics has revealed that they are deficient because they are either confused, fail to make adequate distinctions or are deficient for moral analysis. Thus any such use, even though popular, is an inappropriate use of "quality of life."

7. The second major type of inappropriate use of "quality of life" criteria in contemporary normative argumentation is the "protec-

tionary use." This use is uniquely tied to material well-being and goods. Whereas social goods are distributable without dilution and are extendable without significant cost, material goods are not so abundant nor so easily attainable. If in fact there is some minimal level of material well-being required to live a human quality of life then material goods must be generated in sufficient quantities to guarantee an adequate supply. This involves the development of a theory of productive justice in order to determine not only the desirability of alternative institutions and practices utilized for the generation of wealth, but also the moral tolerability of the limits imposed on production by various constraints such as the efficiency criteria, the rate of resource and energy depletion, and the degree of labor intensivity of various modes of production. Anglo-American moral philosophers have for too long shied away from these questions of political economy in their almost exclusive concern for distribution. Yet this is forgivable. The goal of production is the enhancement of human well-being which is a social goal. Production is but a preliminary to distribution. The equalitarian value of the quality of life clearly makes the generation of wealth social in nature.

However, the inordinate value given to property rights and to exclusive possession of goods which we have inherited from Locke, *et al.*, as a concomitant of liberty conflicts with this equalitarian value has led to the belief that a "quality life" is one of possession, affluence, and consumption. The "quality of life" has now taken on a new eudaimonistic sense—it has been equated with an "affluent lifestyle." This is incompatible with the equalitarian value of providing a minimal level of material goods for all in order to insure a moral community. With the new understanding of quality of life the focus has shifted from the satisfaction

of basic material needs to the satisfaction of wants and desires. Whereas the former is equalitarian at the need level, the latter is eudaimonistic at the want level. This leads inevitably to a scarcity of goods for now—in the wants satisfaction mode—distribution becomes a zero sum game such that for some to have more others must have less. When needs and wants are treated identically the "protectionary" use of "quality of life" appears in normative argumentation. There is no limit to accumulation because increased desire satisfaction indicates a higher "quality of life." But in order to protect my quality of life I am justified in ignoring the claims made by others on "my" goods—my means to happiness—even though others may need these goods to obtain a minimally human level of quality of life. Any redistribution will be seen to diminish my quality of life (my affluence). So I am justified in protecting my "quality of life" against the claims of others.[12]

We can answer this protectionary argument in two ways. One is to simply challenge the conception of eudaimonia operative here. We could cite Aristotle's warning that we must *not* think our needs for external goods "will be great and many in order to be happy,"[13] or we could talk about rich men and eyes of needles. But more important than exposing this misconstrual is again emphasizing the reversal of priority here—that the eudaimonistic use of "quality of life" has been placed above the equalitarian use. This, as was shown earlier, is not warranted, for the former is dependent upon the latter. Our fulfillment as individuals is linked to the maintenance of a kingdom of ends—a world of moral entities—and thus our first priority is to insure a distribution of material goods sufficient to guarantee a minimal level of quality for all. Protection of individual happiness at the cost of maintaining such a community is morally misguided. Yet this type of argument, appealing to the "protectionary" use of quality of life, is popular in practical ethics as the following examples will demonstrate.

Until the recent rise of the Libertarian movement this use was relatively muted by the dominance of welfare economics. But today there is a renewed, and sometimes heated, controversy over the legitimacy of welfare, free health care, guaranteed minimal income, and even over free public education. The protectionary appeal to quality of life is repeatedly used to argue against redistributive taxation.[14]

Similarly, this use has become popular in debates over international justice. If the rich peoples of the world see their material affluence as equivalent to their "quality of life" which they are entitled to protect, then they feel justified in ignoring the claims of the impoverished peoples of the world for emergency relief and developmental assistance. Any international transfer of wealth or the means of wealth generation will be seen as detrimental to the quality of life of the rich.[15] And of course the rich get richer and the poor get poorer—in some cases, devastatingly so.

This protectionary argument is also used in debates over intergenerational justice. The current rate of consumption of nonrenewal energy and other natural resources by the industrialized nations threatens the attainment of even a minimal level of material well-being for future generations of even the next century. If we are justified in protecting our "quality of life," that is affluence, then future generations have no justifiable claim against us in regards to conservation of precious resources.[16]

But, as suggested above, these protectionary uses of "quality of life" fail to recognize the priority of the equalitarian use over the eudaimonistic use and are therefore deficient.

8. In conclusion, the appropriate prescriptive use of the concept "quality of life" was shown to be either absent from or misconstrued by some of the more popular contemporary uses of this concept in ethical arguments. To that extent these arguments often demonstrate not only confusion but also moral deficiency. Solutions to the problems of practical ethics should not be attempted in a vacuum— in total disregard for well-thought-out and time-tested moral traditions. Consequently, bridging the current rift between theoretical ethics and applied ethics should be given more attention.

Notes

1. Plato, *Euthyphro, Apology, Crito,* trans. F. J. Church (New York: Bobbs-Merrill Company, Inc., 1956) p. 57.
2. John Rawls, *A Theory of Justice* (Cambridge, Massachusetts: Harvard University Press, 1971).
3. Gregory Vlastos, "Justice and Equality," in *Social Justice,* ed. Richard Brandt (Englewood Cliffs, N.J.: Prentice-Hall, Inc., 1962), pp. 31–72.
4. Richard Wasserstrom, "Rights, Human Rights, and Racial Discrimination," *The Journal of Philosophy,* 61, no. 20 (October 29, 1964): pp. 628–641.
5. Peter Singer, "Famine, Affluence, and Morality," *Philosophy and Public Affairs,* 1, no. 3 (1972): pp. 229–243.
6. Onora O'Neill, "Lifeboat Earth," *Philosophy and Public Affairs,* 4, no. 3 (1975): pp. 273–292.
7. William Aiken, "The Right to be Saved," in *World Hunger and Moral Obligation,*

eds. William Aiken and Hugh La Follette (Englewood Cliffs, N.J.: Prentice-Hall, Inc., 1977), pp. 86–102. See also my "Starvation, Morality, and the Right to be Saved" (Ph.D. diss., Vanderbilt University, 1977).

8. Jacques Barzun, "In Favor of Capital Punishment," in *Social Ethics,* eds. Thomas Mappes and James Zembaty (New York: McGraw Hill Book Company, 1977). p. 92.

9. William and Paul Paddock, *Time of Famines* (Boston: Little, Brown and Company, 1976), pp. 205–229.

10. This argument is strongly implied by American Friends Service Committee. *Who Shall Live? Man's Control over Birth and Death* (NY: Hill and Wang, 1970). p. 55. It is also discussed by R. B. Brandt, "The Morality of Abortion," in *Abortion: Pro and Con* ed. Robert L. Perkins (Cambridge Mass: Schenkman Publishing Co., 1974). pp. 151–169.

11. See Jonathan Glover, *Causing Death and Saving Lives* (NY: Pelican Books, 1977), pp. 158–162, and H. Tristram Engelhardt, Jr., "ethical Issues in Aiding the Death of Young Children," in *Beneficient Euthanasia,* ed. Marvin Kohl (Buffalo, NY: Prometheus Books, 1975). pp. 180–192.

12. Whether wants and needs can be distinguished is itself highly controversial since economists tend to ignore the difference and use the "neutral" language of "subjective preferences" and "satisfactions." This leaves the point of declining marginal utility as one of the few criteria possible for such a distinction. For an interesting debate on the way the protectionary argument (argued by appeal to property rights) is generated by collapsing this distinction see John Arthur's reply to Peter Singer's essay (cited in footnote 5). "Rights and the Duty to Bring Aid" in *World Hunger and Moral Obligation,* eds. William Aiken and Hugh La Follette (op. cit), pp. 37–48, and Singer's response, *ibid.,* pp. 33–36.

13. Aristotle, *Nicomachean Ethics,* trans. Martin Ostwald (NY: Bobbs Merrill Company, Inc., 1962), p. 193.

14. See for example Robert Nozick, *Anarchy State and Utopia* (NY: Basic Books, Inc., 1974), esp. pp. 167–174.

15. This is usually argued in the context of "survival," for example Garrett Hardin, "Living on a Lifeboat" in his *Stalking the Wild Taboo* (Los Altos, Cal: William Kaufmann Inc., 1978), pp. 220–241 (esp. pp. 223–4). It also seems to underlie his "Tragedy of the Commons" in *Exploring New Ethics for Survival* (NY: Penguin Books, Inc. 1972), pp. 250–264, and is discussed in his "An Ecolate View of the Human Predicament" in *Global Resources: Perspectives and Alternatives,* ed. Clair N. McRostie (Baltimore: University Park Press, 1980), pp. 49–71.

16. Thomas H. Thompson, "Are We Obligated to Future Others?," in *Responsibilities to Future Generations,* ed. Ernest Partridge (Buffalo NY: Prometheus Books, 1980), pp. 195–202.

3

To Save or Let Die

Richard A. McCormick, S.J.

On February 24, the son of Mr. and Mrs. Robert H. T. Houle died following court-ordered emergency surgery at Maine Medical Center. The child was born February 9, horribly deformed. His entire left side was malformed; he had no left eye, was practically without a left ear, had a deformed left hand; some of his vertebrae were not fused. Furthermore, he was afflicted with a tracheal esophageal fistula and could not be fed by mouth. Air leaked into his stomach instead of going to the lungs, and fluid from the stomach pushed up into the lungs. As Dr. André Hellegers recently noted: "It takes little imagination to think there were further internal deformities" (*Obstetrical and Gynecological News*, April, 1974).

As the days passed, the condition of the child deteriorated. Pneumonia set in. His reflexes became impaired and because of poor circulation, severe brain damage was suspected. The tracheal esophageal fistula, the immediate threat to his survival, can be corrected with relative ease by surgery. But in view of the associated complications and deformities, the parents refused their consent to surgery on "Baby Boy Houle." Several doctors in the Maine Medical Center felt differently and took the case to court. Maine Superior Court Judge David G. Roberts ordered the surgery to be performed. He ruled: "At the moment of live birth there does exist a human being entitled to the fullest protection of the law. The most basic right enjoyed by every human being is the right to life itself."

"Meaningful Life"

Instances like this happen frequently. In a recent issue of the *New England Journal of Medicine* (289 [1973], pp. 890–94), Drs. Raymond S. Duff and A. G. M. Campbell reported on 299 deaths in the special-care nursery of the Yale-New Haven Hospital between 1970 and 1972. Of these, 43 (14 percent) were associated with discontinuance of treatment for children with multiple anomalies, trisomy, cardiopulmonary crippling, meningomyelocele

"*To Save or Let Die*" by Richard A. McCormick, S.J. Reprinted with permission of Richard A. McCormick and America 131(July 13, 1974):6–10.

and other central nervous system defects. After careful consideration of each of these 43 infants, parents and physicians in a group decision concluded that the prognosis for "meaningful life" was extremely poor or hopeless, and therefore rejected further treatment. The abstract of the Duff–Campbell report states: "The awesome finality of these decisions, combined with a potential for error in prognosis, made the choice agonizing for families and health professionals. Nevertheless, the issue has to be faced, for not to decide is an arbitrary and potentially devastating decision of default."

In commenting on this study in the Washington *Post* (Oct. 28, 1973), Dr. Lawrence K. Pickett, chief of staff at the Yale-New Haven Hospital, admitted that allowing hopelessly ill patients to die "is accepted medical practice." He continued: "This is nothing new. It's just being talked about now."

It has been talked about, it is safe to say, at least since the publicity associated with the famous "Johns Hopkins Case" some three years ago. (See James M. Gustafson's "Mongolism, Parental Desires and the Right to Life," *Perspectives in Biology and Medicine*, XVI [1973], pp. 529–59.) In this instance, an infant was born with Down syndrome and duodenal atresia. The blockage is reparable by relatively easy surgery. However, after consultation with spiritual advisers, the parents refused permission for this corrective surgery, and the child died by starvation in the hospital after 15 days. For to feed him by mouth in his condition would have killed him. Nearly everyone who has commented on this case has disagreed with the decision.

It must be obvious that these instances— and they are frequent—raise the most agoniz-

ing and delicate moral problems. The problem is best seen in the ambiguity of the term "hopelessly ill." This used to, and still may, refer to lives that cannot be saved, that are irretrievably in the dying process. It may also refer to lives that can be saved and sustained, but in a wretched, painful or deformed condition. With regard to infants, the problem is, which infants, if any, should be allowed to die? On what grounds or according to what criteria, as determined by whom? Or again, is there a point at which a life that can be saved is not "meaningful life," as the medical community so often phrases the question? If our past experience is any hint of the future, it is safe to say that public discussion of such controversial issues will quickly collapse into slogans such as: "There is no such thing as a life not worth saving"; or "Who is the physician to play God?" We saw, and continued to see, this far too frequently in the abortion debate. We are experiencing it in the euthanasia discussion. For instance, "death with dignity" translates for many into a death that is fast, clean, painless. The trouble with slogans is that they do not aid in the discovery of truth; they co-opt this discovery and promulgate it rhetorically, often only thinly disguising a good number of questionable value judgments in the process. Slogans are not tools for analysis and enlightenment; they are weapons for ideological battle.

Thus far, the ethical discussion of these truly terrifying decisions has been less than fully satisfactory. Perhaps this is to be expected, since the problems have only recently come to public attention. In a companion article to the Duff–Campbell report, Dr. Anthony Shaw of the Pediatric Division of the Department of Surgery, University of Virginia Medical Center, Charlottesville, speaks of solutions "based on the circumstances of each case rather than by means of a dogmatic formula approach." Are these really the only options available to us? Dr. Shaw's statement makes it appear that the ethical alternatives are narrowed to dogmatism (which imposes a formula that prescinds from circumstances) and pure concretism (which denies the possibility or usefulness of any guidelines).

Are Guidelines Possible?

Such either-or extremism is understandable. It is easy for the medical profession, in its fully justified concern with the terrible concreteness of these problems and with the issue of who makes these decisions, to trend away from any substantive guidelines. As *Time* remarked in reporting these instances: "Few, if any, doctors are willing to establish guidelines for determining which babies should receive lifesaving surgery or treatment and which should not" (March 25, 1974). On the other hand, moral theologians, in their fully justified concern to avoid total normlessness and arbitrariness wherein the right is "discovered," or really "created," only in and by brute decision, can easily be insensitive to the moral relevance of the raw experience, of the conflicting tensions and concerns provoked through direct cradleside contact with human events and persons.

But is there no middle course between sheer concretism and dogmatism? I believe there is. Dr. Franz J. Ingelfinger, editor of the *New England Journal of Medicine,* in an editorial on the Duff–Campbell–Shaw articles, concluded, even if somewhat reluctantly: "Society, ethics, institutional attitudes and committees can provide the broad guidelines, but the onus of

decision-making ultimately falls on the doctor in whose care the child has been put." Similarly, Frederick Carney of Southern Methodist University, Dallas, and the Kennedy Center for Bioethics stated of these cases: "What is obviously needed is the development of substantive standards to inform parents and physicians who must make such decisions" (Washington *Post,* March 20, 1974).

"Broad guidelines," "substantive standards." There is the middle course, and it is the task of a community broader than the medical community. A guideline is not a slide rule that makes the decision. It is far less than that. But it is far more than the concrete decision of the parents and physician, however seriously and conscientiously this is made. It is more like a light in a room, a light that allows the individual objects to be seen in the fullness of their context. Concretely, if there are certain infants that we agree ought to be saved in spite of illness or deformity, and if there are certain infants that we agree should be allowed to die, then there is a line to be drawn. And if there is a line to be drawn, there ought to be some criteria, even if very general, for doing this. Thus, if nearly every commentator has disagreed with the Hopkins decision, should we not be able to distill from such consensus some general wisdom that will inform and guide future decisions? I think so.

This task is not easy. Indeed, it is so harrowing that the really tempting thing is to run from it. The most sensitive, balanced and penetrating study of the Hopkins case that I have seen is that of the University of Chicago's James Gustafson (the article quoted above). Mr. Gustafson disagreed with the decision of the Hopkins physicians to deny surgery to the mongoloid infant. In summarizing his dissent, he notes: "Why would I draw the line on a different side of mongolism than the physicians did? While reasons can be given, one must recognize that there are intuitive elements, grounded in beliefs and profound feelings, that enter into particular judgments of this sort." He goes on to criticize the assessment made of the child's intelligence as too simplistic, and he proposes a much broader perspective on the meaning of suffering than seemed to have operated in the Hopkins decision. I am in full agreement with Mr. Gustafson's reflections and conclusions. But ultimately, he does not tell us where he would draw the line or why, only where he would *not*, and why.

This is very helpful already, and perhaps it is all that can be done. Dare we take the next step, the combination and analysis of such negative judgments to extract from them the positive criterion or criteria inescapably operative in them? Or more startlingly, dare we *not* if these decisions are already being made? Mr. Gustafson is certainly right in saying that we cannot always establish perfectly rational accounts and norms for our decisions. But I believe we must never cease trying, in fear and trembling, to be sure. Otherwise, we have exempted these decisions in principle from the one critique and control that protects against abuse. Exemption of this sort is the root of all exploitation, whether personal or political. Briefly, if we must face the frightening task of making quality of life judgments—and we must—then we must face the difficult task of building criteria for these judgments.

Facing Responsibility

What has brought us to this position of awesome responsibility? Very simply, the sophistication of modern medicine. Contemporary resuscitation and life-sustaining devices have brought a remarkable change in the state of the question. Our duties toward the care and preservation of life have been traditionally stated in terms of the use of ordinary and extraordinary means. For the moment and for purposes of brevity, we may say that, morally speaking, ordinary means are those whose use does not entail grave hardships to the patient. Those that would involve such hardships are extraordinary. Granted the relativity of these terms and the frequent difficulty of their application, still the distinction has had an honored place in medical ethics and medical practice. Indeed, the distinction was recently reiterated by the House of Delegates of the American Medical Association in a policy statement. After disowning intentional killing (mercy killing), the AMA statement continues: "The cessation of the employment of extraordinary means to prolong the life of the body when there is irrefutable evidence that biological death is imminent is the decision of the patient and/or his immediate family. The advice and judgment of the physician should be freely available to the patient and/or his immediate family" (*JAMA*, 227 [1974], p. 728).

This distinction can take us just so far—and thus the change in the state of the question. The contemporary problem is precisely that the question no longer concerns only those for whom "biological death is imminent" in the sense of the AMA statement. Many infants who would have died a decade ago, whose "biological death was imminent," can be saved. Yesterday's failures are today's successes. Contemporary medicine, with its team approaches, staged surgical techniques, monitoring capabilities, ventilatory support systems and other methods, can keep almost anyone alive. This has tended gradually to shift the problem, from the means to reverse the dying process, to the quality of the life sustained and preserved.

The questions, "Is this means too hazardous or difficult to use?" and "Does this measure only prolong the patient's dying?"—while still useful and valid—now often become: "Granted that we can easily save the life, what kind of life are we saving?" This is a quality of life judgment. And we fear it. And certainly we should. But with increased power goes increased responsibility. Since we have the power, we must face the responsibility.

A Relative Good

In the past, the Judeo-Christian tradition has attempted to walk a balanced middle path between medical vitalism (that preserves life at any cost) and medical pessimism (that kills when life seems frustrating, burdensome, "useless"). Both of these extremes root in an identical idolatry of life—an attitude that, at least by inference, views death as an unmitigated, absolute evil, and life as the absolute good. The middle course that has structured Judeo-Christian attitudes is that life is indeed a basic and precious good, but a good to be preserved precisely as the condition of other values. It is these other values and possibilities that found the duty to preserve physical life and also dictate the limits of this duty. In other words, life is a relative good, and the duty to preserve it a limited one. These limits have always been stated in terms of the *means* required to sustain life. But if the implications of this middle position are unpacked a bit, they will allow us, perhaps, to adapt to the type of quality of life judgment we are now called on to make without tumbling into vitalism or a utilitarian pessimism.

A beginning can be made with a statement of Pope Pius XII in an allocution to physicians delivered Nov. 24, 1957. After noting that we are normally obliged to use only ordinary means to preserve life, the Pontiff stated: "A more strict obligation would be too burdensome for most men and would render the attainment of the higher, more important good too difficult. Life, death, all temporal activities are in fact subordinated to spiritual ends." Here it would be helpful to ask two questions. First, what are these spiritual ends, this "higher, more important good"? Second, how is its attainment rendered too difficult by insisting on the use of extraordinary means to preserve life?

The first question must be answered in terms of love of God and neighbor. This sums up briefly the meaning, substance and consummation of life from a Judeo-Christian perspective. What is or can easily be missed is that these two loves are not separable. St. John wrote: "If any man says, 'I love God' and hates his brother, he is a liar. For he who loves not his brother, whom he sees, how can he love God whom he does not see?" (1 Jn. 4:20–21). This means that our love of neighbor is in some very real sense our love of God. The good our love wants to do Him and to which He enables us, can be done only for the neighbor, as Karl Rahner has so forcefully argued. It is in others that God demands to be recognized and loved. If this is true, it means that, in a Judeo-Christian perspective, the meaning, substance and consummation of life are found in human *relationships,* and the qualities of justice, respect, concern, compassion and support that surround them.

Second, how is the attainment of this "higher, more important [than life] good" rendered "too difficult" by life-supports that are gravely burdensome? One who must support his life with disproportionate effort focuses the time, attention, energy and resources of himself and others not precisely on relationships, but on maintaining the condition of relationships. Such concentration easily becomes overconcentration and distorts one's view of, and weakens one's pursuit of, the very relational goods that define our growth and flourishing. The importance of relationships gets lost in the struggle for survival. The very Judeo-Christian meaning of life is seriously jeopardized when undue and unending effort must go into its maintenance.

I believe an analysis similar to this is implied in traditional treatises on preserving life. The illustrations of grave hardship (rendering the means to preserve life extraordinary and nonobligatory) are instructive, even if they are outdated in some of their particulars. Older moralists often referred to the hardship of moving to another climate or country. As the late Gerald Kelly, S.J., noted of this instance: "They [the classical moral theologians] spoke of other inconveniences, too: e.g., of moving to another climate or another country to preserve one's life. For people whose lives were, so to speak, rooted in the land, and whose native town or village was as dear as life itself, and for whom, moreover, travel was always difficult and often dangerous—for such people, moving to another country or climate was a truly great hardship, and more than God would demand as a 'reasonable' means of preserving one's health and life" (*Medico-Moral Problems,* [1957], p. 132).

Similarly, if the financial cost of life-preserving care was crushing, that is, if it would create grave hardships for oneself or one's family, it was considered extraordinary and nonobligatory. Or again, the grave inconvenience of living with a badly mutilated body was viewed, along with other factors (such as pain in preanesthetic days, uncertainty of success), as constituting the means extraordinary. Even now, the contemporary moralist, Marcellino Zalba,

S.J., states that no one is obligated to preserve his life when the cost is "a most oppressive convalescence."

The Quality of Life

In all of these instances—instances where the life could be saved—the discussion is couched in terms of the means necessary to preserve life. But often enough it is the kind of, the quality of, the life thus saved (painful, poverty-stricken and deprived, away from home and friends, oppressive) that establishes the means as extraordinary. *That* type of life would be an excessive hardship for the individual. It would distort and jeopardize his grasp on the overall meaning of life. Why? Because, it can be argued, human relationships—which are the very possibility of growth in love of God and neighbor—would be so threatened, strained or submerged that they would no longer function as the heart and meaning of the individual's life as they should. Something other than the "higher, more important good" would occupy first place. Life, the condition of other values and achievements, would usurp the place of these and become itself the ultimate value. When that happens, the value of human life has been distorted out of context.

In his *Morals in Medicine* (1957), Thomas O'Donnell, S.J., hinted at an analysis similar to this. Noting that life is a relative, not an absolute, good, he asks: Relative to what? His answer moves in two steps. First, he argues that life is the fundamental natural good God has given to man, "the fundamental context in which all other goods which God has given man as means to the end proposed to him, must be exercised" (p. 66). Second, since this is so, the relativity of the good of life consists in the effort required to preserve this fundamental context and "the potentialities of the other goods that still remain to be worked out within that context."

Can these reflections be brought to bear on the grossly malformed infant? I believe so. Obviously there is a difference between having a terribly mutilated body as the result of surgery, and having a terribly mutilated body from birth. There is also a difference between a long, painful, oppressive convalescence resulting from surgery, and a life that is from birth one long, painful, oppressive convalescence. Similarly, there is a difference between being plunged into poverty by medical expenses and being poor without ever incurring such expenses. However, is there not also a similarity? Cannot these conditions, whether caused by medical intervention or not, equally absorb attention and energies to the point where the "higher, more important good" is simply too difficult to attain? It would appear so. Indeed, is this not precisely why abject poverty (and the systems that support it) is such an enormous moral challenge to us? It simply dehumanizes.

Life's potentiality for other values is dependent on two factors, those external to the individual, and the very condition of the individual. The former we can and must change to maximize individual potential. That is what social justice is all about. The latter we sometimes cannot alter. It is neither inhuman nor unchristian to say that there comes a point where an individual's condition itself represents the negation of any truly human—i.e., relational—potential. When that point is reached, is not the best treatment no treatment? I believe that the *implications* of the traditional distinction between ordinary and extraordinary means point in this direction.

In this tradition, life is not a value to be preserved in and for itself. To maintain that would commit us to a form of medical vitalism that makes no human or Judeo-Christian sense. It is a value to be preserved precisely as a condition for other values, and therefore insofar as these other values remain attainable. Since these other values cluster around and are rooted in human relationships, it seems to follow that life is a value to be preserved only insofar as it contains some potentiality for human relationships. When in human judgment this potentiality is totally absent or would be, because of the condition of the individual, totally subordinated to the mere effort for survival, that life can be said to have achieved its potential.

Human Relationships

If these reflections are valid, they point in the direction of a guideline that may help in decisions about sustaining the lives of grossly deformed and deprived infants. That guideline is the potential for human relationships associated with the infant's condition. If that potential is simply nonexistent or would be utterly submerged and undeveloped in the mere struggle to survive, that life has achieved its potential. There are those who will want to continue to say that some terribly deformed infants may be allowed to die *because* no extraordinary means need to be used. Fair enough. But they should realize that the term "extraordinary" has been so relativized to the condition of the patient that it is this condition that is decisive. The means is extraordinary because the infant's condition is extraordinary. And if that is so, we must face this fact head-on—and discover the substantive standard that allows us to say this of some infants, but not of others.

Here several caveats are in order. First, this

guideline is not a detailed rule that preempts decisions; for relational capacity is not subject to mathematical analysis but to human judgment. However, it is the task of physicians to provide some more concrete categories or presumptive biological symptoms for this human judgment. For instance, nearly all would very likely agree that the anencephalic infant is without relational potential. On the other hand, the same cannot be said of the mongoloid infant. The task ahead is to attach relational potential to presumptive biological symptoms for the gray area between such extremes. In other words, individual decisions will remain the anguishing onus of parents in consultation with physicians.

Second, because this guideline is precisely that, mistakes will be made. Some infants will be judged in all sincerity to be devoid of any meaningful relational potential when that is actually not quite the case. This risk of error should not lead to abandonment of decisions; for that is to walk away from the human scene. Risk of error means only that we must proceed with great humility, caution and tentativeness. Concretely, it means that, if err we must at times, it is better to err on the side of life— and, therefore, to tilt in that direction.

Third, it must be emphasized that allowing some infants to die does not imply that "some lives are valuable, others not" or that "there is such a thing as a life not worth living." Every human being, regardless of age or condition, is of incalculable worth. The point is not, therefore, whether this or that individual has value. Of course he has, or rather *is,* a value. The only point is whether this undoubted value has any potential at all, in continuing physical survival, for attaining a share, even if reduced, in the "higher, more important good." This is not a question about the inherent value of the individual. It is a question about whether this

worldly existence will offer such a valued individual any hope of sharing those values for which physical life is the fundamental condition. Is not the only alternative an attitude that supports mere physical life as long as possible with every means?

Fourth, this whole matter is further complicated by the fact that this decision is being made for someone else. Should not the decision on whether life is to be supported or not be left to the individual? Obviously, wherever possible. But there is nothing inherently objectionable in the fact that parents with physicians must make this decision at some point for infants. Parents must make many crucial decisions for children. The only concern is that the decision not be shaped out of the utilitarian perspectives so deeply sunk into the consciousness of the contemporary world. In a highly technological culture, an individual is always in danger of being valued for his function, what he can do, rather than for who he is.

It remains, then, only to emphasize that these decisions must be made in terms of the child's good, this alone. But that good, as fundamentally a relational good, has many dimensions. Pius XII, in speaking of the duty to preserve life, noted that this duty "derives from well-ordered charity, from submission to the Creator, from social justice, as well as from devotion towards his family." All of these considerations pertain to that "higher, more important good." If that is the case with the duty to preserve life, then the decision not to preserve life must likewise take all of these into account in determining what is for the child's good.

Any discussion of this problem would be incomplete if it did not repeatedly stress that it is the pride of Judeo-Christian tradition that the weak and defenseless, the powerless and unwanted, those whose grasp on the goods of life is most fragile—that is, those whose potential is real but reduced—are cherished and protected as our neighbor in greatest need. Any application of a general guideline that forgets this is but a racism of the adult world profoundly at odds with the gospel, and eventually corrosive of the humanity of those who ought to be caring and supporting as long as that care and support has human meaning. It has meaning as long as there is hope that the infant will, in relative comfort, be able to experience our caring and love. For when this happens, both we and the child are sharing in that "greater, more important good."

Were not those who disagreed with the Hopkins decision saying, in effect, that for the infant, involved human relationships were still within reach and would not be totally submerged by survival? If that is the case, it is potential for relationships that is at the heart of these agonizing decisions.

4

The Quality of Life and Death

Edward W. Keyserlingk

The sanctity of life principle is itself somewhat elusive and indeterminate. It is not however totally without substance and meaning, both in terms of what it means and does not mean. It *does* point to an objective, absolute value of human life and worth, it insists that human life is always worthy of respect and protection, and that it should always be supported without adequate justification to the contrary. Inasmuch as these assertions have always been and still are under attack in open or subtle ways in medical, legal and other debates, the sanctity of life principle continues to require articulate and strenuous defence.

But it does *not* mean vitalism, it does not preclude the need for human decision-making and judgment, for instance in decisions to medically treat or not to treat, to preserve or not to preserve life, in certain circumstances. But if this is so, what exact role has the *kind* of life, the *quality* of life in question to play in that decision-making? The sanctity of life principle is not by itself concrete and determinate

enough to answer all the questions, to solve all the problems. Its primary and indispensable role is to establish parameters and priorities for debates and decision-making involving human life, and to judge and test relevant moral rules. But it needs the moral rules to make it concrete and useful in particular cases. The principle acknowledges that there can be "justifying reasons" for ceasing to preserve human life and (some would say) even for taking it. But it does not indicate clearly what those justifying reasons are. And it does not define for us what human life really is, what its essential qualities or inherent features really are.

Not to face those questions directly would be to avoid doing our "moral homework." To use the sanctity of life principle as a tool to determine all moral decisions in advance without any consideration of further questions and individual circumstances, is therefore to distort the real role of that principle and to use it as a decision-*avoiding*, not a decision-*making* tool.

"The Quality of Life and Death" by Edward W. Keyserlingk in Sanctity of Life or Quality of Life in the Context of Ethics, Medicine and Law (*A study written for The Law Reform Commission of Canada), 1979, pp. 49–72 and 196–199. Reprinted with permission of the Secretary of the Law Reform Commission of Canada.*

But if this is so, how useful and morally legitimate is the "quality of life" concept in helping to shape moral rules, in determining "justifying reasons" for both preserving and ceasing to preserve human life, and in establishing the inherent features of human life?

A. An Elusive Concept—Subjective or Objective? Absolute or Relative? Equal or Unequal?

The answer of course depends upon what is meant, or what meaning *we give* to "quality of life." What makes the question one of practical relevance and not just academic interest is that quality of life concerns are already and long have been influencing medical decisions. But what makes the question an urgent and somewhat worrisome one for society, medicine and law is that quality of life can and does mean many very different things, has no single, generally accepted meaning, and some of its connotations and the uses to which the concept is put are definitely opposed to and in conflict with the sanctity of life principle.

It is probably its very elusiveness which makes the concept so attractive to media and public. It is so vague and glibly used in such quite different contexts (environmental and medical for instance) and in support of such quite different positions (for instance to improve the quality of air, or to cease medical treatment) that the concept seems to commit one to nothing specific, and is seldom given tangible content.

But its very elusiveness encourages as well the polarized, extreme and hostile views about its moral legitimacy and usefulness. There are those who think it answers all questions, and those who think it answers none. There are those who would welcome the replacement of the "traditional" ethic of the absolute value of human life by an ethic of its relative value. There are others who see any recognition of quality of life factors as a danger to be resisted at all costs.

But it is also possible, and in my view legitimate and preferable, to see no need to choose between an old ethic and a new one. Instead, to recognize an urgent need to on the one hand articulate and refine the "old" ethic, and on the other hand to propose a carefully delineated and restricted meaning and purpose for quality of life. The purpose of such an exercise would be to encourage both medical decision-making and (perhaps) law-making to more formally recognize an interest in considering and protecting *both* the intrinsic value of each human life, *and* the quality of those lives, even when this involves a decision to cease or not initiate treatment or life support.

But to make this case successfully depends first of all of course on the meaning we intend for quality of life. The clarification, justification and application of the meaning I intend for this expression will, from various angles, be the task of the remainder of this paper.

I will begin by very explicitly parting company with the most frequently proposed meaning or connotation of quality of life in the medical/health context—namely that it must inevitably and fundamentally involve more or less wholly *subjective judgments about the relative individual or social worth, value, usefulness or equality of the lives of persons*. Both proponents as well as opponents of the quality of life concept generally assume or claim that such notions are at the centre of the concept. There is little doubt that it is exactly that unqualified assumption on both sides of the argument which gives quality of life such a "bad press" and raises fears of "playing God" with human lives. If the concept is to serve the useful function it can and must, it needs rescuing as much from its proponents who claim too much for it as from its opponents who claim too little. Inasmuch as the sanctity of life principle insists that the respect and protection due to human life ought not to be based on judgments of relative worth, value or usefulness, such versions are rightly seen as opposed to and judged wanting by, the sanctity of life principle.

Proponents of such views of the quality of life concept are often well aware of this opposition and applaud it. For instance this editorial entitled, "A New Ethic for Medicine and Society" in *California Medicine,* the official journal of the California Medical Association:

> The traditional Western ethic has always placed great emphasis on the intrinsic worth and equal value of every human life regardless of its stage or condition . . . This traditional ethic is still clearly dominant, but there is much to suggest that *it is being eroded* at its core and may eventually be abandoned . . . there is a *quite new emphasis* on something which is beginning to be called the quality of life . . . It will become *necessary and acceptable* to place relative rather than absolute values on such things as human lives, the use of scarce resources and the various elements which are to make up the quality of life or of living which is to be sought. . . .[1] [emphasis added]

The writer may be correct in observing such a shift in practice and/or values. But one need not agree with him on several other counts—that the shift is a good thing, or that his characterization of quality of life is the only one

possible or that the "traditional ethic" is unconcerned about quality of human life considerations.

Opponents of quality of life considerations in medical life and death decision-making, just as its proponents, generally assume the same reductionist and unqualified meaning of quality of life when they characterize it as opposed to or incompatible with sanctity of life. For instance, this view of a moral theologian:

> The quality of life ethic puts the emphasis on the type of life being lived, not upon the fact of life . . . What the life means to someone is what is important. Keeping this in mind, it is not inappropriate to say that some lives are of *greater value than others,* that the condition or meaning of life does have much to do with the justification for terminating that life. The sanctity of life ethic defends two propositions: 1. That human life is sacred by the very fact of its existence; its value does not depend upon a certain condition or perfection of that life. 2. That, therefore, all human lives are of *equal value;* all have the same right to life. The quality of life ethic finds neither of these two propositions acceptable.[2]

Once again, as stated and without further qualification there may well be opposition between *his* characterizations of sanctity of life and quality of life; at least a difference in stress. But we are not obliged to accept either of his characterizations as the only or most accurate ones possible. One is inclined to classify the above description of that principle as verging on vitalism,—leaving as it appears to, no room for concerns of the "kind," "quality" or "condition" of a life. And below I will attempt to demonstrate that a more qualified and restricted meaning of quality of life than that presented above does not really find those two sanctity of life propositions "unacceptable"—only "insufficient."

B. "Quality of Life" in the Environmental and Medical Contexts —A Comparison

Before coming back to these points and an arguable "definition" of quality of life in greater detail, we should briefly consider the meaning of the concept in another kind of context—that of environmental, ecological or social concerns. Much of the difficulty and ambiguity of the expression in the medical context stems from the fact that we too readily and uncritically use the same expression in two very different circumstances and for two very different purposes. One result is that the concept appears to be positive in one context— the environmental/social, but negative and reductionist in the other—the medical. But another result is that in exaggerating the differences in context and purpose in the use of quality of life, we may overlook some important and useful common denominators and insights.

A brief summary of the state of the quality of life question in contexts other than the medical is therefore in order. First of all, quality of life in those contexts focuses on *improving* the quality of life for members of a society or region—better air, food, privacy, water, education, leisure, working conditions, health and so on.

In those contexts, efforts to measure and improve the quality of life have been generally welcomed as a long overdue corrective to almost exclusive concentration on factors such as production, economic growth and gross national product. "The concept 'Quality of Life' has emerged in the last few years as an undefinable measure of society's determination and desire to improve or at least not permit a further degradation of its condition. Despite its current undefinability, it represents a yearning of people for something which they feel they have lost or are losing, or have been denied, and what to some extent they wish to regain or acquire."[3]

But in the environmental/ecological/social contexts the "life" being evaluated is not "John Smith's" life, but life in a particular society or region. As Kurt Baier points out, quality is a comparative property. It involves comparison with other things. But the things compared are not particular lives, but the "relevant environmental conditions of life" in a certain region. "Those who choose regions on the basis of the quality of life there, will . . . appraise the conditions of this, *i.e.*, the aspects of the physical and social environment which affect how good or bad any person's life is, in so far as that depends on the environment in which he lives. And the aim with reference to which the various types of environments will be appraised is their capacity to make the lives of those living in them as good as possible, or at least enable them to do so."[4]

Appraising, measuring and improving the relevant conditions, depends of course on the determination of and agreement upon social indicators, standards and operational definitions. A difficult if not impossible task, and no effort to establish indicators or an index of quality of life has as yet gained universal support. A number of attempts have been made with more or less success.[5]

Proposed indicators attempt to determine not only environmental factors, but also economic factors and sociopolitical factors (such as health, social relationships, equality, education, community, etc.). Many of the approaches are subjectivist, in that they stress subjective data such as "perceived" happiness, satisfaction or fulfillment in the social indicators stressed, and they attempt to determine the quality of life in that region or society by questioning people about their satisfaction or happiness.[6]

But others convincingly argue for an *objective* approach maintaining, ". . . that it is possible to combine within a single conceptual or methodological framework, the notion of a subjective 'indicator' of the Quality of Life with what is 'constitutive' of the Quality of Life, the latter being wholly non-subjective."[7]

This view defines quality of life and its indicators not just in terms of general average happiness or the sum total of happiness of people in a region or society, or just in terms of tastes or preferences. These are all subjective factors. Central to this view is that quality of life is not just the happiness of a region, but the necessary conditions for happiness. Clearly both objective and subjective factors are relevant to quality of life—for instance salary and satisfaction with salary in the context or working conditions.

But quality of life is not really a combination of objective factors and subjective factors. "We might as well say that the quality of a fabric does not lie in the fabric, but consists, instead, in some esoteric combination of properties of the fabric together with pleasurable feelings on the part of the wearer. No, the quality of a fabric lies in the fabric, and the quality of working life lies in working conditions. The role played by job satisfaction indicators is to indicate 'which' working conditions are important in determining the quality of working life."[8]

The same point can be made from another angle. How are "general happiness requirements" satisfied? Is it by the satisfaction of human needs, or human desires? ". . . we might say that *wanting* and desiring are 'psychological states,' whereas the state of *needing* something is not a psychological state. Combining this result with the one obtained earlier about the non-subjective character of the Quality of Life, we are able to infer something about the general happiness requirements. The Quality of Life, as we have defined it, consists in the fulfillment of the general happiness *requirements*. Since the presence or absence of unsatisfied wants is a mental or 'subjective' phenomenon, fulfillment of the general happiness requirements cannot lie in the satisfaction of human *wants*. If anything, it must lie in the satisfaction of human *needs*."[9] [emphasis added]

And what do humans need in order to be happy? One of the best known attempts to propose a hierarchy of human needs is that of Abraham Maslow.[10] He proposes these five categories:

1. Physiological needs;
2. Safety or security needs;
3. Belongingness needs;
4. Esteem needs;
5. Self-actualization needs.

No argument has yet established that Maslow's list of needs, or some such list, cannot be predicated for all people in all places. That being the case it could provide a good first step to providing objective indicators or criteria for the quality of life.[11]

One last point in this regard, concerning the relevance of "taste" or "personal preference" to quality of life. The fact that different people will have different "optimal lives," different rational goals, is partly due to differences in individual tastes. Yet the determination of what is a person's optimal life is not just a matter of taste and can be given an objective answer.

> Whether the contemplative life is the best life is a matter of taste, but we can in principle tell what sorts of people will have what sorts of taste, and so objectively what sorts of lives will be optimal to them . . . there are some things that can be said about all optimal lives, whatever peoples' talents and tastes. We have as yet no pre-test indicators enabling us to say whether Jones or Smith will find Sacher Torte the best cake, but we can confidently predict such things as that they will not like their favourite dessert laced with DDT or mercury, as some of our foods now come to us.[12]

What has all this to do with quality of life in the medical/health context? A number of things. In the first place it is true that quality of life criteria in the environmental/ecological/social contexts are used for the comparing of *environmental/social conditions* in order to *improve* them; whereas in the medical context they often seem to be used to compare *human lives* but not as grounds for improving, rather for *terminating* them. In the former contexts, quality of life involves a protection and expansion of life in all its forms, styles and levels; whereas in the latter context it suggests a limiting, qualifying, reductive and standardizing impulse.

As used by some in the medical/health context, quality of life suggests that some of the sick and "defective," because they are no longer able, or will not be able to contribute to society, therefore no longer qualify to benefit from the environmental and medical resources as do the rest of us. Quality of life thus compared in the two contexts comes off a very poor second in the medical/health context.

But as stated earlier, what is intended here by quality of life is, among other things, a notion purged of any trace of *relativizing human worth* and the lives of persons, or any hint of "social utility" as a necessary qualification for treatment. And just as in the environmental context it can focus on *objective* factors, criteria and needs, so too in the medical context. Examples of objectivity in criteria, are efforts to "define" person and to formulate criteria for "ordinary" and "extraordinary" treatment, both subjects we will consider below. And just as in those environmental/social contexts, quality of life decisions in the medical context can and should be oriented to *improvement and benefit*—in this case, of the patient.

Quality is a comparative property, an evaluative property. And it is true that quality of life used in environmental/social contexts does essentially involve a comparison with other things—a ranking of the conditions which maximize optimal human life or general happiness requirements of a region. Implicit in the comparison is a readiness to discard or improve certain conditions because of where they rank on the scale.

But in the medical/health context, quality of life *need* not involve a comparison of *different human lives* as the basis for decisions to treat some and not others. Ideally, at the heart of quality of life concerns in this context should be only a comparison of the qualities *this patient* now has with the qualities deemed by *this patient* (or, if incompetent or irreversibly comatose, by the patient's agents) to be normative and desirable, and either still or no longer present actually or potentially.

The real comparison in question is in a sense one between what the patient is and was, is and can or cannot be in the future. The quality of life comparison or evaluation in the medical context need not be a comparison *with others* or a relativizing of persons' lives. And the quality of life norm and decision need not be arbitrary or based upon how treatment or nontreatment will relieve or burden others or society. The norm can and must include whatever the value sciences, medicine and public policy agree upon concerning the essential quality or qualities of a human person; and the decision can and must be in the first instance by, and for the benefit of the patient and no one else.

To include quality of life considerations in life saving or life support decision making by no means must imply *harm* rather than improvement or benefit to the patients. If quality of life is limited only to what is intended here, then quite the contrary is the case and must be the case if the concept is to have any justifiably normative value.

In the first place, investigations, prognoses and conclusions arrived at concerning a patient's actual or potential level of function or degree of suffering, need not inevitably and exclusively lead to decisions *to cease* or *not initiate* life supporting treatment. Given that the sanctity of life principle imposes the burden of proof on those who would cease to support life, the consideration of quality of life factors should more often lead to the opposite decision—to initiate or continue that treatment if there is any realistic hope of minimal human function and controllable pain and suffering.

Secondly, even when quality of life factors do contribute to a decision to cease or not initiate life saving or supporting treatment,

there remains the continuing obligation to seek to improve the newborn's or the patient's *care and comfort*. Neither physician nor patient are usually faced with only two options —to continue or discontinue life support treatment. The third option and continuing responsibility of health care professionals and families, no matter how damaged the patient's condition, is to seek to improve the level of care and comfort of the dying, including being physically present to them. The sanctity of life surely calls for at least the same respect and consideration for dying life as for healthy life. And if greater needs call for greater care and concern, then the dying deserve more, not less of it, than the healthy.[13]

Thirdly, even decisions to cease or not initiate life saving treatments, based partly on quality of life considerations, can and must offer a reasonable hope of *benefit* to the patient. In other words, death should not always be resisted at any cost in terms of present and future suffering and damage, as if anything is an improvement over death. It is an integral part of my thesis that this is not so, that some conditions of human life are so damaged, and will likely remain so or become worse if treatment is continued or initiated, that death can reasonably be seen as beneficial, as an improvement for that patient.

The final weighing and balancing of reasons and criteria normally belongs to the patient, and within morally acceptable parameters different patients may and will weigh the criteria differently and come to different decisions. For the incompetent, the determination of benefit to patient or newborn must be made by proxies. While it remains enormously difficult to make such decisions in the interests and for the benefit of others, it is my contention that they must sometimes be made, and that reasonable and morally justifiable decisions for the benefit of others, based partially at least on quality of life matters, are possible. There will be occasion to come back to the "who decides" question and the other points in more detail as the argument unfolds.

In the light of the above, quality of life in the medical context need not come out the loser when compared to quality of life in the environmental/social context. As noted, there are of course great differences in the contexts and the functions within them of quality of life criteria. But in both contexts the ultimate aim of these criteria is objective improvement and benefit, even if in the medical context that will often be limited to reducing rather than eliminating the patient's discomfort and indignity. In claiming this, the medical cases envisioned are primarily those in which the quality of life criteria are used in decisions made *by others* for the incompetent patient. In such cases the use of these criteria for the patient's objective improvement or reduction of discomfort or some other benefit is a realistic aim. Obviously it may be otherwise for patients able to *themselves* accept or refuse treatment. Since competent patients have the right to refuse treatment on any grounds at all, whether they seem reasonable or foolish to others, there can be no guarantee at all of objective improvement and benefit in the decisions made and criteria used by competent patients for themselves.

Just before attempting to put flesh on the dry bones, to offer more argument for the claims made, the thesis of this quality of life section of the paper should be summarized.

Quality of life need not mean the "relativizing of lives." Excluded here in this paper from that concept and its criteria are considerations such as social worth, social utility, social status

or relative worth. The sanctity of life principle rightly insists on the intrinsic worth and equal value of every life. In excluding these elements from the meaning intended for quality of life, one need not of course deny that they can be ingredients of quality of life in wider contexts than our own. At least some of them are factors which a "general" quality of life theory must consider and weigh in other contexts. I am only excluding these factors from this particular context of medical decision-making in life and death matters, and primarily when such decisions are made by proxies or patients' agents for patients or newborns unable to make these decisions themselves. Whatever the merits and realities of characteristics such as social status in other areas of concern, here I do not believe they should have determinative weight.

New circumstances such as increasingly sophisticated life support systems and treatment have challenged us to recognize in human life a distinction between mere existence and quality with more clarity than previously needed. But that does not mean that in our context the shifting sands of new medical technology, evolving social realities or subjective preferences comprise an adequate source for the meaning and criteria of a quality of life concept, or in themselves validly answer our questions. What is involved here, or should be, is a search for and a weighing of the *inherent features* of human life. That is an objective meaning of "quality" light years away from mere considerations of relative and changing circumstances, facts and values. It does not make the task easier, or ensure an immediate consensus but at least the task is defensible.

In this sense, meaning and criteria for quality of life in life or death decision-making, should focus not on features or conditions which permit patients to act comfortably, well and without burdening others or society, but rather on features and conditions which allow them to act *at all,* even to a minimal extent. The real question and issues raised by considerations of quality of life is not about the value of this patient's *life*—it is about the value of this patient's *treatment.*

The meaning and criteria of quality of life should focus on *benefit to the patient,* and in some circumstances to initiate treatment or prolong or postpone death can reasonably be seen as non-beneficial to the patient. One such circumstance is *excruciating, intractable and prolonged pain and suffering.* Another is the lack of capacity for what can be considered an inherent feature of human life, namely a *minimal capacity to experience, to relate with other human beings.* In such instances to preserve life could in some cases be a dishonouring of the sanctity of life itself, and allowing even death could be a demonstration of respect for the individual and for human life in general.

The above can be clarified and justified from a number of angles. The first point to establish is that there is a distinction to be made between human *biological* life and human *personal* life. On that distinction hang some important conclusions.

C. Life: A Good in Itself? Death: How "Define" It?

In the context of our concerns the question which raises a need to recognize a distinction between human *biological* and human *personal* life is this: is biological or metabolic life (alone) a *good in itself,* a "bonum honestum" to be preserved regardless of any capacity for conscious experience and communication? Or is physical, metabolic life to be seen mainly as a "bonum utile," a *condition* for other capacities such as experiencing and interrelating, and as such a life which has already achieved its potential or never can if those capacities are no longer or never will be possible?

There are many who answer yes to the first question and no to the second. Generally speaking they insist that the real value of human life is in its very *existence,* not in its *capacities or qualities;* and that every life is of equal value. But there are many who hold the second view against the first, arguing for instance that, "Since human life is the condition for the realization of human freedom, it should be prolonged with all appropriate and reasonable means insofar as prolongation according to a competent estimate can serve this goal."[14]

Clearly what is involved here is the need to clarify the ambiguous word, "life." Of humans it can mean two related but very different things. First of all "life" can mean vital or metabolic processes without any specifically "human" function or capacity. This could be called *human biological life,* or human physical life or human "technical" life (the latter if medically life-supported).

Such life is still human in the first sense—it was born of humans and is a potential source of human organs. But such life is no longer, and in some cases never will be human life in a second sense, that is a human life also capable of experiencing, communicating, or being responsible for its actions. This we could call *human "personal"* life. From the ethical/ontological as well as the medical standpoints, the real and crucial question in decision-making is not whether the patients or newborns are human (they are) but whether they are any longer, or can ever be, "persons."

Drawing the line between these two senses of human "life" is not always of course clear or easy. Two related cases in which it is relatively clear and easy (at least in principle if not always in medical diagnoses) are those of brain death in adults or children and cases of anencephalic newborns (those born without a brain). If human personal life is defined as life capable of a minimal function of experience and communication and the brain is what makes that possible, then whole brain death is really equivalent to the death of the person.

A human with whole brain death does not, or should not raise any ethical difficulties as regards initiation or continuation of treatment. Death may be declared in such cases once the standard and careful medical tests have been made, even though other "vital organs" (heart and lungs) may be kept alive to that point (and even after for transplant purposes) by life support systems.[15] As for anencephalic newborns, they too are best classified as instances of human biological, not personal, life and could therefore be deemed "personally" dead at birth. They are generally not in any case paradigmatic cases for cessation of treatment, since such organisms very soon die anyhow, with or without treatment.

Other cases are much more difficult. One in particular is the (apparently) irreversibly comatose patient with massive destruction of the higher brain (cerebral centres), and therefore permanent loss of the ability to experience and relate. Many of these latter are incapable of spontaneous respiration. But far more difficult still are those with the same cerebral (higher) brain damage, but able to breathe spontaneously thanks to more or less undamaged lower brain functions. Are they alive or dead accord-

ing to the above distinction between human *biological* and human *personal* life?

In my view, if the medical tests have in fact determined that there is no potential for spontaneous cerebral brain function, even if spontaneous respiration continues, then the human person is dead. Obviously this view is based on the conviction that man is essentially more than a biological "respiratory" being, and is essentially a rational, experiencing, communicating being. It is based as well on the strong medical evidence that the specific loci in the brain in which these latter functions reside are the cerebral or higher brain centres. From this perspective of course statutes defining death in terms of "whole brain" death (which all of them to date do) do not go as far as they (morally at least) might and perhaps should. In order to legally acknowledge and establish as death this difficult and not infrequent case, statutes would have to require (only) the irreversible cessation of total spontaneous *cerebral* function, instead of the death of the (whole) brain.

On the other hand, from a prudential point of view of course there may well be some good reasons in favour of settling for a whole brain death standard in any proposed statute. There are after all other stances in our society which accept (mere) biological life as personal life, and in an issue as fundamental and contentious as this one, in a pluralistic society like ours, the variety of stances cannot easily be ignored or wished away in the shaping of public policy.

Because of this variety of views it has been suggested that the choice of standards for determining one's death be left to each patient or patient's agent to make, and that legal "definitions" of death be framed with that aim in mind. But in view of the impracticality of such an approach, the best course for now may well be to stay with the generally more acceptable "whole-brain" death standard in present statutes regarding the determination of death.

Another factor which could be advanced against a "cerebral" death criterion is a very practical and frightening one. It is the general and understandable revulsion at the prospect of burying or cremating a body in which respiration and circulation continue, even though cerebral function has irreversibly ceased. To do so would, at the very least, be an act of grave disrespect towards the body and the memory of the person concerned. It is a serious problem, and one seldom dealt with by proponents of a cerebral death criterion.

On the other hand, that understandable revulsion need not be a definitive argument against considering such a person dead and acting accordingly. We say this because "acting accordingly" need not and should not mean burying a body in which the heart is still beating, but could at least involve ceasing treatment, nourishment, resuscitation attempts, infection-fighting and so forth. In short it would mean stopping anything which would uselessly prolong respiration and heartbeat by extending mere biological life in a body now no longer capable of even experiencing pain or comfort.

In this writer's view the best (whole brain) statutory "definition" of death proposed to date is that of Capron and Kass, first proposed in 1972. It states,

> A person will be considered dead if in the announced opinion of a physician, based on ordinary standards of medical practice, he has experienced an *irreversible cessation of spontaneous respiratory and circulatory functions*. In the event that artificial means of support preclude a deter-

mination that these functions have ceased, a person will be considered dead if in the announced opinion of a physician, based on ordinary standards of medical practice, he has experienced an *irreversible cessation of spontaneous brain functions*. Death will have occurred at the time when the relevant functions ceased. [Emphasis added].[16]

This formulation has a number of positive features. Among them are these:

1. It acknowledges the importance and validity of brain death as a criterion of death, even though it could have gone further by acknowledging cerebral death (alone) as personal death. It could probably be adequately amended to that end by changing the word "brain" to "cerebral," and by not limiting the use of this criterion only to instances of artificial means of support. After all, if spontaneous breathing is still possible then presumably at least that function is not being artificially supported.

2. It avoids any suggestion that there are two concepts or kinds of human death—respiratory/circulatory death and brain death. Instead it proposes two alternate criteria for determining the *single* event and phenomenon of personal death. From a moral perspective it is incorrect to argue or suggest that there are different human deaths, or that because different cells and organs die at different times death is a continuing process or that the moment of death is arbitrary. Terms such as "brain death" or "cerebral death" therefore do not (or should not) suggest only the death of that organ or part of it, but the altered moral status— from personal life to personal death—of the entire individual human being.

3. It recognizes that in most instances of death the usual criteria (respiratory and circula-

tory functions) remain applicable, and that it is in relatively rare and special circumstances that the direct determination of brain death becomes necessary.[17]

By way of an aside, it should be acknowledged that increasingly death in practice *appears* to be anything but a "single" and "personal" event. This is especially so in the hospital context. As Philippe Ariès writes,

> Death in the hospital is no longer the occasion of a ritual ceremony, over which the dying person presides amidst his assembled relatives and friends. Death is a technical phenomenon obtained by a cessation of care . . . Indeed in the majority of cases the dying person has already lost consciousness. Death has been dissected, cut to bits by a series of little steps, which finally makes it impossible to know which step was the real death, the one in which consciousness was lost, or the one in which breathing stopped. All these little silent deaths have replaced and erased the great dramatic act of death, and no one any longer has the strength or patience to wait over a period of weeks for a moment which has lost a part of its meaning.[18]

My major point is that once the distinction between human *personal,* and human *biological* life is made and the line drawn, neither moral theology nor moral philosophy require us to maintain human biological or metabolic life for its own sake as a "good in itself," as if its condition or quality were irrelevant.

In a sense, despite the ambiguities, complexities and debates which persist, that distinction is probably the easiest of all issues with which to establish the principle that human life is not always a "good in itself." But cessation of treatment in the face of and because of personal death is one thing. We have yet to argue

in detail (though we began to in the previous section) that sometimes the prolonging of life is not a good or a benefit to the subject even when human personal life does exist, and this because of the degree of handicap and/or level of suffering and/or irreversible imminence of death.

A great deal of experience and even some empirical data[19] suggest that it is not so much life in itself which we desire, but bearable, enjoyable and worthwhile experiences and satisfactions. We want life for what can be done with it, not for what it is in itself. "It always seems to be assumed that life, of whatever quality, is the most priceless of possessions. Physicians often assume that patients would always prefer life no matter how handicapped, to death. The opposite is often the case."[20]

But does not this view and the general use of quality of life language imply that there is an *inequality* between lives, and in the degree of protection they therefore merit? "Can one really use a condition of life criterion and still insist that every life is of equal value regardless of condition? . . . does not one statement cancel out the other in the actual ethical climate in which today's debate is taking place?"[21]

Again, the answer to this objection depends upon the meaning we give to the word "life." If "life" means "person" or personal life, then there is no inconsistency or inequality. All *persons* are of equal value no matter what their condition. But not all *lives* in the biological sense are equally of value to the individual person concerned, particularly (though not only) those alive merely in a vegetative or metabolic state.

Because of different (biological, physical) conditions and in respect to decisions about whether and how to treat, all lives are *not* equal if equal means "identical." "What the 'equal value' language is attempting to say is legitimate—we must avoid *unjust* discrimination in the provision of health care and life supports. But not all discrimination (inequality of treatment) is unjust. *Unjust* discrimination is avoided if decision-making centres on the benefit to the patient, even if the benefit is described largely in terms of quality of life criteria."[22]

D. Death with Dignity

Is there any help to be found for our case in the expression and meaning of the oft heard phrase "death with dignity"? Is the reality it indicates a compelling argument for the use of quality of life criteria for the benefit of the patient? Many think it is, and write of the basic indignity done to patients for whom the end comes, "while comatose, betubed, aerated, glucosed, narcosed, sedated, not conscious, not even human anymore."[23]

These views usually identify the indignity in both the patient's helplessness, and in the mechanical substitutes which act for and on the patient. "There is an implicit indignity in the conception of the meaning of life revealed by over-vigorous efforts to maintain its outward, visible and entirely trivial signs. It is not breathing, urinating and defecating that makes a human being important even when he can do these things by himself. How much greater is the indignity when all these things must be done for him, and he can do nothing else. Not only have means been converted into ends; the very means themselves have become artificial. It is simply an insult to the very idea of humanity to equate it with these mechanically maintained appearances."[24]

But if restraining these so-called "heroic" means lessens at least to some degree death with *indignity,* is the more "natural" dying and death which remains therefore a dying and death with *dignity?* Again, many would say, yes. A certain dignity in dying is professed to be inevitable and essential. To accept it is to accept the natural world, life and death the way they are for all contingent beings. Human death is for the good and progress of the group, the larger community, both its biological and societal good.

The community requires continuing rejuvenation, and it is in the enduring human community, not in the transient, contingent individual, that unities and values of the spirit continue. Such for instance was the view of Hegel and is the view of many contemporaries of many disciplines. Not that he and others today claim death of individuals is a dignity, a benefit only for the larger community of man. In old age for instance, the loss of vitality and creativity, as well as the increase of disease and of monotony underline the limits of finitude and make of death a necessary, natural and welcome culmination to the individual.

In this view death itself is neither unnatural nor the real enemy of medicine. In the natural order of things, physical immortality would be an absurdity and decidedly non-beneficial to both individual humans and the community. The natural enemy of medicine is not death itself, but "... it does make sense to see a painful death or a premature death (less than the usual life span) as 'unnatural' in the sense of violating a reasonable human hope—for a painless death and an average life span."[25]

But there is another side of the issue which deserves consideration. Some aspects of this other argument draw attention to important qualifications in the "death with dignity" position. First of all it must be admitted that the "naturalness" and "dignity" of death is often more compelling a view to the non-religious than to the Christian. The Christian view is somewhat ambivalent about death. On the one hand death is seen as a punishment for original sin and not at all natural.

But on the other hand, Christians believe in salvation and immortality which should endow death with a dignity and even a certain attraction. Yet as one theologian writes, "How striking it is that those who profess faith in personal survival after biological death are often the ones who hang on most grimly and desperately to biological life in spite of the end of personal integrity."[26]

Part of the answer to that observation comes largely from testimony of the dying themselves and those with most experience with the dying. The answer is simply that while death may be natural, necessary and dignified looked at communally or religiously or from the long range and evolutionary standpoint, the actual individual *experience* of it is more often that of varying degrees of *indignity*. And this includes so-called "natural" death.

Dying can be peaceful, dignified and noble, but this is probably more because of what the dying persons and those who assist them bring to the experience in terms of convictions, insights and empathies than what the experience of itself and by itself provides.

As Elisabeth Kübler-Ross writes, though learning to look at and prepare for death and dying from the right perspective remains essential and long overdue for most of us, nevertheless, "It *is* hard to die, and it will always be so, even when we have learned to accept death as an integral part of life, because dying means giving up life on this earth."[27]

She and others write of how the dread of death involves for many the fear of oblivion and the loss and separation from all one's loved ones, and one's own self, one's experiences and the possibility of any new experiences in the future. For some the consuming dread includes expected punishment in the afterlife. For most, fear of death is fear of the unknown. But whatever one's particular reason for fearing death, the fear is there in all of us at one level of consciousness or another, and it may very likely serve a positive function: "Such constant expenditure of psychological energy on the business of preserving life would be impossible if the fear of death were not as constant. The very term 'self-preservation' implies an effort against some form of disintegration; the affective aspect of this is fear, fear of death."[28]

In the light of these existential observations it may be both unrealistic and unhelpful to the dying to pretend that "indignity" can ever be fully refined out of the experience of death. "We do not begin to keep human community with the dying if we interpose between them and us most of the current notions of 'death with dignity.' Rather do we draw closer to them if and only if our conception of 'dying with dignity' encompasses—nakedly and without dilution—the final indignity of death itself, whether accepted or raged against."[29]

A further qualification of the "death with dignity" thesis deserves attention here. It should not be forgotten either by physicians who use life support systems and treatment, or those who argue against their use, that the primary, original and laudable purpose in their development and use is that of "buying time," so that careful diagnoses and prognoses of the patient's illness can be made.

They were not and (in principle) are not intended to serve as permanent substitutes for all the patient's own vital functions. As such it would be unreasonable to argue that the dignity of all those on life supporting systems is inevitably being violated. Several good medical reasons might justify even the protracted use of such life supporting treatment.

First of all a diagnosis or prognosis might not yet have been completed. Secondly, there may be good reasons to hope for a return of spontaneous functions and consciousness. Thirdly, if the patient is conscious he or she may prefer to fight on even though there are tubes in every orifice and hardly a shred of hope of staving off imminent death. Fourthly, if the patient is in a coma, proxies and attending physicians may believe that the patient indicated before becoming comatose that he or she wanted to be "artificially" supported to the end, no matter what.

In other words, the mere fact of life support systems and their paraphernalia being used need not necessarily imply an indignity to the patient. "Certainly such a state as the one described is not very pretty, nor is it comfortable for any of the parties concerned. But that is not really the issue, unless we let a question of aesthetics rule the issue of life and death. The issue is whether it is undignified for an individual in the throes of death to fight by any means at his disposal . . ."[30]

In the light of both sides of the "dignity of death" thesis, what is its relevance for or against quality of life considerations?

First of all, none of the views considered above argued that there are no cases where life support systems or treatment constitute an indignity to the patient. It is generally agreed that there are cases which can constitute an unnecessarily undignified dying, particularly when the treatment involves discomfort, offers no hope of even a minimal recovery, is no longer serving its diagnostic function, and the patient has not requested it. This point was forcibly made by the theologian Karl Barth, one of the strongest defenders of the sanctity of life. He wondered whether, ". . . This kind of artificial prolongation of life does not amount to human arrogance in the opposite direction, whether the fulfillment of medical duty does not threaten to become fanaticism, reason folly, and the required assisting of human life a forbidden torturing of it."[31]

Secondly, the mere removal and withdrawal of tubes and respirators does not in itself effect a "death with dignity." The final indignity of dying and death itself remains. It would probably be more accurate to speak of such patients as "dying with *less indignity.*" If there is to be dignity it will be because the conscious patient, hopefully now less encumbered, more accessible and able to communicate is assisted and comforted by others in dying.

Thirdly, the brief analysis of the "death with dignity" concept reaffirms the centrality of the "benefit to patient" criterion in such quality of life considerations. Only a reasonable application of that criterion, ideally by the patient himself or herself, or by the reasonable judgment of proxies if the patient is incapable of making a choice, can determine how the patient's interest, wishes or "dignity" would be best served in a given instance.

In one case patient benefit may best be served by an unsupported but more comfortable last few hours in a terminal illness; or in another case by continuing to fight against death until the last moment with all the medical hardware and software available; or in still another case, by coming to a decision that though death is not imminent, the likely condition or quality of life on recovery will not be sufficient to justify continuation of treatment now.

E. Conclusions: Equal Lives and Objective Criteria

(1) The indeterminate sanctity of life principle alone cannot be used to determine in advance all treatment decisions, without consideration as well of the quality of the lives in question. To do so would be to use that principle as a "decision-avoiding" not a "decision-making" guide.

(2) The meaning of quality of life in the medical context need not mean wholly subjective judgments about the relative worth, value, utility or equality of the lives of persons. Purged of connotations of "relative worth" or "social utility," the function of quality of life thinking in this context (as in the environmental context) can be one of improving and benefiting the patient, and can focus on objective criteria and needs.

(3) In particular there are two such quality of life criteria relevant to decisions to treat, or to continue treatment or to stop treatment. The first considers the capacity to experience, to relate. The second considers the intensity and susceptibility to control of the patient's pain and suffering. If despite treatment there is not and cannot be even a minimal capacity to experience, and to relate, or if the level of pain and suffering will be prolonged, excruciating and intractable, then a decision to cease or not initiate treatment (of for instance a comatose patient) can be preferable to treatment.

(4) The word "life" can mean two things in this context. It can mean vital or metabolic processes alone, a life incapable of experiencing or communicating and one which therefore could be called "human biological life." Or it could mean a level or quality of life which includes *both* metabolic functions and at least a minimal capacity to experience or communicate, which together could be called "human personal life."

(5) Those with whole brain death are dead as persons, even if biological life (alone) can be maintained externally. It could be convincingly argued as well that those who are (only) cerebrally dead are also dead as persons.

(6) Death is best spoken of as a *single* event occurring when the brain dies. It would be incorrect to say there are different human deaths or that the moment of death is arbitrary even though different cells and organs die at different points on the dying continuum, or because hospitals often are able to "draw out" death and make possible a sort of "technical life" even after real (personal) death has occurred.

(7) If by "life" here is meant personal life, then the use of quality of life language and criteria need not imply or assume *inequality* between lives. All *persons* are equal in value no matter what their condition or quality. But not all lives in the biological sense are of equal value to the patients in question. To cease medical treatment in some of these cases is not unjust discrimination as long as the decision-making focuses on benefit to patient. Death need not always be resisted as if anything is an improvement over death.

(8) Given that the sanctity of life principle imposes the burden of proof on those who would cease to support the lives of others, the consideration of quality of life criteria should not inevitably and exclusively lead to decisions to cease or not initiate life supporting or saving

treatment. Quite the opposite should just as often or more often be the case.

(9) While a degree of "indignity" is an inescapable element of death and dying, and while not every instance of a patient's life being externally supported is thereby undignified, there are cases in which the refusal to consider and weigh the patient's quality of life can result in a prolongation of treatment to the point that a real and further indignity is being done.

(10) Both medical decision-making and law should continue to protect the intrinsic sanctity and value of each human life. But medicine (and perhaps law as well) should formally acknowledge that in some cases the quality or conditions of a patient's life can be so damaged and minimal that treatment or further treatment could be a violation precisely of that life's sanctity and value.

(11) Even in those cases for which it is decided to cease or not initiate external life supporting *treatment*, there always remains a continuing obligation no matter how damaged the patient's condition, to provide whatever amount of *care and comfort* is needed and possible.

Notes

1. Editorial, *California Medicine*, Sept. 1970, pp. 67–68.
2. Weber, Leonard J., *Who Shall Live?* Paulist Press, N.Y., 1976, pp. 41–42.
3. *The Quality of Life Concept*, U.S. Environmental Protection Agency, Washington, D.C., 1973, p. iii.
4. Baier, Kurt, "Towards a Definition of Quality of Life," in Peter C. List and Ronald O. Clarke (editors), *Environmental Spectrum*, D. van Nostrand Co., N.Y., 1974, p. 67.
5. See for instance, U.S. Environmental Protection Agency, *Quality of Life Indicators*, 1972. Also, Dillman, Don A., and Tremblay, Kenneth R., "The Quality of Life in Rural America," *The Annals of the American Academy of Political and Social Science*, 429, Jan. '77, 115–129.
6. See for instance, Office of Management and Budget (U.S.), *Social Indicators*, Washington, 1973, p. xiii, also, *Perspective Canada*, Ottawa, 1974, p. xxii.
7. McCall, Storrs, "Human Needs and the Quality of Life," in John King-Farlow and William R. Shea (editors), *Values and the Quality of Life*, Canadian Contemporary Philosophy Series, Science History Publications, N.Y., 1976, p. 14.
8. Ibid., p. 15.
9. Ibid., p. 18.
10. Maslow, Abraham, *Motivation and Personality*, N.Y., 1954, pp. 35–47, as cited by McCall, op. cit., p. 19.
11. This is a suggestion convincingly argued by Storrs McCall, op. cit., note 84, pp. 20–21.
12. Baier, Kurt, "The Sanctity of Life," *Journal of Social Philosophy* 5, (2), April '74, p. 5.
13. For probably the best treatment of the obligation and significance of "Care," see Paul Ramsey, "On (Only) Caring for the Dying," ch. 3 of his *The Patient as Person*, Yale University Press, New Haven, 1970, pp. 113–164.
14. Kautzky, R. "Der Arzt," *Arzt und Christ* 15 (1969), 138, (as cited by R. McCormick, "The Quality of Life, The Sanctity of Life," *Hastings Center Report*, 8, 1, Feb. '78, p. 34).
15. One can think of no compelling moral or medical reason why, once death has been declared, such "unburied corpses" cannot continue to be maintained biologically alive for any length of time as "vital organ banks" or "tissue banks." As one

moralist puts it, "it seems to me that one should not speak in such cases of having maintained 'life.' For what is really maintained is merely certain limited biological functions. To put it more pointedly, there has been a preservation of the vitality of specific organs of an unburied corpse . . . the organism as a whole has ceased to be . . ." Thielicke, Helmuth, in Kenneth Vaux (ed.) *Who Shall Live? Medicine, Technology, Ethics,* Fortress Press, Philadelphia, 1970, p. 176.

16.   Capron, A. M. and Kass, L. R., "A Statutory Definition of the Standards for Determining Human Death: an Appraisal and a Proposal," *U. of Penn. Law Review,* 121, Nov. 1972, p. 111.

17.   The major such test would be the presence of a flat EEG (Electroencephalogram). Because some brain activity can apparently still remain even if the EEG indicates no electrical activity, it can be only of confirmatory value for the determination of *whole brain* death. But because it measures mainly neocortical or higher brain activity, it can be the central and major test for *cerebral* death. Its reliability for that purpose has been strongly supported by medical evidence. See D. Silverman *et al.,* "Irreversible Coma Associated with Electrocerebral Silence." *Neurology,* 20, 1970, 525–533. For a fuller discussion of brain death and cerebral death, see: Veatch, Robert, "The Whole-Brain-Oriented Concept of Death: An Outmoded Philosophical Formulation," *Journal of Thanatology* 3, 13 (1975) and his, *Death, Dying and the Biological Revolution,* Yale U. Press, New Haven, 1976, pp. 21–76; Brierley, J. B. *et al.,* "Neocortical Death after Cardiac Arrest," *Lancet,* Sept. 11, 1971 pp. 560–565; Capron, Alexander Morgan and Kass, Leon R., "A Statutory Definition

of the Standards for Determining Human Death: An Appraisal and a Proposal," *U. of Pennsylvania Law Review,* 121, Nov. 1972, p. 97. For further proof (if any is required) that this paper's discussion of death and brain death has merely skimmed the surface of a very complex, long debated and fascinating subject, see the collection of readings edited and introduced by Antony Flew in his, *Body, Mind and Death,* Macmillan, N.Y., 1964. The readings, ". . . have been selected in the light of the editorial conviction that the fundamental issues outstanding are primarily philosophical rather than scientific. Yet, equally certainly, they are issues that can be resolved satisfactorily only by a philosophy receptive to a scientific outlook, and informed by scientific knowledge." (p. 2). For a scientific (but very readable) history of the human brain, see Carl Sagan's, *The Dragons of Eden,* Ballantine Books, N.Y., 1977.

18.   Ariès, Philippe, *Western Attitudes Toward Death, from the Middle Ages to the Present,* Johns Hopkins U. Press, Baltimore, 1974, p. 88.

19.   Diggory, J. C., and Rothman, D. Z., "Values Destroyed by Death," *Journal of Abnormal and Social Psychology,* 63, 1961, 205–210.

20.   Gellman, Derek, M.D. *Dimensions in Health Services* 52, Nov. '75, p. 23.

21.   Weber, Leonard J., op. cit., (note 79) p. 83.

22.   McCormick, Richard A., "The Quality of Life, The Sanctity of Life," *Hastings Center Report* 8(1), 1978, p. 35.

23.   Fletcher, Joseph, "The Right to Live and the Right to Die," *The Humanist,* 34(4), Aug. '74, p. 13.

24.   Morrison, Robert S., "The Dignity of the Inevitable and Necessary," in Peter

Steinfels and Robert Veatch (editors) *Death Inside Out,* Harper and Row, 1974, p. 98.

25. Englehardt, H. Tristram, "The Counsels of Finitude," in *Death Inside Out,* op. cit. (note 101), p. 124.

26. Fletcher, Joseph, op. cit., (note 100) p. 13.

27. Kübler-Ross, Elisabeth, *Death, The Final Stage of Growth,* Prentice Hall Inc., Englewood Cliffs, N.J., 1975, p. 6.

28. Zilboorg, G., "Fear of Death," *Psychoanalytic Quarterly,* 12, 1943, p. 467.

29. Ramsey, Paul, "The Indignity of Death with Dignity," in *Death Inside Out,* op. cit. (note 101), p. 82.

30. Kluge, Eike–Henner W., *The Practice of Death,* Yale University Press, New Haven, 1975, p. 155.

31. Barth, Karl, *Church Dogmatics,* Vol. 3, Part 4, T. Clark, Edinburgh, 1961, p. 246.

5

Quality of Life

John R. Connery, S.J.

In recent years, due to advances in medical sciences, the capability of prolonging life has been dramatically enhanced. While this is generally considered a blessing, it may also add to already existing problems. Human beings have always had to face decisions about preserving or prolonging their lives. This is not new. What is new is the relative frequency with which such decisions must be faced today . . . at both ends of life. But there is another dimension to the problem which is new today. It is the introduction of a quality of life consideration into the discussion. The question is: What effect does the quality of a patient's life have on his duty to preserve it? Can it be so low that it affects the obligation to preserve this life . . . even to the point of removing all obligation?

In the past, moral theologians have always admitted that the obligation to preserve or prolong life was not an absolute one; it had its limits. They discussed this duty and its limits in terms of a distinction between ordinary and extraordinary means. The obligation to pro-

long life would not go beyond the use of ordinary means. Generally speaking, these were means which would not be too burdensome and which would actually prolong life in a significant way. If means were excessively burdensome, or if they would not prolong life in any appreciable way, one could not impose an obligation on a person to use them.

As already pointed out, this decision must be faced with greater frequency today than in the past, since there are ways and means of preserving life today that were simply not available in the past. While some of these treatments would be classified as extraordinary, because they are very burdensome or offer no hope of benefit, some would be considered ordinary (at least for short term use), and therefore obligatory. It is the increased availability of these means that has raised the quality of life issue. Many patients who simply would have died in the past may now continue to live. The question is: Must they? Or may they forego treatment available today, even though it is not excessively burdensome and will pro-

"Quality of Life" by John R. Connery, S.J. Reprinted with permission of Linacre Quarterly 53(February, 1986):26–33.

long life, because of their quality of life? Obviously, they cannot retreat into the past and pretend such means do not exist. But may they appeal simply to quality of life considerations in assessing their duty to preserve their lives?

Among Catholic moral theologians in this country, this question was raised initially by Richard McCormick, S.J., regarding infants born with serious defects.[1] The question was, at least in part, occasioned by an account in the *New England Journal of Medicine* of 43 seriously defective infants for whom treatment was rejected because of a poor prognosis for *meaningful* life.[2] McCormick accepted the basic quality of life approach but was attempting to produce more precise, and hence more secure, guidelines for making such decisions. He arrived at the following norm: if the defects were so severe that the child would never have the capacity for establishing human relations (a specifically human function), or would at least find it morally impossible to do so, the child would not be obliged even to the use of ordinary means. McCormick was speaking of infants, but the norm would obviously have to apply even to those who had reached the age when the capacity for establishing human relations should have been reached. Logic would demand that such incapacity even at this stage would remove any obligation to preserve life.

But the allowance would not apply to children with lesser defects. The obligation to use ordinary means could prevail in such cases. Thus it might prevail in the case of the ordinary retarded child, or the child with lesser physical defects.

McCormick Used Pius XII's Argument

In support of his position, McCormick used the argument Pius XII made to justify omission of extraordinary means, namely that an obligation to use extraordinary means "would be too burdensome for most men and would render the attainment of the higher, more important good too difficult."[3] The Pontiff was explaining why one could not oblige a person to use extraordinary means, but McCormick took it to mean that if the patient himself or herself would not have either the physical or even moral capacity to achieve what he considered to be the higher good (establish human relations) to which the Pontiff was referring, there would be no obligation to preserve his life. In so doing he was adding a *quality of life* norm to the traditional *quality of treatment* norm already in place. This went radically beyond anything the Pontiff had in mind.

The practicality of McCormick's norm has been questioned, since in many cases it would be most difficult to make a very precise judgment at time of birth about the eventual capability—or lack of it—of a seriously defective infant for human function. This would be even more true of a prediction of moral incapacity. In the latter case, the physical potency would be present but the handicapped person would be so distracted by his handicap that it would be extremely difficult to relate to others in a human way. Indeed it would be difficult to make such a judgment of a person at the appropriate age. The added problem of prediction doubles the difficulty. Our primary concern here is with the acceptability of the norm, rather than its practicality. Even if it was a very practical norm, we hope to show that there are serious reasons to question its acceptability.

More recently, in an article in the *NEJM*, a quality of life norm was applied to a third trimester termination of pregnancy.[4] The assumption in a third trimester pregnancy is that the fetus is viable, and that therefore, termination of the pregnancy is not automatically a lethal procedure. In a particular case, however, a doctor may judge that termination of a third trimester pregnancy would be lethal. In that case we are presuming that the authors would not allow termination. We are not discussing the allowance of a lethal procedure on the basis of quality of life considerations. We are dealing only with the duty to preserve life.

In the past, termination of pregnancy right after viability was allowed only if the life of the mother (or the fetus) was at stake. It was not allowed on the basis of the quality of life of the fetus. One of the theses of the above article is that it would be permissible to terminate a third trimester pregnancy if there is total or virtual absence of cognitive function in the fetus. The authors felt that this condition was verified in the case of a fetus diagnosed as anencephalic. The article speaks of the benefits that might come to the mother from such a termination, but these do not seem to be the primary consideration. It seems clear that the basic justification for terminating the pregnancy and the risk to the fetus involved is the quality of life judgment made about the fetus.

While the wording of the condition these authors use is different, the meaning of the requirement would seem to be close to McCormick's lack of capacity for human relations. His allowance even for the lack of moral potency may go beyond what is allowed in this case, since it would include even a person who was conscious, but so obsessed by some handicap that it would be very difficult to establish human relations. It should be pointed out, however, that the authors of the article allow termination of pregnancy where there is "virtual" absence of cognitive function. This may approximate the moral impotency of the McCormick norm, but since the authors do not elucidate the meaning of virtual, we are not sure whether it does.

In practice, McCormick's norm might, in some sense, be less difficult to apply, since the ability to establish human relations would seem to call for some ability to communicate externally. One who could not do so would not be able to establish such relations. But cognition can be present without communication. So one cannot conclude with certainty to the absence of cognition from the fact that a person cannot communicate (e.g., a person in a coma). Admission of this would seem to be implied in extending the allowance of termination of pregnancy even to the case where there is "virtual" absence of cognition.

In recent times also, the same question has been raised regarding patients in an irreversible coma (or a persistent vegetative state). If, indeed, the case is terminal (the patient will die shortly whether the treatment is used or not), since treatment will be useless, it cannot be obligatory. But in a case where treatment will prolong life and will not be excessively burdensome, it will be obligatory according to traditional norms. Some want to argue that even in this case, if the treatment does nothing more than prolong comatose life, it may still be omitted. In other words, the quality of life of a person in an irreversible coma automatically releases him or her from any obligation to preserve it. So if a treatment, even the most ordinary kind, will do nothing more than prolong life, they will argue that there is no obligation to use it. Briefly, there is no obligation to preserve this kind of life in itself.

Norm Applied in California Court

This norm was applied practically in a California court hearing to the case of Clarence Herbert, a 54-year-old man declared to be in an irreversible coma as the result of cardiac arrest. John J. Paris, S.J., an expert witness in the case, argued that there was no obligation to keep this person alive because he was in an irreversible coma.[5] We cannot go into this case, but the appeals judge ruled in favor of a previous decision to stop treatment of Herbert on this score. We are not interested in the legal ramifications of the case, but the judge cited as the source of his decision the position taken by the President's Commission for the Study of Ethical Problems in Medicine and Biomedical and Behavioral Research in a publication entitled *Deciding to Forego Life-Sustaining Treatment*. The judge's statement read as follows:

> ... proportionate treatment is that which, in the view of the patient, has at least a reasonable chance of providing benefits to the patient, which benefits outweigh the burdens attendant to the treatment. Thus, even if a course of treatment might be extremely painful, it would still be proportionate treatment if the prognosis was for complete cure or significant improvement in the patient's condition. On the other hand, a treatment course which is only minimally painful or intrusive may nonetheless be considered disproportionate to the potential benefits if the prognosis is virtually hopeless for any significant improvement in condition.[6]

The judge traces this opinion to pp. 82–90 of the Commission's report. It is obviously a summary statement, so it will not be found verbatim in this report. The following sentence from that section comes closest to the judgment of the court:

> So long as a mere biological existence is not considered the only value, patients may want to take the nature of that additional life into account (p. 88).

I am not sure that I could successfully interpret this sentence, but the judge seemed to feel that he was interpreting the mind of the Commission. Briefly, according to the judge, the opinion of the Commission seemed to be that life as such (what the report calls "biological existence") is not a sufficient value to warrant the imposition of any duty to preserve it. In the present case, this means that since there is no chance to return the patient to a cognitive state, there is no obligation to keep him alive. Since this is an ethical commission, and the language used is basically ethical, one must conclude that it was not dealing on the level of legislation alone.

The judge puts the obligation in terms of proportionate/disproportionate treatment. In the Declaration on Euthanasia, the Sacred Congregation for the Doctrine of the Faith (1980) says that some use this distinction in preference to the traditional ordinary/extraordinary distinction to avoid the confusion caused by the latter.[7] The Congregation has nothing against the change in terminology, but insists that the underlying principle still holds good. In other words the criterion is still the benefit or burden of the treatment.

What is ethically objectionable in the court decision is that it departs from this principle in two critical respects: (1) it seems to make benefit the sole consideration, and (2) it makes it depend on quality of life considerations. If a treatment will be effective, the court considers it obligatory even if "extremely painful." But more relevant to our discussion is the judgment that prolonging the life of a person in an irreversible coma is not considered enough of a benefit to make any treatment (even minimally painful or intrusive) obligatory. In other words, the quality of life of this person is so low that there is no obligation to preserve it. As far as any obligation to preserve life goes, such a patient is like a dead man. In taking this stand the Court was departing not only from the distinction between ordinary/extraordinary means, but also from the principle underlying it. In making this point, however, we are not making a judgment about the rightness or wrongness of withdrawing treatment in the case involved. We have dealt with this issue elsewhere.[8] Here we are simply questioning the reason the Court gave to justify withdrawal. Our concern is that it approved withdrawal of treatment for the wrong reason.

In all of the cases described above the basic consideration in discerning the duty to prolong life was the quality of life the patient was leading. The argument is that life itself can be so burdensome or so empty that it ceases to be of value, or at least that its value is not sufficient to impose an obligation on the victim to preserve it.

From what we have seen, it seems clear that in the past, the duty to preserve life was related to respect for life itself as a basic good. All life deserved this respect, and it was to be shown as long as life was present. No limitation was put on the duty in this regard. No one ever suggested that the duty pertained only to those who enjoyed a certain quality of life or that it did not pertain to those who did not have that quality. The duty was the same for all.

At times the position of those who oppose quality of life considerations is classified pejoratively as "vitalism" or "biologism." I think this charge may well apply to those who make life a supreme value to which everything else must yield and who hold, consequently, that all possible means to preserve it must be used. But to use the term of the position of those who oppose quality of life considerations is to misuse it. Those who hold this latter position in no way subscribe to the opinion that all means must be used to preserve life. They ad-

mit that there is a limit to the obligation to preserve life. They simply deny that this limit is based on quality of life as such.

In two (termination of pregnancy, irreversible coma) of the three instances mentioned in which quality of life was appealed to, little argumentation was offered to substantiate the positions taken. As we have seen, McCormick, in the case of the seriously defective infant, constructed an argument from the reason given by Pius XII to show why one could not impose an obligation to use extraordinary means, but he changed the whole context of that argument, and in doing so, undermined any claim he might make to support from the Pontiff's statement. So what we have are three instances in which quality of life was appealed to with little or no supporting reason.

McCormick attempts to show that his position is in continuity with past tradition by offering examples of cases in which quality of life was a consideration even in the past. It is quite true that, in the past, if quality of life affected the means or treatment, it became a factor in assessing the duty to use the means. Thus, the quality of life resulting from a quadruple amputation would affect the duty to undergo this kind of surgery. Similarly, if the patient was dying, it would frequently render the means to preserve life useless. McCormick would argue that he is simply extending the use of quality of life to another situation.

Writer Explains Contention

It is the contention of this writer that moving the criterion from *quality of treatment* to *quality of life* as such is not just another step in the same direction. It is a quantum leap. As pointed out, in the past, quality of life was considered only in reference to means. It might make a means burdensome, or it might make it useless. In the present usage it becomes the basic consideration. Even if it does not make the means burdensome or useless, it is appealed to in order to justify what is done or not done. This involves a whole new attitude toward this issue, and one which raises serious questions.

This can be illustrated very simply with the Quinlan case. The intention in that case was to relieve the girl of the burden of long-term dependence on a respirator. It was not to bring on the death of the girl. This was made clear by the efforts (successful) to wean her from the respirator. And the goal (removing the burden constituted by the respirator) was achieved even though she lived.

When quality of life is in itself the basic consideration, the entire approach is different. The intention is not to free the patient of the burden of using some means, but the burden (or the uselessness) of the life itself. The only way to achieve this goal is by the death of the patient. So when one foregoes means because of quality of life considerations in this sense, the intention is the death of the patient. In this respect it differs vastly from the traditional approach. In the traditional approach, death was an unintentional side-effect of foregoing the treatment. In the current use, it is the intention in foregoing the treatment. Put briefly, in the traditional approach, one was making a legitimate application of the principle of double effect. In the present approach, one of the conditions for the legitimate use of that principle is violated (the evil effect is intended), so no such justification is available.

On the contrary, given the intention of bringing on death, one is forced to the conclusion that an independent quality of life norm involves euthanasia by omission (or by act, in the case of the pregnancy termination). The recent *Declaration on Euthanasia* by the SCDF (1980) defines euthanasia as an act or omission which either by nature or intention brings on the death of the patient (out of mercy). Since death is intended in quality of life decisions of this kind, they fulfill the definition of intentional euthanasia by act or omission.

An additional problem in the use of quality of life norms is that, up to the present, no norm has been suggested that would clearly define the cases to which it would apply and exclude those to which it would not apply. In the present discussion we have seen it applied e.g., to a person in an irreversible coma, or in a persistent vegetative state, but there is no way to limit it to those cases. Tomorrow, it could be applied to someone with Alzheimer's disease, the next day to a person with some other serious mental or physical handicap. In other words, it puts us on a slippery slope with no braking power. This kind of norm, even if it were legitimate, would end up a menace to society because of its lack of precision.

There are those who fear that if the withdrawal of treatment is not allowed on the basis of a quality of life criterion, we will be overwhelmed with people living in institutions at a very low level of existence. Even if this were the case, it would not of itself justify withdrawing treatment on a quality of life basis, any more than it would justify simply inflicting a painless death on them. However beneficial this might be to society, it would not be permissible. But I do not think this would happen. My judgment is that many, if not most, of the decisions that are made to withdraw treatment could be justified because burdensome means are involved. Many of the means in question, even if ordinary in a crisis situation, can become burdensome when used on a long term basis. If a judgment can be made that long term use will be required, such treatment may become optional. Certainly, death is the result in any event. But it is important that it should not result from the use of a criterion as objectionable and as open to abuse as quality of life.

In brief, then, an independent quality of life norm represents a radical departure from the past which put the emphasis on the quality of the treatment. The basic difference is in the intention. In the traditional quality of treatment norm, death is not intended but a side effect of a decision to spare the patient the burden of a difficult treatment. In an independent quality of life norm, death is intended, and this is basically what makes it objectionable. It is intentional euthanasia by omission (or by act in the termination of a third trimester pregnancy). But even if a quality of life approach could be justified in itself, the norms suggested up to the present carry with them inherent risk of abuse because of their imprecision. Adoption will put one on a slippery slope with no braking power.

Notes

1. "To Save or Let Die." *America* (1974) pp. 6–10.
2. "Moral and Ethical Dilemmas in the Special-Care Nursery. *New England Journal of Medicine,* 289 (1973) pp. 890–94.
3. Address to an International Congress of Anesthesiologists. *The Pope Speaks* (1958) pp. 393–98.
4. "When is Termination of Pregnancy During the Third Trimester Morally Justifiable?" *New England Journal of Medicine,* 310 (1984) pp. 501–04.
5. People v. Barber-Nejdl, Reporter's Transcript of Preliminary Hearing, Jan. 25, 1983.
6. Decision of California State Court of Appeals, Oct. 12, 1983.
7. Declaratio de Euthanasia (1980) pp. 10–12.
8. "The Clarence Herbert Case: Was Withdrawal Justified?" *Hospital Progress,* 65 (1984) 31–35.

6

"Quality of Life" and the Analogy with the Nazis

Cynthia B. Cohen

Human beings who are critically ill are being allowed to die or caused to remain alive with increasing frequency on the basis of poorly understood "quality of life" judgments. These are viewed as pernicious by some who take them to deny the equal value of all human beings as such and to presuppose that some human lives are not "worthy to be lived." Proponents of "quality of life" assessments claim that they are based on recognition of the value of human beings, and maintain that this very value entails that individuals ought not be subjected to a life that is below that of minimal human well-being. This disagreement about "quality of life" considerations raises basic questions concerning the foundation of the value of human beings and of their lives, the relation of the condition of an individual's life to its value, and the priority that should be given to human life as a good.

Discussion of these issues, however, has been impeded by an analogy that is sometimes drawn between the use of "quality of life" considerations in decisions about whether or not to treat individuals and the Nazi practice of exterminating those whom they took to fall below certain standards. This analogy has played a major role in the opposition to such disparate proposals as those for "Living Will" legislation (Dunphy, 1976; Keene, 1978), the selective treatment of impaired newborns (Kelsey, 1975; Koop, 1977; Ramsey, 1978, p. 211), legalized euthanasia (Kamisar, 1958; Dyck, 1973, pp. 107–108), and triage for admission to and retention in intensive care units.[1] Each of these has been charged with the implicit adoption of Nazi-like judgments that correlate the value of human beings with the quality of their lives. The analogy is one that needs to be analyzed seriously, both to determine whether policies and programs based on "quality of life" assessments are morally ac-

---

" 'Quality of Life' and the Analogy with the Nazis" by Cynthia B. Cohen. Reprinted with permission of The Journal of Medicine and Philosophy *8(1983):113–135.*

61

ceptable on these grounds, and also to assist us to understand what is meant by the "quality of life" and how this relates to the value of human beings and their lives.

I will argue that the analogy at issue is mistaken, for it misconstrues and assimilates the senses of "value" and "quality" that figure in the Nazi ideology and a "quality of life" position. This leads the analogizers to claim incorrectly that both views measure the value of human beings according to the relative quality of their physical and mental condition as this is determined by social utilitarian standards. I will suggest that a coherent "quality of life" position is grounded in a theory of the value of humans as beings with a capacity for self-reflective deliberation and action. It explicates the meaning of the "quality of life" of human beings in terms of standards of individual well-being, rather than in terms of social worth. It is premised on respect for individual autonomy and principles of compensatory justice. Finally, I will propose that we must carefully develop criteria of minimal well-being or "quality of life" for the voiceless in order to ensure that they will not be subjected to a life that denies all that is distinctively valuable about human beings.

I

At the end of October, 1939, an order was officially promulgated by Hitler that "persons who, according to human judgment, are incurably ill may, upon the most serious evaluation of their medical condition, be accorded a mercy death" (Nürnberg, 1949–53). Six units were set up in which medical personnel carried out what came to be known as the "Euthanasia Program." This was, in effect, a program of

mass murder, in which accurate medical diagnoses and humane considerations played no part (Dawidowicz, 1975, pp. 834–844). The killings, which had begun earlier in secrecy with mentally and physically impaired children, now engulfed adults who were ill or disabled. Ultimately, they consumed a wider range of people including those who were "useless eaters," Jews, Gypsies, foreigners, "deviants" of a conscientious nature, and those simply labelled as "undesirable" (Mitscherlich and Mielke, 1949; Krausnick, 1965; Gorlitz, 1960). Untold numbers of human beings were murdered before the termination of the Third Reich. They were killed on grounds that they were "devoid of value" and *unlebenswertig* or "unworthy of life" (Broszat, 1960).

The theoretical basis of the Nazi belief that some human beings are without value is not readily explicated, as it was not clearly formulated. This was not an oversight. Hitler viewed attempts to provide a clear and consistent exposition of Nazi tenets as amusing (Picker, 1963, p. 275). He declared that:

> What is necessary is that some few, really great ideas be made clear to every individual . . . and that the essential fundamental lines be burned inextinguishably into him, so that he is entirely permeated by the necessity of the victory of his movement and its doctrine (Hitler, 1943, p. 456).

The result of his exaltation of minimal theory was an ideology that was incoherent at its very core. Nazi theory consisted of a group of ideas strung together without heed to their internal consistency.

A leading notion that Hitler used to explain the ultimate source and criterion of value was the *Volk*. He conceived of the *Volk* as a creative, eternal, primordial being, a boundless, expanding force that incorporated a certain racial type within itself. It was not the sum of the collection of individuals who belonged to this type, but an organic whole that surpassed and completely defined each one of them. There were no distinctions among individuals of this type or between individuals and the *Volk*. Only the *Volk* was a true individual and the full reality; it had a life and a will of its own (Stuckgart and Globke, 1966). It was the ultimate value and the perfect end toward which all of life was directed. It could not be evaluated by external criteria; its very existence provided its justification.

There were many different qualitatively unequal racial types, each of which was related to the *Volk* in a different way. Only the "pure-blooded" Aryan type, the highest, was essential to the organic whole. The Aryan race was "the Prometheus of mankind from whose bright forehead the divine spark of genius has sprung at all times . . ." (Hitler, 1943, p. 290). The immutable laws of racial type guaranteed the survival and predominance of the Aryan race (Picker, 1963, pp. 494–495). Non-Aryan types were sub-human and degenerate accretions which were ranked biologically between human beings and chimpanzees (Ivy, 1977). They were described by the S.S. Main Office as "a creation of nature, apparently completely similar biologically to the human with hands, feet, and a sort of brain, with eyes and mouth, which is, however, completely different, a horrible creature who is only an attempt at being human . . ." (Hofer, 1957). The "sub-human" types were of unequal value. The Slavs, for instance were of sufficient worth to the *Volk* to be used as slaves. The Jews had to be isolated and, ultimately, destroyed since they had lost their territory due to their weak character and could only survive by posing a serious threat to Aryan soil (Dawidowicz, 1975, pp. 114–115; Jäckel, 1975, pp. 101–105).

Behind Hitler's views about human quality and value was his perception of the mass of people as stupid, treacherous, and weak-willed (Hitler, 1943, pp. 237, 240–241, 374–375, 379, 381). Individuals were moved by biological instincts and drives grounded in race. Since the behavior of each individual was predetermined by race, and the goal of each individual was the survival and success of his race (Mosse, 1966), race had to be the primary factor by which the value of each individual was assessed. Further, since most people were cowardly and bestial, every trace of their individuality had to be eradicated for the sake of an unimpeded *Volk*. Within the Aryan race, there were some individuals who were of distinctive value due to their creative achievements and capacity for vigorous leadership. Still, even they were expendable. It was the life, freedom, and will of the *Volk*, not that of the individual, that had to be ensured. Individuals were not entitled to fulfill their needs, to claim their rights, to shape their future. Their task was to ensure the well-being of the *Volk*.

The highest expression of the will of the *Volk* was war; violence and conflict were essential to its nature. The Nazi "higher ethic" maintained that the better and stronger were locked in "the bitter struggle for existence" against the "sub-humans" who occupied their living-space. This putative law of nature was transformed into a law of higher moral necessity. The Aryans had to conquer all who resisted them, for what was not given to them had to be taken by force (Hitler, 1943, pp. 8, 244–245, 393; Jäckel, 1972, pp. 93–95). Each Aryan was obliged to engage in the struggle for existence and to devote his or her life to the enhancement of the *Volk* by whatever means necessary. Hitler's call to violence was clear: "Those who want to live, let them fight, and those who do not want to fight in this world of eternal struggle, do not deserve to live. Even if this were hard—that is how it is!" (Hitler, 1943, p. 397). Conscience was only a weakness that could erode the life of the *Volk*. Each Aryan had to overcome moral scruples and squeamishness to enforce the bioracial laws that governed the nature of things.

The view that emerges from the Nazis' concatenation of ideas is that no particular value accrued to individual human beings as such. It was the value of a people (*Volkswert*), of a living race, that was the basic unit of measurement of worth for Hitler. The members of the Aryan race were considered fully human; yet even their individual value was derived from their intimate fusion with the *Volk*. Individual "sub-humans" of sufficient racial quality to be of service to the *Volk* had some derivative value. It was race, the "central principle of human existence," that provided the basic criterion for the classification of the value of an individual. The higher the racial type of an individual, the greater his or her worth. Racial membership and value were assumed to be correlative by the Nazis.

The postulation of an entity such as the *Volk* as the ultimate source of all value and arbiter of worth is fraught with conceptual difficulties. The notion of the *Volk* as the living essence of the Aryan race is incoherent. It is unclear in what sense an abstract racial classification can be a living creature. We are given no explanation of how the various attributes of the *Volk* interrelate or how they affect the nature of individual Aryans. We are told that this "higher entity" separated into distinct individuals who thereafter struggled for extinction

through reunification, but we are not informed about how and why the mutilation of the *Volk* occurred or whether the individuals spewed forth in the process were illusory appearances or real beings. Since individuals are completely defined by their racial type, it is not clear how there could be a distinction between certain individuals within the Aryan race who are of greater value to the *Volk* than others. That the powerful *Volk* could be threatened by submissive and ineffectual weaklings appears inconceivable. Scientifically, the view that there are static, ideal racial types was a fiction in Hitler's time, and has received no subsequent validation. The incoherence of the notion of the *Volk* and the lack of substantiation of Hitler's racial views in fact undermine Naziism as a credible theory.

Nazi thought about the value and quality of human beings founders on an incoherent and unverified germinal notion; the ethical framework built up from this notion is vague and often incoherent. It is dangerous to draw an analogy from a paradigm with these defects, for it cannot provide the perspicuous model necessary for adequate comparison. It is not only the inconsistency and lack of justification for Nazi thought that makes it so susceptible to misapplication in an analogy, but also its terrible simplicity. Hitler's "few, really ideas" could be put into effect only through brutal murders, war, and the abolition of individual rights. If a "quality of life" position is to serve as a credible view, it cannot match the simplicity of Naziism with an equally terrible simplicity of its own.

II

A "quality of life" approach has been said to replace the traditional "sanctity of life" position (Anon., 1970; Diamond, 1976) with a view that does not respect the value of human life (Robertson, 1975, p. 242; Weber, 1976; Ramsey, 1978, pp. 177–178) but "demeans" it (Superintendent, 1977). It has been claimed that a "quality of life" position accepts that some human beings are less valuable than others (Lebacqz, 1973; Ramsey, 1978, pp. 172, 178) and that those of lesser worth do not deserve to live (Alexander, 1949, p. 44; Dyck, 1973, p. 111). There is no one fully developed "quality of life" position that its critics cite. Indeed, those whose descriptions of such a position have been conjoined above may not agree with each other's version of it. Rather than deal with a straw man, it behooves us first to present a clear and consistent "quality of life" view and then to evaluate the analogy between it and Naziism.

Although ours is a pluralistic society in many senses, a basic moral premise that underlies and allows this pluralism is that human beings are of value as such. This is not a simple narcissistic generalization derived from the fleeting preferences of human beings. It is a judgment that can be defended in terms of that which is both distinctive and essential to human beings. Human beings possess not only certain distinctive physiological, anatomical, and other biophysical functions and features, but many capacities not encompassed within the province of explanation of any one of the sciences. Human beings have the capacity to conceptualize, classify and generalize; to act for reasons; to will to bring about certain ends; to create new ends and purposes; to develop emotions that are both self- and other-directed. These capacities together constitute a higher order human capacity for self-reflective evaluation and action (Nagel, 1970; Frankfurt, 1971; Taylor, 1976; Warnock, 1978). Human beings have the capacity to shape their lives according to their own critically assessed long-term goals and values. It is this characteristic higher order capacity that is distinctively human.

Evidence appears to indicate that some animals can use means-ends reasoning, and can act to achieve goals. As Aquinas points out, however, they cannot be aware of ends *as* ends or of the *relationship* of means to an end (Aquinas, 1945). Not even the strongest admirers of animals maintain that they have a higher capacity to make distinctions and judgments according to reflectively formulated concepts of means and ends and to act on these in order to achieve long-range goals and values. We do not hold animals responsible for their actions on grounds that they could have acted for better reasons, and should have chosen otherwise. It is, however, a central feature of the very *concept* of what it is to be human that human beings have the capacity to shape their own lives in the light of self-reflective deliberation and evaluation. They are the kinds of beings who are not simply victims of overpowering drives and instincts, as the Nazis insisted, but beings with the capacity to originate action grounded in qualitative and reasoned appraisals of themselves, others, and the nature of things (Cohen, 1980). A capacity, rather than its vehicle or exercise, is taken as a distinctive and essential feature of what it is to be human. It is this characteristic capacity of human beings that provides the basis for their value.

The kind of value that is possessed by human beings as such stands in a unique relationship to other kinds of value. As beings with the capacity to determine, critically assess, and act to achieve values, human beings possess a higher order value that is possessed by no other known natural beings. In order to determine and live according to a particular ordering of values, it is logically necessary to have the capacity to assess, adopt, and act upon values. This capacity is itself of value just because it is a prerequisite for the determination and ordering of all values. Those who possess this capacity are in a unique position of value, for they can formulate the very questions of how values should be prioritized and how beings ought to act. Thus, possession of this capacity which is characteristically human, imbues human beings with a higher order value that is prior in value to all first order values.

Despite its difference from the Nazi view, it may be argued against this position that it leaves a subtle opening for a Nazi-like distinction between humans and "sub-humans." By specifying a certain higher order capacity as important to human status, the view outlined will lead to the categorization of those with an impaired distinctively human capacity to evaluate as "sub-human." In the way that the Nazis claimed that only those with certain racial characteristics could have value, so this position implies that only those with certain intact human capabilities have value. It may therefore lead to the diminution of both the humanness and the value of some whom we would ordinarily take to be valuable human beings.

This concern rests on certain misconceptions. To classify according to kind is to classify according to certain distinctive sorts of properties, capacities, and dispositions possessed by individuals of that kind *without regard to the degree* to which they are possessed or developed. To be human is to have human characteristics, capacities, and dispositions to any degree whatsoever. The genius is no more

human than the slow learner; the Olympic medalist is no more human than the paraplegic. There are no degrees of humanness (Chisholm, 1977), any more than there are degrees of treeness. Those who are ill or disabled, and who have diminished distinctively human capacities as a result, are not to be defined as lesser humans or "sub-humans"; they are fully human beings who are ill or disabled. Those who may have lost their higher order capacity to evaluate due to untoward circumstances present difficult borderline cases. It is reasonable to take such individuals as the newborn hydrocephalic with spina bifida or the elderly, bed-ridden person suffering from senile dementia as human until and if good reason is produced against so doing. This precludes the possibility of defining those who may well be human out of human existence.

Although there are not degrees of humanness, there are degrees of some kinds of value. A dollar bill is more valuable than a quarter; a sharp knife is more valuable than a dull one. It would seem that in the same way, a human being with an unimpaired capacity for reflective choice of priorities is of more value as a human being than one who is impaired in this respect. To explain why this is not the case, we must look more carefully at the different kinds of value involved. A dollar bill is more valuable than a quarter in terms of buying power, and so is of greater functional value as a matter of fact. Yet the numerical value of the dollar bill *as such* does not change, even though the amount and quality of what it can buy does change. The value of a dollar bill in itself will never be equivalent to or less than that of a quarter. A sharp knife is more valuable than a dull one in functional terms; it can cut more cleanly. This value does not belong to it as a knife by definition, for it is not a conceptual truth that all knives are sharp. The functional value of the knife belongs to it as a matter of fact for practical purposes. This value will change when the knife becomes dull. Things, therefore, can have a certain functional value in fact, as a sharp knife has value for cutting cleanly, and they can have distinctive kinds of value by definition, as a dollar bill has a certain numerical value. The value of the dollar bill as a matter of kind cannot vary in degree. The value of the knife for practical purposes as a matter of fact can vary in degree.

What it means to be human is conceptually dependent upon the distinctively human capacity for self-reflective evaluation and action. This capacity is valuable primarily because it is a logical precondition for the assessment of and action upon all values. Logical priority does not vary in degree. Either X is logically prior to Y or it is not; it cannot be more or less logically prior, no matter how much X may vary in degree as a matter of fact. This means that the priority in value of the human capacity for making critical evaluative judgments is unvarying as a matter of conceptual necessity. Its value is a matter of kind that cannot vary in degree. To have value *as a human being* is to have unchanging value as one who possesses a higher order capacity for evaluation and action to any degree. Therefore, the value of an unimpaired human being is not greater than that of a human being who is impaired. Both are human beings, and so of unvarying value as such.

Yet clearly it is more valuable *as a matter of fact* to be unimpaired with respect to this and other essential human capacities than to be impaired. The functional value of the condition of a human being does vary in degree. It is better to be conscious, rather than comatose, to be well, rather than ill, to be ambulatory, rather than bed-ridden for all practical purposes. This does not mean that the value of being human is relative to the "quality" of an individual's life (Gustafson, 1973, p. 537). When we say that it is better to live in a certain way, we mean that it is of greater value *to the individual involved* to live in that way as a matter of fact. We do not mean that the person who lives in that way has somehow become of greater value as a human being, for this is not logically possible. The value of a particular status of a human being, as this is measured according to standards of well-being of and for that individual, is distinct from the value of that same individual as a human being. The value of an individual's condition, as this is viewed in terms of its possible contribution to his well-being, is of importance *just because* that person is a human being and so is of value. Those who are critically ill or severely impaired and unable to achieve a high degree of well-being are of great value as human beings, but their "quality of life" is not of the high functional value that they and we would wish for them.

The "quality" of an individual's life refers to the degree to which that life possesses certain kinds of properties and characteristics related to its goodness. This "quality" is not itself a simple property, as is the quality of redness of an apple, but it is a measurement of the extent to which a certain complex of kinds of properties related to well-being is present in an individual's life. Those who have a certain "quality of life" have capacities, conditions, and characteristics that will contribute to their good to a certain degree. There is no specific degree of well-being that is indicated by the term, "quality of life"; the "quality" of an individual's life can be high or low, depending on whether basic needs that beings of that kind have are met for this individual and, when appropriate, whether his reflectively prioritized values definitive of his unique good can be achieved. The determination of an individual's "quality of life" involves consideration of his unique set of priorities whenever this is possible. It does not require the assessment of his social utility, as some critics assume (Robertson, 1975, pp. 261–262, f.n. 259; Kass, 1980, p. 1948). This is not to say that in considering the "quality of life" of an individual, we must conceptually isolate that individual from his or her social relations and resources. It is to say that the value *to* others of an individual is irrelevant to the determination of that individual's "quality of life." Those who are unable to make a positive contribution to society or who represent a drain on others may be in this position due to their poor "quality of life." That their "quality of life" is poor, however, is not determined by their effect on others, but by the low degree to which their lives possess certain properties necessary for their own well-being.

That the "quality of life" of a human being is to be defined in terms of individual well-being, rather than social worth, is confirmed by the current usage of representative medical professionals. When Shaw (1977, 1978), for instance, evaluates the "quality of life," he takes it to involve consideration of the patient's mental and physical condition, his or her home situation, and the societal resources available to that patient. He chooses these as relevant factors because they have an effect on the well-being of the patient. When Shaw brings in questions of family and societal resources, he weighs these as they can benefit the patient, not as the patient detracts from them.

Although some may disagree with the opening that Shaw leaves for poor home and societal support to weigh against active treatment, this disagreement is about specific factors that should enter into the determination of a minimal level of well-being below which active treatment is not morally required, rather than with his basic conception of the "quality of life."

In a second case, it appears initially that Duff and Campbell (1973) do not similarly place individual well-being at the heart of the meaning of the "quality of life," for at times they allow the damaging effect of the patient on the family to serve as a determining factor in decisions not to treat. Yet when their discussion is examined carefully, it becomes clear that they maintain that the needs and interests of the family constitute different grounds from "quality of life" grounds for non-treatment decisions. They do not attempt to define the concept of the "quality of life" in terms of the well-being of anyone other than the individual under consideration. Although many may not accept their introduction of the well-being of others into treatment decisions for an individual patient, this must not obscure the fact, recognized by Duff and Campbell themselves, that when this basis for choice is used, it is not a "quality of life" basis.

The well-being of a human being takes as its end the good of the individual. The presentation of a general theory of human well-being that includes the necessary and sufficient conditions for the minimal well-being of any human being is not within the scope of this paper. A "quality of life" theory of well-being would posit those basic goods without which a human being could not achieve minimal well-being. Such goods could include basic integrated physical and mental functioning, some form of communication with others, and freedom from severe pain and suffering. Basic universal human needs related to well-being would then be defined in terms of such factors. In addition, the unique priorities of individuals would be taken into account in a general "quality of life" theory of well-being. Human beings define themselves by their reflectively developed interests and values. Their distinctive and essential capacity for reasoned consideration of their own and others' good enables them to select those ends that are definitive of their own well-being. It is essential to a "quality of life" position to respect the autonomy of each human being as an individual with the right to shape his life according to his conception of his own well-being. A "quality of life" position by definition does not override the freedom of the individual to choose how he will live and die for the sake of some greater social good.

III

A basic objection to "quality of life" determinations is that they necessarily involve an inequitable social utilitarian comparison and choice from among individual human beings. Ramsey believes that the introduction of "quality of life" considerations requires comparison of "patient-persons" and thereby runs the risk of failing to extend treatment to the abnormal that would be provided to the normal (Ramsey, 1978, pp. 172, 177). Robertson also assumes that the introduction of "quality of life" assessments would involve comparisons of the utility or relative social worth of normal and defective persons (Robertson, 1975, p. 252). Reich objects to a proposed criterion for minimal "quality of life" on grounds that it is unjust to allow someone to die who

does not have a specific quality that most others have (Reich, 1978). Their criticisms presuppose that inter-personal comparability is a necessary feature of "quality of life" judgments.

However, comparisons with others are not empirically or logically necessary to the development of the concept of an individual's well-being. In the course of formulating their own standards of well-being, individuals can, but need not as a matter of fact, make evaluative distinctions based on comparisons with others. A person facing amputation of all four extremities at great risk may, as a matter of fact, compare his view of the minimally good life with that of his neighbors, but this is not empirically necessary to the formulation of his notion of well-being. Nor is an individual's conception of his own good logically dependent on that of another. That is, a comparison of the state of well-being of one person with that of another is not built into the very concept of individual well-being. Therefore individuals are not subjected to inequitable relativizations when their concept of well-being provides the basis for a decision about whether or not they should be treated.

The concern about unjust comparisons raised by these authors does have a basis in decisions that have been made about treatment of the voiceless person by others. Waldman finds

> the ethics and morality of the neonatal intensive care unit a total enigma. In some places the neonatal intensive care unit is committed to the role of salvaging every infant regardless of outcome. In other places, I find neonatologists making no effect to resuscitate a baby who, in their opinion, is hopeless, weighing less than

1,000 gm. with an Apgar score of 1 and no heartbeat (Waldman, 1976).

In a Seattle study, it was found that persons in nine extended-care facilities did not necessarily receive active treatment for fever (Brown and Thompson, 1979). Factors such as marital status, degree of pain, or a feeding problem showed a significant association with treatment decisions. Although the nontreatment of more than 42 per cent of febrile patients was "part of an intentional plan," it is difficult to determine from the data just what the plan could have been. In some cases, a standard of normality has been established as the minimally acceptable degree of well-being for such persons. An infant born at Johns Hopkins University Hospital in 1971 with Down's Syndrome and operable duodenal atresia was allowed to die, apparently because it could never achieve some semblance of normality (Gustafson, 1973). Certain controversial degrees of well-being have been assumed as the minimally acceptable "quality of life" for non-competent human beings who cannot decide for themselves in several of these instances. It is this that is at issue.

Those concerned about the possible relativization of the value of voiceless individuals in "quality of life" judgments believe that we ought to treat the ill, impaired, and incompetent person as we would the normal, competent person in our proxy judgments. This is correct, but needs clarification. We cannot pretend that an individual is not ill and impaired and that his degree of well-being is not severely diminished. Indeed, to do so would make us culpable of neglect. The respects in which we ought to treat the ill, impaired, and incompetent person like the person who is not are grounded in both need, a material principle

of compensatory justice, and in the right to self-determination, a basic human right. It is precisely because an individual has a poor "quality of life" that we ought to give special consideration to his fundamental needs as a valuable human being and when possible, to his self-chosen values. Justice and autonomy require that we consider not only whether the institution of active treatment would meet his basic human needs and fulfill his unique set of values, but also whether the non-institution or cessation of active treatment would recognize his value as human by acknowledging that his fundamental needs cannot be met and that his value priorities cannot be fulfilled.

We cannot escape from the moral necessity of making proxy judgments in such circumstances, even though there are difficult questions to be answered about who should make them and how (McCormick, 1975; Freedman, 1978; Baron, 1978, 1979; Relman, 1978; Buchanan, 1979; Gutheil and Appelbaum, 1980). If we provide active therapy on grounds that we ought always preserve life for as long as possible, regardless of considerations of justice and autonomy, we are making a proxy judgment. If we do not provide therapy on "quality of life" grounds that to do so would prolong a human life of intolerable suffering or would violate an individual's known standards of minimal well-being, we are also making a proxy judgment. There is as much moral onus on us to determine that life-saving treatment is required in a particular instance as there is to determine that it is not. The use of "quality of life" criteria in such situations by others is morally required to ensure that the needs and values of impaired individuals provide the primary basis for the decision.

The spectre of Naziism still troubles some. The very question of whether an individual will be able to achieve at least a minimal degree of well-being, some critics of the "quality of life" view suggest, presumes that some human beings do not "deserve" to live (Dyck, 1975), that "some lives are not worth living and can be taken" (Davis and Aroskar, 1978), and that we are moving toward acceptance of the Nazi notion that there is such a thing as "life not worthy to be lived" (Alexander, 1949). It is not the value of human beings as such, but of their lives, with which such critics are concerned. To allow individuals to die, they suggest, is to say that the lives of some human beings have become valueless.

Human biological life, as we know it, is a necessary condition for the exercise of all human capacities and for the achievement and recognition of all other goods (McCormick, 1974; Frankena, 1975). Life is not, however, an absolute good that must be created, maintained, and perfected *for its own sake*. As McCormick (1978) points out, we are not vitalists. Nor need we be to distinguish ourselves morally from the Nazis. It is neither logically nor morally necessary to declare human life to be the supreme value because the Nazis took it as a relative value. We recognize that such values as freedom of choice, liberty of movement, justice, religious belief, and friendship can have moral priority over life. There are heroes, saints, and martyrs who have knowingly given up their lives for the sake of such values. That life is not an absolute value is further confirmed by our practice regarding rights. We do not compel persons to donate organs to those in need of life-saving organ transplantations on grounds that the right to life of the ill outweighs the right to bodily integrity and self-determination of the healthy. We do not maintain that the person in danger of death necessarily has a right to the life-saving goods

of others on the basis that the right to life has precedence over the right to property. Human life is extremely valuable and the right to life a most important right, but human life does not take moral precedence over all other values, nor does the right to life outweigh all other rights (Cohen, 1977).

We do not require that each human life achieve a high level of excellence as measured by some qualitative or quantitative standard. We do not contend that each human life must perfectly exemplify the species or that each must be patterned after that of some great moral or political leader to have any value. It is not morally necessary to create as much human life as possible on grounds that the kind of value with which human life is suffused is increased by its quantity. Nor is it a moral obligation to extend individual lives for as long as possible. It is not morally required that we fly those in the throes of death across the country for therapy in recognition of the value of human life. That the lives of human beings are valuable does not entail that their quality must be high or that their numbers and individual duration must be extended as much and as long as possible.

Further, human life can end without diminishment of its previous value. An individual may determine that although his life has been good in the light of his self-reflectively chosen long-term goals, it will not continue to be at least minimally good if it suffers a certain kind of irremediable impairment. There is nothing self-contradictory about a valuable human life that has no reasonable possibility of being minimally good and fulfilling to its possessor in the future. Further, that a life will be drained of that which enables it to contribute to an individual's well-being in the future does not reflect negatively on the merit or desert of that individual, as the Nazis claimed. The person is not to be blamed for his poor condition and deemed "unworthy of life." Due to circumstances that cannot be controlled and that no one wants, an individual's condition will make it impossible for him to lead a life conducive to minimal well-being.

The refusal to accept that there can be a life that has no reasonable possibility of reaching minimal well-being is as erroneous as is the refusal to accept that there can be a condition that is terminal. Death is viewed as such a misfortune that it is difficult to accept its inevitability at times. It is equally a misfortune to face a life devoid of all that makes it at least minimally good, and yet this is equally inevitable at times. There is no devaluation of a critically ill individual as a human being when it is determined that treatment or its results would constitute excessive hardship to him and a form of "extraordinary" care. Similarly, there is no devaluation of an individual as a human being when it is determined that treatment would create a condition below that individual's standards of minimal well-being. "Quality of life" considerations are grounded in the recognition that in some tragic instances the lives of valuable human beings can regress to a state in which they bear no reasonable promise of reflecting their self-chosen values. If we insist that such persons must be given intensive medical treatment, we are violating our very belief in the immense value of human beings as reflective deliberators with the capacity to direct their lives according to their conception of well-being.

IV

There are at least three major respects in which similarities and differences between the Nazi and the "quality of life" positions are incorrectly perceived by the analogizers. First, what it meant to be human on each view is misconstrued. According to the Nazis, to be human was to have a certain racial quality as this was putatively revealed by physiognomy. Those who were born into the Aryan race automatically qualified as human. All others were "only attempts at being human," even though the Nazis admitted that they had all the biological characteristics of human beings. There is a self-contradiction in the Nazi notion of fully human beings as independent *Uebermenschen* who have the strength and will to conquer all who stand in their way and the same beings as passive, threatened nonentities manipulated by the *Volk* through the necessary laws of nature. These two views of the nature of human beings are never satisfactorily reconciled within Nazi thought. What it is to be human, for the Nazis, is therefore never clearly developed and defended.

The "quality of life" view, in contrast, explains what it means to be distinctively human in terms of an essential capacity for self-reflective deliberation and evaluation, and acknowledges the human status of all those who possess this capacity to any degree. Certain impaired individuals are not selected as lesser human beings. It envisions fully developed human beings as self-determining moral agents who can move toward their ends by means of reasoned evaluation and choice. Considerations of justice and autonomy require that those who cannot exercise this capacity due to untoward circumstances are to be cared for by others in the light of that which is conducive to meeting their fundamental needs and self-developed priorities. The views of human nature propounded by the two putative analogues are wholly disparate and cannot be appropriately set side by side in an analogy.

A second basic difference between the two positions lies in their conceptions of human value and quality. For the Nazis, human beings had only functional value for some purpose extrinsic to themselves. Any putative distinctive features possessed by human beings were irrelevant to their worth. Quality was a two-part accolade bestowed on those who passed the initial racial screening process and then performed in ways that were useful to the *Volk*. The grant of quality could be rescinded from those who did not perform well or who lost their usefulness. Quality correlated with value for the Nazis; those of high quality were also of high value. The grounds for establishing criteria of value were not susceptible to explanation according to principles of reason; value was based on predetermined racial instincts and by explosions of will-power of the *Volk*.

For the "quality of life" view, in contrast, the quality of an individual is defined in terms of that person's conception of well-being, rather than in terms of racial type or social usefulness. Quality and value do not stand in some simple correlation, for the value of human beings can be assessed in two wholly different senses. Human beings, as such, have necessary, unvarying value that is grounded in their essential capacity for deliberating, evaluating, and acting. Human lives, however, have contingent, changing value as a matter of fact; this is assessed according to standards of well-being chosen by individuals. When an individual's condition is below that of minimal well-being, the value of his life is severely diminished. However his value as a human being is not. This value is respected when he or his proxies are allowed to exercise the very capacities on which it rests in order to determine his appropriate care. The value of a human being as such is not negated if he is not given intensive medical treatment in such circumstances. The concepts of quality and value presumed by a

"quality of life" view stand in radical contrast with those of the Nazis, and cannot be appropriately drawn into an analogy with them.

Third, it follows from the above distinctions that these two positions are not alike with regard to their conceptions of well-being. The Nazi notion of well-being was defined solely in terms of the aggrandizement of the *Volk*. Since human beings had no necessary value as independent moral agents with self-selected purposes and ends, their wishes and long-term goals were of no importance. The concept of individual "quality of life" would have been a self-contradictory notion in the context of Nazi thought, for the Nazis maintained that well-being could only be defined in terms of the good of the only true being, the *Volk*. The difference between the two analogies in this respect is clear. A "quality of life" position defines well-being in terms of the goals and long-term priorities of individual human beings. The distinctive value of human beings entitles them to determine criteria for their own well-being. The views of the two positions with regard to what is meant by well-being therefore differ crucially.

It is because human beings are of unique value as self-reflective beings with the capacity to shape the direction of their lives that their degree of well-being or "quality of life" is of great importance. When the "quality of life" of a human being is considered in medical treatment decisions, it is the degree to which the basic human needs and priorities of the person are met that is of concern. The use of such "quality of life" considerations cannot and does not follow a well-beaten path established by Naziism, for *such "quality of life" considerations were wholly absent from Nazi thought*. Concern about the well-being of individual human beings and their unique priorities had no place in an ideology devoted to the advancement of a transcendent

Volk and the negation of that which is distinctively human. An analogy that attempts to draw on a purported similarity between Nazi thought and a "quality of life" position falls prey to several of the errors possible in the formulation of an analogy. It partially misconstrues the beliefs of both the Nazi paradigm and the "quality of life" analogue, and it misjudges certain similarities between the two, while overlooking their differences. These difficulties lead to the misapplication of Nazi thought and to a misunderstanding of the meaning and implications of a "quality of life" position. Any analogy, therefore, that attempts to illuminate a parallel between the two positions is seriously misdirected.

V

"Quality of life" decisions are made in medical centers every day. "Physicians have always taken into account, among other factors, the quality of life in making decisions and giving advice" (Relman, 1978). It is not possible to avoid "quality of life" assessments, for not to make them is to allow a particular degree of well-being or "quality of life" to prevail. Many physicians verbally acknowledge that they do not recommend the active treatment of life-threatening illnesses in situations in which the "quality of life" prognosis for patients is extremely poor. This occurs not only in highly controversial publicized cases, but also in circumstances that are not well known. It occurs according to no consistent and generally discussed reflections or guidelines.

If we continue to make difficult "quality of life" decisions on an *ad hoc* basis, we will undoubtedly allow valuable human beings to live and to die for the wrong reasons. If we allow care to cease without any coherent account of why we are doing this, we may misjudge the minimal level at which a human being can achieve some degree of well-being. If we provide active therapy in other circumstances, and have no clear reflective grounds for so doing, we run the risk of unjustly keeping some valuable human beings in a state that makes a mockery of this very value. The lack of "quality of life" guidelines of any sort means that ill, impaired, suffering, and comatose patients are forced to live and to die in violation of the very concept of the value of human beings.

The spectre of Naziism hangs over us in a way that the critics of a "quality of life" position overlook. The very humanity and value of human beings as reflective agents was denied by the Nazis and subverted to a form of vitalism that made the life of the *Volk* an absolute good that had to be preserved at any cost. We run the risk of similarly denying the very humanity and value of human beings as reflective agents and subverting this to a form of biological vitalism that makes human life an absolute good that must be preserved at any cost to its possessor.

Note

1. A concern expressed to me verbally by medical personnel.

References

Alexander, L.: 1949, "Medical science under dictatorship," *The New England Journal of Medicine* 241, 39–47.

Anon.: 1970, "A new ethic for medicine and society," *California Medicine* 113, 67–68.

Aquinas, T.: 1945, *Summa Theologica*, A. C. Pegis (ed.), Random House, New York, II, pp. 228–229 (Ia, IIae 6, 3).

Baron, C. H.: 1978, "Assuring 'detached but passionate investigation and decision,'" *American Journal of Law and Medicine* 4, 111–130.

Baron, C. H.: 1979, "Medical paternalism and the rule of law," *American Journal of Law and Medicine* 4, 338–365.

Broszat, M.: 1960, *Der Nationalsozialismus: Weltanschauung, Programm und Wirklichkeit*, Deutsche Verlags-Anstalt, Stuttgart, pp. 31–33.

Brown, N. K. and Thompson, D. J.: 1979, "Nontreatment of fever in extended-care facilities," *The New England Journal of Medicine* 300, 1246–1250.

Buchanan, A.: 1979, "Medical paternalism or legal imperialism," *American Journal of Law and Medicine* 5, 97–117.

Chisholm, R. M.: 1977, "Coming into being and passing away; Can the metaphysician help?," in S. F. Spicker and H. T. Engelhardt, Jr. (eds.), *Philosophical Medical Ethics: Its Nature and Significance*, D. Reidel, Dordrecht, pp. 169–182.

Cohen, C. B.: 1977, "Ethical problems of intensive care," *Anesthesiology* 47, 217–227.

Cohen, C. B.: 1980, "The trials of Socrates and Joseph K.," Philosophy and Literature, 212–227.

Davis, A. and Aroskar, M.: 2978, *Ethical Dilemmas in Nursing Practice*, Appleton-Century-Crofts, New York, p. 120.

Dawidowicz, L.: 1975, *The War Against the Jews, 1933–1945*, Holt, Rinehart and Winston, New York.

Dennett, D. C.: 1973, "Mechanism and responsibility," in T. Honderich (ed.), *Essays on Freedom of Action*, Routledge and Kegan Paul, London, pp. 169–173.

Diamond, E. F.: 1976, " 'Quality' versus 'sanctity' of life in the nursery," *America* 135, 396–398.

Duff, R. S. and Campbell, A. G. M.: 1973, "Moral and ethical dilemmas in the special care nursery," *The New England Journal of Medicine* 289, 890–894.

Dunphy, J. E.: 1976, "On caring for the patient with cancer," *The New England Journal of Medicine* 295, 313.

Dyck, A.: 1973, "An alternative to an ethic of euthanasia," in R. H. Williams (ed.), *To Live and to Die: When, Why and How?*, Springer-Verlag, New York, pp. 107–111.

Dyck, A.: 1975, "Beneficent euthanasia and benemortasia: Alternative views of mercy," in M. Kohl (ed.), *Beneficent Euthanasia*, Prometheus Books, Buffalo, p. 127.

Frankena, W. K.: 1975, "The ethics of respect for life," in O. Temkin (ed.), *Respect for Life in Medicine, Philosophy and the Law*, Johns Hopkins University Press, Baltimore, pp. 53–54.

Frankfurt, H.: 1971, "Freedom of the will and the concept of a person," *Journal of Philosophy* LXVIII, 5–20.

Freedman, B.: 1978, "On the rights of the voiceless," *The Journal of Medicine and Philosophy* 3, 196–210.

Gorlitz, W.: 1960, *Adolf Hitler*, Musterschmidt-Verlag, Göttingen, p. 140.

Gustafson, J.: 1973, "Mongolism, parental desires, and the right to life," *Perspectives in Biology and Medicine* 16, 529–557.

Gutheil, T. G. and Appelbaum, P. S.: 1980, "Substituted judgment and the physician's ethical dilemma," *Journal of Clinical Psychiatry* 41, 303–305.

Hitler, A.: 1943, *Mein Kampf*, R. Manheim (tr.), Houghton-Mifflin, Boston.

Hofer, W.: 1957, *Der Nationalsozialismus: Dokumente 1933-1945*, Fischer Taschenbuch Verlag, Frankfurt, pp. 280-281.

Ivy, A. C.: 1977, "Nazi war crimes of a medical nature," in S. J. Reiser (ed.), *Ethics in Medicine*, M.I.T. Press, Cambridge, pp. 267-268.

Jäckel, E.: 1972, *Hitler's Weltanschauung*, H. Arnold (tr.), Wesleyan University Press, Middletown.

Kamisar, Y.: 1958, "Some nonreligious views against proposed 'mercy killing' legislation," *Minnesota Law Review* 42, 969-1042.

Kass, L.: 1980, "Ethical dilemmas in the care of the ill, II. What is the patient's good?," *Journal of the American Medical Association* 244, 1946-1949.

Keene, B.: 1978, "The natural death act: A well baby check-up on its first birthday," *Annals of the New York Academy of Sciences* 315, 379.

Kelsey, B.: 1975, "Which infants should live? Who should decide?," *The Hastings Center Report* 5, 5-8.

Kenny, A.: 1975, *Will, Freedom, and Power*, Basil Blackwell, Oxford, pp. 18-22.

Koop, C. E.: 1977, "The slide to Auschwitz," *Human Life Review* III, 109-113.

Krausnick, H.: 1965, "Judenverfolgung," *Anatomie des SS-States*, Walter-Verlag, Olten and Freiburg im Breisgau, pp. 360-380.

Lebacqz, K.: 1973, "Prenatal diagnosis and selective abortion," *Linacre Quarterly* 40, 109-127.

McCormick, R.: 1974, "To save or let die: The dilemma of modern medicine," *Journal of the American Medical Association* 229, 175-176.

McCormick, R.: 1975, "Fetal research, morality, and public policy," *The Hastings Center Report* 5, 26-31.

McCormick, R.: 1978, "The quality of life, the sanctity of life," *The Hastings Center Report* 8, 32-36.

Mitscherlich, A. and Mielke, F.: 1949, *Doctors of Infamy, The Story of the Nazi Medical Crimes*, Henry Schuman, New York, pp. 90-130.

Mosse, G.: 1966, "Introduction," in G. Mosse (ed.), *Nazi Culture*, Grosset and Dunlap, New York, p. xxviii.

Nagel, T.: 1970, *The Possibility of Altruism*, Princeton University Press, Princeton, New Jersey, pp. 29, 64-69, 81.

Nürnberg Military Trials: 1949-1953, *Trials of War Criminals Before the Nurnberg Military Tribunals Under Control Council No. 10*, Washington, D.C., Green Series, Case No. 1, The Medical Case, Vol. 1, Doc. 630PS, p. 848. The order was predated to September 1, 1939.

Picker, H.: 1963, *Hitlers Tischgespräche im Führerhauptquartier 1941-42*, P. E. Schramm (ed.), Degerloch, Stuttgart.

Ramsey, P.: 2978, *Ethics at the Edges of Life*, Yale University Press, New Haven.

Reich, W. T.: 1978, "Quality of life and defective newborn children: An ethical analysis," in C. A. Swinyard (ed.), *Decision Making and the Defective Newborn*, Charles C Thomas, Springfield, pp. 489-511.

Relman, A. S.: 1978, "The Saikewicz decision: A medical viewpoint," *American Journal of Law and Medicine* 4, 234-242.

Robertson, J.: 1975, "Involuntary euthanasia of defective newborns: A legal analysis," *Stanford Law Review* 27, 139-195.

Shaw, A.: 1977, "Defining the quality of life," *The Hastings Center Report* 7, 11.

Shaw, A.: 1978, "The ethics of proxy consent," in C. A. Swinyard (ed.), *Decision Making and the Defective Newborn,* Charles C Thomas, Springfield, Illinois, pp. 589–597.

Stuckgart, W. and Globke, H.: 1966, "Civil rights and the natural inequality of man," in G. Mosse (ed.), *Nazi Culture,* Grosset and Dunlap, New York, pp. 328–329.

Superintendent of Belchertown State School v. Saikewicz, 1977, 370 N.E. 2d 417.

Taylor, C.: 1976, "Responsibility for self," in A. Rorty (ed.), *The Identities of Persons,* University of California Press, Berkeley, pp. 282–285.

Waldman, A. M.: 1976, "Medical ethics and the hopelessly ill child," *The Journal of Pediatrics* 88, 891.

Warnock, G. J.: 1978, "On choosing values," *Midwest Studies in Philosophy, Vol. III: Studies in Ethical Theory,* pp. 28–34.

Weber, L. J.: 1976, *Who Shall Live?,* Paulist Press, New York, pp. 41–42.

7

The Meaning and Validity of Quality of Life Judgments in Contemporary Roman Catholic Medical Ethics

James J. Walter

One of the most controversial and vexing issues in contemporary Catholic medical ethics concerns the validity of what are called quality of life judgments in deciding whether to forego or withdraw treatment from patients. Scarcely a week goes by that we do not hear or read about cases of severely handicapped neonates or patients in a persistent vegetative state having all treatment, including nutrition and hydration, removed from them. Some Catholic ethicists and physicians view these judgments as just one more step toward an inevitable slide down the slippery slope toward the euthanasia of those who are the most vulnerable in society, viz., the dying, the comatose, the

handicapped and the incurably demented.[1] A growing number of theologians, on the other hand, argue that making quality of life judgments is fully consistent with the substance of the longstanding Catholic tradition on the distinction between ordinary and extraordinary means of preserving life.[2]

My intent is to locate and analyze a few of the definitional and ethical issues that are at stake in the discussion over the legitimacy of quality of life judgments. Though I cannot address the legal questions that the topic has raised, the seemingly intractable nature of this issue has been further complicated in the United States by the intervention of the courts[3] and some governmental agencies[4] dur-

"The Meaning and Validity of Quality of Life Judgments in Contemporary Roman Catholic Medical Ethics" by James J. Walter. Reprinted with permission of Louvain Studies *13(Fall, 1988):195–208.*

ing the past decade to decide patient treatment or non-treatment.

I. Some Preliminary Distinctions and the Goals of Medicine

Statements about the "quality" or "qualities" of life can be descriptive, evaluative or morally normative.[5] Descriptive statements about a quality of life are morally neutral in that they only make reference to the fact that a patient possesses a certain characteristic quality, e.g., cognitive capacity. Evaluative statements, on the other hand, indicate that some value or worth is attached to a life that possesses the quality, and so evaluative statements assess that the quality (and thus the life) is desired, appreciated or sacred. Finally, morally normative (prescriptive) statements about a quality of life always entail a moral judgment on the valued quality. These latter statements, then, presume that a quality is valued (e.g., cognitive capacity) but also involve judgments whether, and under which conditions, one *ought* to support or protect the life which possesses the quality or qualities (e.g., "Life that has cognitive capabilities always ought to be given all medical treatment"). Though descriptive and evaluative statements definitely come to bear on clinical and ethical decision-making, all would agree that the key issue concerns the meaning and validity of morally normative claims about the quality of life.

When one makes either an evaluative or a normative claim about a quality of life, it is not altogether clear what the meaning of the word "life" is. Is one referring to life as mere physical or biological existence, or is one making a claim about life as personal existence (personhood)? At least part of the ambiguity or confusion in the discussion results from not clearly distinguishing life as mere biological existence from life understood as embodied personal existence. Anencephalic neonates and patients in a persistent vegetative state certainly have biological existence, but neither will ever experience personal existence as most of us understand that notion, i.e., life with sapient consciousness and personal freedom.[6] By making this distinction we can become clearer about both what we value about physical life (evaluative claims) and what our duties and their limits are to preserve mere biological existence (morally normative claims).

Surely one of the key factors that has provoked this debate over quality of life has been the tremendous advancement of medical technology during the past several decades. Not to take this technology seriously in one's analysis is both to misread the "signs of the times"[7] and to expect that traditional moral principles, which could not have anticipated these developments, can be equally applicable today as they were when they were conceived. We now have the capability of keeping patients biologically alive who would have certainly died only a few years ago.[8] These advancements in technology are well known and do not need to be detailed here. However, what this technology has done is to call into question the traditional goals of medicine. No doubt, medicine rightfully seeks to prevent death (especially an untimely death), to alleviate pain and physical suffering, and to promote health. Though these are important goals in the application of medical knowledge and skill, I would argue that they must be viewed as subordinate to the more encompassing goal of serving the purposefulness of personal existence.[9] Physicians promote health, prevent death, perform surgery, relieve pain, etc. on behalf of others *in order that* we as patients might continue in some fashion to pursue values (material, moral and spiritual) that transcend physical life. Pain, disease, general ill health and death either frustrate our desires to pursue these values or make it impossible to pursue them at all. As a consequence, when medicine cannot any longer promote this goal for a patient at all, or when, by its interventions, medicine will place a patient in a condition that makes the pursuit of purposefulness too burdensome, then medicine has reached its limits *on the basis of its own principal reason for existence.*[10]

II. Definition of "Quality" of Life

One of the more difficult problems in assessing the validity of quality of life judgments concerns the definition of the word "quality." Because this word is ambiguous, the entire phrase "quality of life" is subject to expansion to include just about anything, and so its use in medical decision-making is open to serious abuse. Consequently, those who are entirely opposed to quality of life considerations in the medical environment have good reason to be concerned.[11] However, because there are ways to control the definition of the term and thus to restrict the range of its application, I will argue that the issue is not *whether* we should employ this type of judgment but rather *how* do we circumscribe the limits of the judgment.

It is not infrequent in our consumerist society to link the word "quality" to the idea of excellence. So it is not unusual for us to talk about quality hotels, quality meals, and even quality medicine.[12] If "quality" is defined by reference to excellence, then the meaning of the term will be bounded only by the horizons of our imaginations and desires, and no doubt we will find it very difficult to find objective criteria by which to assess these judgments. One's worst fears about quality of life judgments will be realized because all patients who cannot live an excellent life, and they will surely include the handicapped and dying, will either not be given treatment or will be actively killed.

Another possibility is to define "quality" as a property or as an attribute. The attribute or property at issue is an attribute or property of physical and/or personal life. I find that most authors who argue against quality of life judgments, and even some who argue for their validity, will define the term in this way. There are a number of complex issues at stake once "quality" is so defined, but I will only have space to analyze two of them: first, the evaluative status of physical life which does not possess the valued property and, second, the origin of and the limits to our obligations to preserve biological life (normative status).

A. *The Evaluative Status of Life*

When quality of life is defined by reference to an attribute or property of physical life, then basic questions are raised about the fundamental value of physical life (evaluative status) and the origin of this valuing. What is it that we value about physical life? Do we value physical life in and for the sake of itself, or do we value life because of some property that life possesses, e.g., cognitive capacity? What philosophical or theological justifications can be offered for this valuing of life? Unfortunately, answers to these questions have led some to frame the contemporary debate in terms of a "quality of life ethic" versus a "sanctity of life ethic." I say unfortunately, because it is quite possible that this entire discussion about the evaluative status of human life may be misplaced.

Those who have argued for a sanctity of life ethic[13] over and against a quality of life ethic are aware that physical life is not an absolute value. On this point they are in total agreement with the proponents of the quality of life ethic. However, they maintain that those who support a quality of life ethic accord either no value or varying degrees of value to physical life contingent on the presence of some property that life possesses.[14] Such a view, they argue, is intolerable because: (1) it denies the equality of physical life and the equality of persons, and thus it is a violation of justice; (2) it denies that all lives are inherently valuable, and so some lives can be truly "not worth living"; and (3) it denies the Christian (especially Roman Catholic) theological position that human life is valued holistically as body-spirit life by adopting a bi-level anthropology that is committed to sustaining physical life only as an instrumental value.[15] These authors conclude that a sanctity of life ethic is superior because it can affirm the equality of life on the grounds that physical life is truly a *bonum honestum* (a good or value in itself) and not a *bonum utile* (a useful or negotiable value that is dependent on some other intrinsically valuable property). Some argue the origin of this valuing philosophically by reference to a theory of goods that are incommensurable,[16] and others argue it theologically by reference to persons as created in the image of God.[17]

At first sight, these arguments against the so-called quality of life ethic seem formidable. In some ways, those who have supported the validity of quality of life judgments have not been as clear as they might be on the evaluative status of physical life, and in some instances they might have even poorly stated their own case. First, as I indicated above, it is necessary to distinguish clearly and consistently between physical or mere biological life and personal life (personhood). When this important distinction is not made, the opponents of quality of life judgments are prone to move back and forth between the value of biological life and the value of personhood.[18]

Second, those who support quality of life judgments should state explicitly and unequivocally that physical life is indeed a value that is not conditioned on any property. Some proponents, like Kevin O'Rourke and Dennis Brodeur, have stated, inappropriately in my mind, that "Mere physiological existence is *not* a value if no potential for mental-creative function exists."[19] Richard McCormick, who is one of the strongest supporters of quality of life judgments, has himself vacillated somewhat between claiming that physical life is a *bonum utile* and a *bonum honestum*.[20] David Thomasma *et al.* have also described physical life as a *conditional* value.[21] These ways of phrasing the issue of the evaluative status of physical life have led opponents of the position to the criticisms noted above. Unless I misunderstand what the proponents of quality of life judgments are driving at, I would suggest that it would be better to claim that physical life is a *bonum onticum*, that is, a true and real value, but by definition a created and therefore a limited good.[22] By so arguing, one can now affirm that all physical lives are of equal *ontic* value and that all persons are of equal *moral* value.

This leads me to my final suggestion, which I will not develop until later. It is possible that the issue of the evaluative status of physical life is misplaced from the start. Despite some possible misstatements on the part of the proponents of quality of life judgments and misunderstandings on the part of the opponents, the word "quality" in the phrase quality of life does not and should not primarily refer to a property or attribute *of life*. Rather, the quality that is at issue is the quality *of the relationship* which exists between the medical condition of the patient, on the one hand, and the patient's ability to pursue life's goals and purposes (purposefulness) understood as the values that transcend physical life, on the other.[23] "Quality of life" may be an unfortunate phrase not only because it leaves the word "life" ambiguous (mere biological life as distinguished from personal life) but also because the word "quality" will tend to be construed as a property or an attribute which gives life its inherent meaning and value. Nonetheless, if we understand the phrase to refer to the quality of a relation and not to a quality of life itself, then the evaluative status of physical life is no longer a central issue in the debate. As a result, the formidable character of the arguments, if not the substance of the arguments, against the so-called quality of life ethic at this level loses its force.

B. The Normative Status of Life

Those who are opposed to the quality of life ethic believe that such an ethic logically entails a moral judgment on the valued qualities of life. Since morally normative judgments are statements about our moral duties and their limits toward supporting and protecting life, these authors fear that life and death decisions will be made solely on the presence or absence of certain qualities (properties) that a patient's life possesses. The result will be that our duties toward protecting life, especially those whose lives are most vulnerable, will be seriously eroded in society. The response to this erosion, and to the ethic which has precipitated it, is once again to argue for a sanctity of life ethic that refuses to ground our moral obligations on some valued quality, i.e., property or attribute, of life.

There are multiple issues involved in this discussion, but three particular questions clearly emerge at the heart of the matter. The first involves an attempt to define the normatively human, the second concerns the norma-

tive moral theory that underlies and grounds our moral obligations, and the third is concerned with how to establish limits and/or exceptions to our obligations and the justifications for such limits. Thus, the first issue is definitional in nature, though it also entails normative considerations; the second turns on the well-worn debate over the grounding of our moral obligations either deontologically or teleologically; and the last issue involves an assessment of the adequacy of the Catholic tradition's distinction between ordinary and extraordinary means of preserving life.

To define "quality" as a property of life (physical or personal) entails defining explicitly or implicitly what is called the normatively human. A number of years ago Joseph Fletcher attempted to isolate what he called the "indicators of humanhood."[24] He listed fifteen positive criteria (e.g., minimal intelligence, self-control, sense of futurity, concern for others, and curiosity) and five negative criteria (e.g., humans are not essentially parental, not essentially sexual, and not essentially worshipers) to define the normatively human. What he was doing in this essay was defining those qualities (positive and negative) which not only define who is human but also who is morally entitled to our care. The problem with Fletcher's position is that it falls into what William Aiken calls the "eudaimonistic" use of quality of life judgments, that is, it seeks to define the "good life" at its upper limits and then seeks to provide knowledge of both the necessary and sufficient conditions for its attainment.[25] The eudaimonistic use then becomes entrapped within what Aiken calls the "exclusionary" use of quality of life in which one cites the lack of certain qualities as a means of excluding potential patients from the normal standards of medical and moral treatment.[26] Thus, a judgment is made that, because a patient's quality of life is below the desirable level, i.e., it lacks a certain property, that patient's life is not worth living and we are morally justified in treating them accordingly. The opponents of the quality of life ethic have rightfully perceived the problem of falling into the eudaimonistic and exclusionary uses of quality of life judgments, but, as I will show below, the mistake they make is to attribute this problem to contemporary Catholic theologians who have argued for the legitimacy of quality of life judgments.

Normative moral theories are concerned with establishing standards for the moral evaluation of actions and a rationale for our moral obligations. To my knowledge, all the proponents of the so-called sanctity of life ethic subscribe to either a rights[27] or rule[28] deontology and accuse those who adopt a quality of life ethic of grounding moral obligations in some form of personal or social consequentialism.[29] In other words, in the sanctity of life ethic the duty to preserve physical life is grounded either in the patient's right to life or in the rules that require respect for life, justice or care for another. This position contends that if our duties to preserve life are based on a prior judgment of whether a specific quality or property of physical life will result in benefits or good consequences to the patient him/herself (personal consequentialism) or to society (social consequentialism), then our duties to preserve life are improperly grounded in what the patient earns through accomplishments to society or by means of the potentialities that the patient's life might possess.

This critique of a consequentialist grounding of our obligations to protect and preserve life is correct as far as it goes. It is true that the Christian tradition in general and the Roman Catholic tradition in particular have not based our duties simply on the presence of certain qualities or properties of physical life or on the contributions that a person has made or might make to society. Beyond any doubt, a critique should be leveled against any moral position that purports such a normative theory. The problem is that I remain unconvinced that this critique can really be applied to what many contemporary Catholic theologians have held on the validity of quality of life judgments. Though there might be some ambiguities in these theologians' positions on the evaluative and normative status of physical life, one could interpret their position as deriving our *prima facie* duties to preserve life from the ontic value of life and as deriving our actual *moral* obligations[30] from a teleological, but not *consequentialist,* assessment of the quality of the relationship that exists between the patient's medical condition and the ability to pursue life's goals and purposes.[31]

Because physical life is not an absolute value, those who argue for a sanctity of life ethic admit that there are definite limits to our obligations to preserve life. As a matter of fact, several authors admit that these limits and/or exceptions to our duties are controlled by "quality of life" considerations that are embodied in the traditional Catholic distinction between ordinary and extraordinary means of treatment. For example, John Connery,[32] Warren Reich[33] and Brian Johnstone[34] all concede that "qualitative" factors or contingent qualities of life, such as the pain associated with using a certain medical treatment or the burden associated with the attainment of medical treatment, limit the duty to preserve life either on the part of the patient or on the part of health-care providers. Thus, they argue that the distinction between ordinary means (morally obligatory) and extraordinary means (optional and not morally obligatory) of treatment remains essentially valid and applicable today.

The crucial point is not that the proponents

of the sanctity of life ethic reject all quality of life factors; what they reject at the level of normative theory is the derivation of our duties from the presence of certain properties of physical or personal life, e.g., the capacity for human relationships. In other words, "quality of life" judgments, which are judgments strictly circumscribed by an assessment of the benefits and burdens of medical treatment considered in itself and/or of those benefits and burdens that will accrue to the patient as a result of treatment, function appropriately in this ethic as ways of limiting or of making exceptions to our duties, which themselves are priorly grounded on deontological considerations, e.g., the right to life or respect for life. Thus, as long as the equality of both physical life and personhood is assured at the evaluative and normative levels, this ethic does in fact recognize the relative importance of "quality of life" judgments in medical decision-making.

III. An Argument for Quality of Life Judgments

The debate among contemporary Catholic theologians over the validity of quality of life judgments in the medical environment has reached an impasse as long as the terms of the debate continue to revolve around the opposition between two types of ethics, viz., sanctity of life ethic versus quality of life ethic. A successful negotiation of the impasse, but surely not the resolution of all the problems, will depend, at least in part, on the admission of the insights of the other's approach. Thus, in this final section I want to offer in broad strokes an outline to support the validity of quality of life judgments, while at the same time recognizing and admitting the insights of those who have opposed the use of such judgments.

One of the items that most often remains on a hidden agenda behind this debate concerns the goals and limits of medicine. In effect, a stalemate on almost all fronts, i.e., moral, legal and medical, exists because there is little or no agreement at this important level of discussion. I have already proposed above that the central and over-arching end of medicine is to promote and enhance the purposefulness of physical and personal life. Such a proposal about the goal of medicine does not at all address the worth or value of physical or personal life. What the proposal does do is to state the *raison d'être* of medical interventions and its limits, on the one hand, and to give us some insight into what is meant *in a general way* by the terms "benefits," "burdens" and "best interests" of a patient, on the other hand.

As I have already noted, quality of life judgments should not be construed as judgments about the value of either physical or personal life. They are not concerned with assessing qualities or properties that, when present, make life itself valuable. Rather, these judgments are evaluative and normative claims or assessments about the relation between the patient's medical condition and the patient's ability to pursue material, moral and spiritual values which transcend physical life but do not give that life its very meaning and worth. As such, they specify *concretely* the meaning of the terms "benefits," "burdens" and "best interests" of a patient as well as the limits of medical interventions within a given historical and cultural situation.

Whereas all physical life is of equal ontic worth and all personal life is of equal moral value, the quality of the relation between these lives and the pursuit of values is not equal. Due to multiple factors, a number of which have to do with genetic endowment and the ways in which we live our lives and a number of which are dependent on the nurturing and accessibility of values in culture, some people are fortunate enough to attain a high quality of life. Other individuals, regrettably, are not as fortunate, and they must live most of their lives pursuing life's purposes at a less than optimal level. But some have no discernible or such a minimal qualitative relation between their medical condition and the pursuit of values that a growing number of theologians have argued that those in this last category have no moral obligation to prolong their physical lives and thus that all treatment, including artificial nutrition and hydration, can be withdrawn from them. In the past, most, if not all, these lives in such conditions would have been mercifully ended by the underlying pathology, but the intervention of modern medical technology today has not been as merciful.

Two things are important to note here. First, none of the theologians proposing this view has accepted the active killing of patients. Second, this view does not fall into either a eudaimonistic or an exclusionary use of quality of life judgments. These theologians have not drawn a line at the upper limits of pursuing life's purposes (eudaimonistic use), but they have sought to establish the lowest possible limits of what reasonable people would judge bearable and acceptable vis-à-vis the qualitative relation under consideration.[35] Furthermore, this position does not employ the exclusionary use because it does not exclude those who fall below these limits from our ordinary moral obligations not to kill them or to care for them.

The duties and their limits to prolong life that bear on health-care professionals are correlative to the patient's obligations and their limits.[36] When it is determined that a patient no longer has an obligation to prolong physical or personal life, e.g., when the pursuit of values is too burdensome due to an underlying fatal pathology that cannot be removed, then medical personnel do not exclude the patient from *their* obligations to offer treatment but acquiesce to the limits of the *patient's* obligations. Thus, other things being equal, when medicine can intervene to ameliorate the quality of the relation between the patient's condition and the pursuit of life's goals, then such an intervention can be considered a benefit to the patient and is in his/her best interests. However, *because of the condition of the patient*, when a proposed intervention cannot offer the patient any reasonable hope of pursuing life's purposes at all or can only offer the patient a condition where the pursuit of life's purposes will be filled with profound frustration or with utter neglect of these purposes because of the energy needed merely to sustain physical life, then medical intervention: (1) can only offer burden to the life treated, (2) is contrary to the best interests of the patient, (3) is harmful to the patient, and (4) medicine has reached its limits on the basis of its own reason for existence and thus should not intervene except to palliate or to comfort the patient.

What should be obvious is that quality of life judgments are concerned with what the Vatican "Declaration on Euthanasia"[37] called the assessment of a due proportion between benefits and burdens. However, the proportionality referred to is not about the benefits/burdens of the treatments considered *in themselves* apart from the patient; rather, the assessment is concerned with the proportionality of benefits/burdens (considered teleologically) that will affect the quality of the relation between the patient's medical condition and his/her pursuit of values. By adopting this view of what quality of life judgments are concerned with, it seems that the so-called "two ethics of life" are not two but really one.

Notes

1. For example, see John R. Connery, S.J., "Quality of Life," *Linacre Quarterly* 53 (1986) 26–33; Daniel Callahan, "On Feeding the Dying," *The Hastings Center Report* 13 (1983) no. 5, 22; Eugene F. Diamond, M.D., "Nutrition, Hydration and Cost Containment," *Linacre Quarterly* 53 (1986) 24–34; and New Jersey State Catholic Conference, "Providing Food and Fluids to Severely Brain Damaged Patients," *Origins* 16 (1987) 582–584.

2. For example, see Richard A. McCormick, S.J., *How Brave A New World? Dilemmas in Bioethics* (Washington, D.C.: Georgetown University Press, 1981), esp. pp. 339–351 and 393–411; *idem,* "Notes on Moral Theology: 1980," *Theological Studies* 42 (1981) 100–110; John J. Paris, S.J. and Richard A. McCormick, S.J. "The Catholic Tradition on the Use of Nutrition and Fluids," *America* 156 (1987) 356–361; Kevin O'Rourke, "The A.M.A. Statement on Tube Feeding: An Ethical Analysis," *America* 155 (1986) 321–323 and 331; and James J. Walter, "Food and Water: An Ethical Burden," *Commonweal* 113 (1986) 616–619. For a summary of these and other positions that have been taken recently, see Lisa S. Cahill, "Notes on Moral Theology: 1986," *Theological Studies* 48 (1987) 105–123.

3. The number of court cases during the past decade and a half is almost staggering. Some of the more publicized cases would include: Karen Quinlan, Claire Conroy, Paul Brophy, Bro. Fox, Joseph Saikewicz and Nancy Ellen Jobes.

4. The Department of Health and Human Services (DHHS) originally intervened after the Bloomington, IN "Baby Doe" case (April, 1982). Since that time, DHHS has issued a number of regulations governing the treatment of neonates who are severely handicapped. The final regulations were published in the *Federal Register* 50 (1985) 14887–14889.

5. Warren T. Reich, "Quality of Life," in Warren T. Reich (ed.) *Encyclopedia of Bioethics,* Vol. 2, (New York: The Free Press, 1978) pp. 830–831.

6. For a description of patients who are in a persistent vegetative state (PVS), see The President's Commission Report entitled *Deciding to Forego Life-Sustaining Treatment: A Report on the Ethical, Medical, and Legal Issues in Treatment Decisions* (Washington, D.C.: U.S. Government Printing Office, 1983) esp. pp. 171–181.

7. *Pastoral Constitution on the Church in the Modern World (Gaudium et Spes)* in Walter M. Abbott (ed.) *The Documents of Vatican II* (New York: Association Press, 1966) no. 4.

8. The longest case of coma on record is that of Elaine Esposito. She never recovered consciousness after receiving general anesthesia for surgery, and therefore she had to be fed and hydrated artificially. She remained in this condition for 37 years and 111 days before dying. See The President's Commission Report, *Deciding to Forego Life-Sustaining Treatment,* p. 177.

9. Albert R. Jonsen, "Purposefulness in Human Life," *The Western Journal of Medicine* 125 (July 5–7, 1976) 5–7.

10. For a similar view, see David Roy, "Issues in Health Care Meriting Particular Christian Concern—A Priority Issue: The Severely Defective Newborn," *Linacre Quarterly* 49 (1982) 60–80.

11. For example, see Mark Siegler, M.D. and

Alan J. Weisbard, J.D., "Against the Emerging Stream: Should Fluids and Nutritional Support be Continued?" *Archives of Internal Medicine* 145 (1985) 129–131; Patrick G. Derr, "Why Food and Fluids Can Never Be Denied," *Hastings Center Report* 16 (1986) no. 1, 28–30; and John R. Connery, S.J., "The Clarence Herbert Case: Was Withdrawal of Treatment Justified?" *Hospital Progress* 65 (February, 1984) 32–35 and 70.

12. Jonsen, "Purposefulness in Human Life," p. 5.

13. For example, see Warren T. Reich, "Quality of Life and Defective Newborn Children: An Ethical Analysis," in Chester A. Swinyard (ed.) *Decision Making and the Defective Newborn: Proceedings of a Conference on Spina Bifida and Ethics,* (Springfield, IL: Charles C. Thomas, 1978) pp. 489–511; and Brian V. Johnstone, C.S.S.R., "The Sanctity of Life, the Quality of Life and the New 'Baby Doe' Law," *Linacre Quarterly* 52 (1985) 258–270.

14. Johnstone, "The Sanctity of Life," p. 263.

15. Reich, "Quality of Life and Defective Newborn Children," p. 504.

16. For example, see William E. May, *Human Existence, Medicine and Ethics* (Chicago: Franciscan Herald Press, 1977) p. 10.

17. Reich, "Quality of Life and Defective Newborn Children," p. 504.

18. For example, Warren Reich's theological position grounds both the value and the equality of "human life" on the belief that "all men are created as persons in the image of God." *Ibid.* His use of the phrase "human life" is ambiguous here and therefore misleading. Though the context of his argument is a critique of what he believes to be McCormick's position on the inherent value of *physical* life, he completes his argument by referring to *persons* and their nature and value as images of God.

19. Kevin D. O'Rourke, OP and Dennis Brodeur, *Medical Ethics: Common Ground for Understanding* (St. Louis, MO: The Catholic Health Association of the U.S., 1986) p. 213 (emphasis added).

20. Richard A. McCormick, S.J., *How Brave A New World,* pp. 405–407; and *idem, Health and Medicine in the Catholic Tradition: Tradition in Transition* (New York, Crossroad, 1984) p. 148.

21. David Thomasma *et al.,* "Continuance of Nutritional Care in the Terminally Ill Patient," *Critical Care Clinics* 2 (1986) 66.

22. For two important articles on the distinction between the ontic and the moral levels in moral analysis, see Louis Janssens, "Ontic Evil and Moral Evil," *Louvain Studies* 4 (1972) 115–156; and *idem,* "Ontic Good and Evil—Premoral Values and Disvalues," *Louvain Studies* 12 (1987) 62–82.

23. Richard McCormick has proposed that the minimal potential for human relationships is one of the central criteria in quality of life judgments. It is probably the case that McCormick intended "potential for human relationships" to mean a property or attribute *of life* in his quality of life criterion. (See his *How Brave A New World,* pp. 339–351 and 393–411.) Whereas this may be true, I think that the basic thrust of McCormick's position is to assess the quality *of the relation* between the patient's medical condition and the pursuit of life's purposes. For McCormick, the fact that a patient does not possess any capacity for relationality means that the patient will not have any qualitative relation between his/her medical condition and the pursuit of life's values. Indications of my interpretation can be found throughout his more recent writings. For example, see his "The Best Interests of the Baby," *Second Opinion* 2

(1986) esp. p. 23. For my earlier interpretation and evaluation of McCormick's position, see James J. Walter, "A Public Policy Option on the Treatment of Severely Handicapped Newborns," *Laval Théologique et Philosophique* 41 (1985) 239–250.

24. Joseph Fletcher, "Indicators of Humanhood: A Tentative Profile of Man," *The Hastings Center Report* 2 (November, 1972) 1–4.

25. William Aiken, "The Quality of Life," *Applied Philosophy* 1 (1982) 27.

26. *Ibid.,* p. 30.

27. For example, see Reich, "Quality of Life and Defective Newborn Children," pp. 491–492.

28. For example, see Connery, "Quality of Life," pp. 31–32; Johnstone, "The Sanctity of Life," pp. 264–265; and Paul Ramsey, *Ethics at the Edges of Life: Medical and Legal Intersections* (New Haven: Yale University Press, 1978), esp. pp. 153–188.

29. Reich, "Quality of Life," p. 833; and *idem,* "Quality of Life and Defective Newborns," pp. 503–504.

30. For the distinction between prima facie and actual moral obligations, see W.D. Ross, *The Right and the Good* (Oxford: Clarendon, 1930).

31. McCormick himself argues that we have a prima facie obligation to preserve *physical* life. To my knowledge, none of his critics has pointed out this fact about his position. See McCormick, "The Best Interests of the Baby," p. 21.

32. Connery, "Quality of Life," p. 31.

33. Reich, "Quality of Life and Defective Newborns," pp. 506–509.

34. Johnstone, "The Sanctity of Life," pp. 265–269.

35. For McCormick's formulation of his "reasonable person" standard, see his *How Brave A New World,* pp. 383–401.

36. The substance of my position is based on Pius XII's allocution "The Prolongation of Life," *The Pope Speaks* 4 (1958) 393–398.

37. "Declaration on Euthanasia," *Origins* 10 (1980) 156. It seems to me that the Pontifical Academy of Sciences departs from the essential substance of the "Declaration on Euthanasia" when it requires that food and water must always be given (regardless of the proportionality between the benefits and burdens?) to patients who are in a persistent vegetative state. See "The Artificial Prolongation of Life," *Origins* 15 (1985) 415.

MEDICAL ISSUES

8

Defining the Quality of Life

Anthony Shaw

Many of the difficult ethical choices in medical decision making revolve around assessments of actual or potential quality of life. Attempts to reach decisions in medical cases in which quality of life considerations appear to be relevant founder on the difficulty of defining a life of good or bad quality.

Physicians and other medical professionals often tend to think of the quality of life of patients in terms of their measurable or quantifiable physical and mental characteristics. Such a view of quality of life, expressed in mathematical terms, might read as follows:

$QL = NE$; where (QL) represents quality of life and (NE) represents the patient's natural endowment (physical and intellectual).

The problem with this formulation is that it fails to take note of those ingredients which, along with physical and intellectual capacity (NE), determine quality of life, that is, the aptitudes, motivation, skills and pleasure, physical and intellectual, which the individual acquires as a result of efforts made on his behalf by his *family* and by *society*.

Thus a more accurate formulation of quality of life might be represented as follows: $QL = NE \times (H + S)$ in which (H) represents the contributions made to that individual by his home and family and (S) represents the contributions made to that individual by society.

The actions of medical or societal decision makers toward an individual handicapped by congenital or acquired disease might be different if they perceive that $QL = NE \times (H + S)$ rather than $QL = NE$ alone.

It is obvious that (QL) may be improved for many individuals with an impaired (NE) by increasing the contributions of (H) and/or (S). Given an (NE) greater than 0, the (QL) will depend to varying degrees on the contributions home and society are willing to make to that individual.

Under what circumstances does quality of life = 0? First consider an anencephalic newborn infant, insensible and unresponsive. No matter how much his family and society pour into this baby in terms of love, medication, special education and so on, the infant's qual-

"Defining the Quality of Life" by Anthony Shaw. Reprinted with permission of Anthony Shaw and The Hastings Center Report 7(October, 1977):11.

ity of life will not be measurably improved. Indeed for such an infant, no matter what the amount of (H) *and* (S), $QL = 0 \times (H + S) = 0$.

Now look at a child born normally formed but one who has the misfortune of being born in an urban ghetto to an unwed teenage drug addict. (NE) may be a respectable quantity but (H) is likely to equal 0. If society turns its back on this child, $QL = NE \times (0 + 0) = 0$.

Bedside medical conferences at which attempts are made to assess actual or potential quality of the lives of patients often tend to shift focus (inadvertently or intentionally) from the quality of life of the individual patient at issue $(QL)_i$ to that of the quality of life of those in his household $(QL)_h$ or to that of society at large $(QL)_s$. (This shift of emphasis away from the patient to others affected by him seems more likely to occur if the term "meaningful life" is used. The use of the term "meaningful" tends to move a discussion easily from $(QL)_i$ to $(QL)_s$—a shift from the value of his life to the individual himself to the value of his life to society.)

If we are considering the potential quality of life of a newborn infant with Down's Syndrome, factors dealing with the willingness of the parents to keep the baby at home, to love him, to enroll him in preschool stimulation classes, to train him to the extent to which he is educable—all influence the quality of life *of the baby*, $(QL)_i$. Factors such as the contributions the infant will make to the understanding and maturing of his siblings, to what extent he

will give pleasure to his parents and other members of the family, the financial burdens of medical care and special education—such factors belong in a calculation of the quality of life of the infant's *family*, $(QL)_h$. Proper application of the formula excludes potential contributions to or detractions from society and family when considering any individual's potential quality of life, i.e., $(QL)_i \neq NE \times (H + S)$ when H and S represent contributions *by* not *to* the individual (except, of course, insofar as the contributions he makes to his family and society support his own self-esteem).

I do not propose this formula as a method of calculating the numerical value of a human life. Nor do I propose it as a guide to a definition of humanhood or personhood, or as a way of assigning points to decide whether lifesaving efforts should be made or discontinued in a particular case. Rather the formula shows simply and dramatically, in terms a schoolchild can readily grasp, that a person's quality of life, whether it be a baby born with intestinal obstruction, a depressed adolescent, a father of three with intractable angina or an octogenarian with terminal cancer, may be determined to a significant degree by factors physicians frequently fail to consider. The (QL) formula identifies, in broad terms, those factors which affect quality of life. Moreover the equation format may help clarify the issues involved by focusing sharply on exactly whose life is under consideration—a necessary precondition, I submit, for decision making.

9

The Use of Quality of Life Considerations in Medical Decision Making

Robert A. Pearlman and Albert Jonsen

In recent months there has been considerable attention in the medical literature on life-sustaining treatments for chronically ill patients.[1-9] In several of these articles, the patient's quality of life is discussed as a factor affecting medical decisions.[5-9]

The traditional pressures in acute care facilities for aggressive treatment and the uncertainties of diagnosis and prognosis may make it difficult to predict the quality of a patient's life with or without treatment.[10,11] Other factors also may make quality of life difficult to predict. These include the physician's subjective values relative to the patient's characteristics, inadequate communication between physicians and patients, and problems with the measurement of quality of life.[3,10,12] The extent to which the patient's quality of life is considered in medical decisions and the variability in judg-ments among physicians have not been well defined in the literature.

This study was designed to provide a better understanding of physician consideration (mention) of patient quality of life in medical decisions. We studied the explicit mention of "quality of life" as an influential factor in a patient management problem (PMP) pertaining to the use of mechanical ventilation to sustain life. This paper presents the results of this research, defines quality of life, and provides guidelines for physician consideration of patient quality of life.

Methods

After the nature of the patient management problem was explained and informed consent

Reprinted with permission from the American Geriatrics Society and Robert A. Pearlman, "The Use of Quality of Life Considerations in Medical Decision Making," by Robert A. Pearlman, M.D., M.P.H. and Albert Jonsen, Ph.D. (The Journal of the American Geriatrics Society, Vol. 33, No. 5, pp. 344–350, May, 1985).

was obtained, the patient management problem was presented to 205 physicians specializ-
ing in internal medicine or family medicine in
King County, Washington. The physicians
performed several tasks during this exercise,
including (1) indication of a treatment preference after the initial reading of the case description, (2) indication of the potential value
of available (but unknown) case information,
(3) selection of a limited amount of case information to acquire more detailed data about
the clinical situation, (4) indication of a treatment decision as to whether to use intubation
or current therapy without intubation after ac-
quiring the additional case knowledge, (5) explanation of the rationale for the treatment
decision, and (6) prognostication regarding the
patient's expected survival time. In a previous
article, the precise details of the selection of
subjects, the PMP, the management of case
information, and the interview were presented.[13] In this paper we describe and discuss
physicians' expressed consideration of the "patient's quality of life" as a reason for the treatment decision.

Case Description

The patient management problem was mod-
eled after American Board of Internal Medicine certification examination questions. It
was developed to explore physicians' decisions
to withhold mechanical ventilation.

The case presented a male patient with an
acute exacerbation of his chronic obstructive
pulmonary disease. The patient was an elderly-
looking 69-year-old who lived in a nursing
home, was easily incapacitated by shortness of
breath, and had recently had a prolonged hospitalization (2 months) because of a similar
episode. His forced expiratory volume in one
second was 0.38 liters (12 per cent), his forced

expiratory volume in one second/vital capacity ratio was 0.22, and his forced expiratory
flow (0.25–0.75 seconds) was 0.17 liters (9 per
cent). He had never expressed to his physician
his view on conditions in which withholding
therapy might be desirable, nor had he offered
his own assessment of his quality of life. His
physician had never inquired about these
points. At this hospital admission he expressed
concern about the possible need for intubation. However, a precise plan for dealing with
worsening respiratory failure was not defined.
Despite treatment with oxygen, antibiotics,
bronchodilators, and steroids, the patient deteriorated into profound respiratory failure.
This life-and-death situation forced the studied physicians to decide between intubation
(life prolonging) and the currently administered drug regimen without intubation (allowing to die).

Additional information about the patient's
physical and functional status while residing in
the nursing home was available. However, the
patient management problem required physicians to seek further information that was not
provided initially in the case description. Available data about the patient's baseline, precrisis
level of function included slight forgetfulness,
mild depression, and inability to walk more
than halfway across a room because of worsening shortness of breath.

Data Analysis

Statistical analyses were accomplished with
univariate and multivariate methods (SPSS).[14]
Significance values are reported in the text
with the name of the test statistic. Stepwise
discriminant analysis was used to select and
combine into an index a limited number of
measures to best predict use of quality of life.
The predictive ability of this index was vali-

dated by developing it on one-half of the data and using it to predict the use of quality of life in the other half of the data.

Results

Thirty-seven per cent of all physicians justified their clinical decisions, at least in part, by explicit references to the "patient's quality of life." Forty-nine per cent of those who decided not to withhold mechanical ventilation (nonintubators) volunteered quality of life as a rationale for their decision. In contrast, 29 per cent of those who chose to intubate (intubators) mentioned quality of life as an influential factor affecting their treatment choice ($0.005 < p \leqslant 0.01$, unpaired t-test). Among nonintubators, approximately 87 per cent indicated that the patient's quality of life positively supported their treatment decision. Among intubators, approximately 82 per cent indicated that the patient's quality of life positively supported their treatment decision. This was determined by asking the physician how each factor affecting the therapeutic choice influenced their decision; that is, whether it supported, militated against, or had no impact. It is noteworthy that these divergent evaluations of an individual patient's quality of life were used to justify polar treatment decisions of clinical significance.

There was no appreciable difference in consideration of "quality of life" between specialities (39 per cent for family medicine and 36 per cent for internal medicine). However, residents in training programs considered quality of life more often than did attending physicians and private practitioners (47 per cent for residents, 33 per cent for attending physicians, 31 per cent for private practitioners). The comparison between residents and other physicians was statistically significant, $0.025 < p \leqslant 0.05$ (χ^2, 2 degrees of freedom). These data are presented in Table 1. Physicians who indicated that quality of life was a consideration thought it was an important factor. This was noted on a scale of increasing importance from 1 (unimportant) to 10 (very important). These results are diagrammed in Figure 1.

Physician consideration of "quality of life" as a factor influencing the treatment decision was associated with consideration of available specific case information and with several other volunteered explanations. Table 2 outlines the statistically significant correlates of quality of life consideration. Physicians who requested information either from the social worker or from the nurse at the nursing home and learned either that the family finances were depleted or that the patient was only able to walk halfway across the room, respectively, were more inclined to use quality of life as a justification for their treatment decisions ($p \leqslant 0.05$). Other expressed explanations, such as cost-benefit factors, the expected survival time (if intubated) for the patient, the patient's right to determine his own therapy, the physician's responsibility to sustain life, and the patient's prior hospital experience with respirator dependence, were significantly associated with the consideration of quality of life as a partial justification for the treatment decision ($p \leqslant 0.05$). Nonintubators cited the right of the patient to determine his own therapy and his prior hospital experience as a rationale along with consideration of quality of life ($p \leqslant 0.05$). On the other hand, intubators cited the patient's expected survival time and their own responsibility to sustain life ($p \leqslant 0.05$).

Physician consideration of quality of life was not associated with medical specialty (internal medicine or family medicine), religion, degree of faith, or estimates of the patient's

TABLE 1. Quality of Life Rationale

	Physicians Mentioning Quality of Life	Physicians Not Mentioning Quality of Life
Treatment decision		
Intubators*	34 (29%)	85
Nonintubators*	42 (49%)	44
Specialty		
Internal medicine	48 (36%)	85
Family medicine	28 (39%)	44
Role		
Residents†	34 (47%)	38
Attending physicians†	18 (33%)	37
Private practitioners†	24 (31%)	54

* $p \leq 0.01$.

† $p \leq 0.05$ (residents versus others).

survival time (if intubated). The relationship between quality of life consideration and a measure of moral judgment was also examined. Moral judgment was assessed by administering Robert Hogan's Survey of Ethical Attitudes to each physician.[13] This test explores the effects of the difference between an ethic of social responsibility and an ethic of personal conscience.[15-18] Use of quality of life as a factor in this treatment decision was not significantly associated with either ethical stance.

Table 2 shows a large number of variables that are significantly related to the consideration of quality of life as a justification for the treatment choice in this case management problem. One could predict, to some extent, use of quality of life by assessing any one of these measures. Using stepwise discriminant analysis, an index was developed that identified a limited number of measures that would best predict the mention or nonmention of quality of life. Table 3 reviews the important

discriminate variables that were used in the stepwise analysis. The management of case information and other volunteered explanations appeared to significantly account for or explain the use of quality of life as a consideration in decision making. The measures identified in Table 3 correctly predicted the consideration of quality of life in this therapeutic decision (justifying intubation or current therapy without intubation) with a probability greater than 80 per cent.

Discussion

Consideration of "quality of life" in medical decision-making was systematically observed in a PMP. It was commonly voiced as a rationale for the medical decision by physicians inclined to withhold mechanical ventilation, physicians who considered the patient's survival time, and physicians who extensively fo-

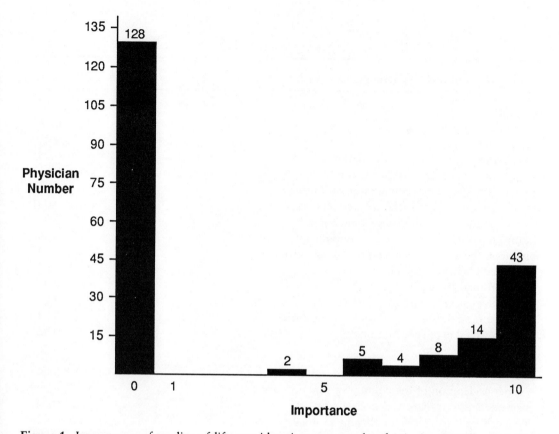

Figure 1. Importance of quality of life considerations on a scale of 1 (unimportant) to 10 (very important); 0 represents physicians who did not express an opinion.

cused on social information about the patient. However, the marked variation in perceptions of quality of life for a given patient gives rise to serious concerns about how physicians use this term.

The greater consideration of quality of life by residents may reflect several factors. The residents focused more on socioeconomic case information, which may have influenced their consideration of quality of life. However, it is also possible that residents are more harshly judgmental about an older person's

quality of life or more concerned with this issue than attending physicians or private practitioners. Whether this will change as the residents advance in their professional lives is unknown. Their consideration of quality of life may represent a cohort effect caused by recent changes in medical education or a temporary phenomenon due to their current age and experience.

The lack of association between consideration of quality of life and an ethical stance (based on Hogan's Survey of Ethical Attitudes)

TABLE 2. Correlates of Quality of Life Consideration

Reasons for Considering Quality of Life	*p* Values
All subjects	
Preference for nonintubation	0.01
Residency status (role)	0.05
Valuation of physiologic information*	0.03
Valuation of professional information*	0.01
Valuation of socioeconomic information*	0.01
Consideration of the social worker's report†	0.001
Consideration of the nursing home report†	0.03
Consideration of general socioeconomic information†	0.04
Nonconsideration of general physiologic information‡	0.04
Costs and benefits rationale§	0.04
Survival time rationale§	0.02
Patient's right to determine therapy rationale§	0.004
Physician responsibility to sustain life rationale§	0.04
Prior hospital experience rationale§	0.02
Nonintubators	
Valuation of general professional information*	0.04
Nonconsideration of the pulmonary function data‡	0.006
Consideration of the social worker's report†	0.002
Patient's right to determine therapy rationale§	0.02
Prior hospital experience rationale§	0.001
Intubators	
Valuation of general physiologic information*	0.02
Valuation of general socioeconomic information*	0.04
Nonconsideration of the repeat chest x-ray data‡	0.03
Survival time rationale§	0.02
Physician responsibility to sustain life rationale§	0.04

* Valuation refers to attributing a value to categories of information in terms of importance to the therapeutic choice.

† Consideration here refers to selection of case information to obtain detailed data.

‡ Nonconsideration refers to nonselection of detailed case information.

§ Rationale refers to a volunteered explanation.

TABLE 3. Significant Variables in a Discriminant Analysis Predicting
Consideration of Quality of Life*

Preference for nonintubation
Valuation of general professional information†
Consideration of the social worker's report‡
Nonconsideration of complete blood chemistry data§
Nonconsideration of theophylline level report§
Survival time rationale¶
Nonmention of rationale concerning the patient's social attributes¶

---

* Split-sample analysis correctly predicted use of quality of life 80.9 per cent of the time.

† Valuation refers to attributing a value to categories of information in terms of importance to the therapeutic choice.

‡ Consideration refers to selection of case information to obtain detailed data.

§ Nonconsideration refers to nonselection of detailed case information.

¶ Rationale refers to volunteered explanations.

may reflect the ambiguous nature and the unprincipled use of the concept. If consideration of quality of life were a clearly defined professional responsibility, it might have correlated with the ethic of social responsibility. And if the consideration of quality of life represented attempts to avoid patient harm or promote patient well-being, it might have correlated with the ethic of personal conscience. However, as neither ethical stance appeared to be associated with consideration of quality of life, the principled rationale for such consideration is yet undefined.

The explicit consideration of quality of life in the case management of a nursing home patient with an acute exacerbation of chronic obstructive pulmonary disease reflects a more general and pervasive consideration of quality of life in health care decisions. In rheumatology, oncology, and geriatric medicine, quality of life is becoming a common measure of outcome and health status.[19-22] It would be extremely unusual for physicians not to be concerned about the quality of their patients'

lives. Physicians, after all, work to diagnose and treat the medical causes of impaired quality of life in hopes of improving that quality. However, in recent years the term "quality of life" has taken on a more specific and problematic meaning in medicine.

Quality of life has come to serve as a criterion for the utility of intervention in many clinical situations, including those involving life-and-death decisions. However, there are some individuals who reject quality of life as an important determinant of the value of life. They consider life to have intrinsic worth and regard prolongation of life as the overriding determinant of the utility of an intervention. From this point of view, quality of life is a moot issue in clinical decision making. In contrast, many individuals consider quality of life to be a vague complex of personal characteristics and social accidents and feel that medical interventions are worthwhile only to the extent that they can promote this beneficial state. In these situations, physicians actually may cite quality of life as their primary or one of several standards for treatment, as this study demonstrates. In situations in which quality of life connotes a vague set of attributes and conditions, the variability of perceptions of a patient's quality of life may be great, as this study suggests. The methods used in this study may have introduced other reasons for the variability in citing quality of life. These might include the limited amount of patient information given, the variability in the physicians' consideration of additional case information, and the possibility of idiosyncratic responses by physicians to a PMP that involves an open-ended interview.

Medicine abounds in clear and safe criteria for medical intervention—for instance, a symptomatically low serum sugar concentration (hypoglycemia) indicates a need for administration of glucose, and severely elevated blood pressure indicates a need for administration of an antihypertensive regimen. When physicians move beyond these to such general criteria as quality of life, prudent use is required. Quality of life is a particularly imprecise criterion subject to misinterpretation and variable application. This does not imply that such a criterion is illegitimate; it does imply that its meaning should be as clear as possible and its use as responsible as can be.

Meaning

The term "quality of life" has no obvious meaning; it is not clear to which empirical states the term refers, nor is it manifest how any particular person will evaluate those states. A major result of this study is the demonstration that physician evaluation of a patient's quality of life is variable and can lead to diverse conclusions about treatment. A significant minority of the physicians studied considered the patient's quality of life sufficiently poor to withhold additional treatment, whereas other physicians considered it sufficiently good to justify implementing additional therapy. These results highlight the inherent ambiguity of the term "quality of life."

Three possible definitions recently have been proposed to minimize the ambiguity in the term "quality of life."[19] Quality of life may reflect the subjective satisfaction by an individual with his or her own personal life (physical, mental, and social situation). Several authors who have written about quality of life in medical decisions have used this definition.[1,3,4,6,8,10] Another definition is that quality of life represents an evaluation by an onlooker of another's life situation. Two authors modified this definition for use with seriously ill, incompetent patients by recommending guidelines for considering patient quality of life. One author recommended judgment by "reasonable measures," whereas another author accepted the Canadian Law Reform Commission recommendation that evaluation of quality of life be made by competent patients of the same age and condition.[7,8] The third definition is that quality of life is the achievement of certain attributes highly valued in our society.

A common, clinical context in which the first definition occurs is when a patient presents a physician with a concern or complaint and the physician intervenes to diagnose and treat. In this situation, the most frequent paradigm of the physician/patient interaction, the patient has evaluated his or her own life and found it in some way unsatisfying.

The second definition finds common use in clinical settings when a physician or a patient's family member or friend makes an evaluative judgment about the patient's condition that reflects his or her own personal views about what the condition *must* be like. This often occurs in clinical discussions concerning the initiation or continuation of life-sustaining procedures for a patient incapable of making or expressing a personal evaluation. It may also occur when a seriously impaired patient could be queried about personal satisfaction but the reluctance or inhibition of others, including the physician, prevent this approach to the patient. Although these evaluations may be thoughtful and compassionate, they may not necessarily reflect the patient's own views on the condition. This second definition of quality of life may lead to inter-rater variability because of differences in values. This operational definition probably was used by the physician respondents in this study.

The third definition is less obvious, but it is still influential in medical situations. Clinicians' perceptions of a patient's quality of life may be influenced by their perceptions of the difference between a patient's conditions and the achievement of certain attributes that the culture deems necessary or contributory to a life of good quality. Here, invidious prejudices may be hidden below the surface of apparently benign judgments. It has been demonstrated that these prejudices, often deeply buried, can strongly affect the treatment plans of physicians for these sorts of patients.[12,23-26]

Responsible Use

Responsible use of the inherently ambiguous concept of quality of life occurs when clinicians attune their interactions with patients to the values and goals of the patient. In these contexts, a patient's own evaluation of the quality of personal life may affect the nature of the clinician-patient relationship, the schedule for a diagnostic evaluation, the choice of a therapeutic intervention, and the determination of patient benefit or best interest. A common example in geriatric medicine is when a

clinician recommends a walker rather than a nursing home for a patient with irreversible gait instability and the desire to remain independent. A less common example is when a clinician accepts a competent elderly patient's refusal of treatment because the proposed intervention will not improve the patient's overall quality of life in the patient's view. When consideration of a patient's quality of life is grounded in the patient's self-evaluation, it is important and relevant for good patient care. This use rarely poses an ethical concern. Ethical problems appear only when a patient's competency is in doubt or an incompetent patient's family proposes that the patient's quality of life does not justify a medical intervention.

The common use of quality of life as a factor in making a decision on withholding or withdrawing life-sustaining procedures represents a crucial ethical concern in patient care.[19] With an informed, competent patient who is able to communicate his or her feelings, respect for patient autonomy should foster respect for the patient's attitudes about the use of life-sustaining procedures. The underlying rationale is that this type of patient is able to determine what is beneficial for himself or herself (on the basis of his or her perceived current or future quality of life). This situation requires that a clinician's subjective evaluation of the patient's quality of life generally be relegated to the patient's opinions.[27] When a patient is unable to communicate his or her feelings about life-sustaining procedures, quality of life may be considered a decisive factor only if the patient's quality of life falls below a minimum standard and the intervention would only preserve this condition or maintain organic life.[19] One recommendation for minimal threshold is extreme physical debilitation and a complete loss of sensory and intellectual activity.[19] This threshold should be kept extremely low to ensure specificity. Only when the qualities common to human interaction have been irreversibly lost should the clinician's assessment of the patient's quality of life determine withholding of life-supporting therapy. Specificity is particularly important in avoiding the potential use of subjective judgments of poor quality of life based on socioeconomic or other value-laden attributes ("false positives").

This minimum standard reflects respect for personal function, cerebration, and the essential qualities of being human.[28,29] This standard shows respect for the sanctity of human life and the need to safeguard this principle. These guidelines attempt to protect patient autonomy, to ensure justice by preventing capricious decision making based on personal preferences, to promote beneficial results for patients, and to prevent doing harm.

In summary, in this study a PMP was used to demonstrate the use of quality of life considerations in medical decision making. In clinical usage, quality of life is an ambiguous term. Quality of life may refer to a patient's subjective satisfaction with his or her life or a subjective evaluation by an observer of the patient's life. When quality of life is considered by the patient, responsible use of this evaluation helps clarify the "best interests" of the patient as well as what is beneficial for that patient. An ethical problem arises in situations in which clinicians consider withholding or withdrawing life-sustaining procedures without knowledge of the patient's preferences. In this context, it is responsible to include consideration of a patient's quality of life in medical decision making only under the following conditions: the qualities of human interaction must be lacking, the patient must be unable to express his preferences, and the situation must be such that life-sustaining procedures serve only to prolong a life that is only biologically functional.

There are no current guarantees that the subjective evaluation by a clinician of a patient's quality of life will result in the evaluation's ethically responsible use. Responsible use occurs when a clinician's subjective evaluation (projection) concerning a patient's quality of life assists him or her in communicating with the patient and in giving compassionate care. Responsible use also occurs when clinicians analyze their own values to prevent personally biased judgments. As Fletcher has written, "A person's values, therefore, are the key to his or her ethical position. Failure to state one's values whether through dishonest camouflage or lack of self-knowledge is a source of much more heat than light in ethical discourse."[28]

Notes

1. Bayer R, Callahan D, Fletcher J, et al: The care of the terminally ill: morality and economics. N Engl J Med 309:1490, 1983

2. Wanzer SH, Adelstein SJ, Cranford RE, et al: The physician's responsibility toward hopelessly ill patients. N Engl J Med 310:955, 1984

3. Bedell SE, Delbanco TL: Choices about cardiopulmonary resuscitation in the hospital: when do physicians talk with patients? N Engl J Med 310:1089, 1984

4. Wagner A: Cardiopulmonary resuscitation in the aged. N Engl J Med 310:1129, 1984

5. Avorn J: Benefit and cost analysis in geriatric care: turning age discrimination into health policy. N Engl J Med 310:1294, 1984

6. Watts DT, Cassel CK: Extraordinary nutritional support: a case study and ethical analysis. J Am Geriatr Soc 32:237, 1984

7. Besdine RW: Decisions to withhold treatment from nursing home residents. J Am Geriatr Soc 31:602, 1983

8. Thomasma DC: Ethical judgments of quality of life in the care of the aged. J Am Geriatr Soc 32:525, 1984

9. Stollerman GH: Quality of life treatment decisions and the third alternative. J Am Geriatr Soc 32:483, 1984

10. Pearlman RA, Speer JB: Quality of life considerations in geriatric care. J Am Geriatr Soc 31:113, 1983

11. Thibault GE, Mulley AG, Barnett GO, et al: Medical intensive care: indications, interventions and outcomes. N Engl J Med 302:938, 1980

12. Eisenberg JM: Sociological influences on decision-making by clinicians. Ann Intern Med 90:957, 1979

13. Pearlman RA, Inui TS, Carter WB: Variability in physician bioethical decision making: a case study of euthanasia. Ann Intern Med 97:420, 1982

14. Nie NH, Hull CH, Jenkins JG, et al: SPSS: Statistical Package for the Social Sciences. New York, McGraw-Hill, 1975

15. Hogan R: A dimension of moral judgment. J Consult Clin Psychol 36:205, 1970

16. Hogan R, Johnson J, Emler N: A socioanalytic theory of moral development. New Directions for Child Development 2:1, 1978

17. Hogan R, Dickstein E: Moral judgment and perceptions of injustice. J Pers Soc Psychol 23:409, 1972

18. Lorr M, Zea R: Moral judgment and liberal-conservative attitude. Psychol Rep 40:627, 1977

19. Jonsen AR, Siegler M, Winslade WJ: Clinical Ethics. New York, Macmillan, 1982, pp 109–38

20. Spitzer WO, Dobson AJ, Hall J, et al: Measuring the quality of life of cancer patients. J Chronic Dis 34:585, 1981

21. Oliver H, Blum MH, Roskin G: The psychiatrist as advocate for post surgical "quality of life." Psychosomatics 27:157, 1976

22. Poe WD: The physician's dilemma: when to let go. Forum Med 3:163, 1980

23. Crane D: The Sanctity of Social Life: Physicians' Treatment of Critically Ill Patients. New York, Russell Sage Foundation, 1975

24. Sudnow D: Passing On. Englewood Cliffs, NJ, Prentice-Hall, 1967

25. Uhlmann RF, McDonald WJ: An empiric study of nonresuscitation. Clin Res 30:45A, 1982

26. Shaw A, Randolph JG, Manard B: Ethical issues in pediatric surgery: a national survey of pediatricians and pediatric surgeons. Pediatrics 60:588, 1977

27. President's Commission for the Study of Ethical Problems in Medicine and Biomedical and Behavioral Research: Making Health Care Decisions: The Ethical and Legal Implications of Informed Consent in the Patient—Practitioner Relationship. Washington, DC, Library of Congress, 1982, p 38

28. Fletcher J: Humanhood: Essays in Biomedical Ethics. Buffalo, NY, Prometheus Books, 1979, p 122

29. Fletcher J: Four indicators of humanhood: the enquiry matures. Hastings Cent Rep 4:4, 1974

Part 2

APPLICATIONS

part 2

Introduction

The application of quality of life considerations to the clinical setting has been vigorously debated over the past several years. The purpose of this part will be to illustrate how quality of life has been applied to several areas of contemporary medical practice. No doubt, one of the significant reasons why quality of life has become such an important concept is due to the tremendous advancements in medical science and technology.

Physicians now have the ability to diagnose many debilitating genetic diseases while the fetus is *in utero*, and under liberalized abortion laws parents can now make decisions whether to abort their offspring who have these diseases. Neonatology and geriatric medicine have become sophisticated medical specialties, and the technical advancements in these areas have given medical personnel the tools to save severely ill newborns and to prolong the lives of very elderly patients. Unconscious patients who once died within a few days because they could not ingest food and liquids by mouth now can live for decades in a persistent vegetative state by inserting tubes directly into their gastrointestinal systems. For some, the development and use of these medical technologies have been acclaimed because they have prevented an untimely death or they have healed a mishap due to nature or an accident; for others, their use has only continued an unfortunate existence or has consigned the patient to a chronic state of ill-health without any hope of a cure or relief of suffering.

Many important issues are at stake in the application of quality of life considerations to the medical setting. The definition of quality of life again surfaces in this discussion, and the question of the limits of such considerations now becomes particularly relevant. Because some of these technologies have become so routine in medical practice today, should they not be looked upon as ordinary means of preserving life? If they are indeed ordinary ways of treating patients with certain kinds of diseases, then are not patients or those who must decide or care for them morally obliged to use the technologies? Furthermore, should not a calculation of the benefits and burdens which will accrue to patients and to those who must care for them be part of the very definition of quality of life? When patients cannot be cured, can medical personnel actively kill or assist in the death of these patients? What are the proper goals of medical practice, and do these goals help to clarify when and how medical technology should be used? Is it ever possible to say that a person's existence possesses such a minimal quality of life that it is not worth saving?

The five areas of application we present in this part only begin to illustrate the range of questions that can and must be asked. These areas are particularly significant because a quality of life decision in any one of these clinical settings could result in the death of the patient. What is important at a conceptual level, however, is the realization that each position taken in the debate does imply theological, ethical, medical, social and political considerations that lie behind and justify the application of quality of life.

Further Readings

Arras, John D.; Asch, Adrienne; Macklin, Ruth; O'Connell, Larry; Rhoden, Nancy K.; and Weisbard, Alan J. "Imperiled Newborns: Standards of Judgment for Treatment," *Hastings Center Report* 17(December, 1987):13–16.

Cohen, Howard. "Abortion and the Quality of Life," in *Feminism and Philosophy,* eds. Vitterling-Braggin et al. (Totowa, NJ: Rowman and Littlefield, 1977), pp. 429–440.

Johnstone, Brian V., C.S.S.R. "The Sanctity of Life, the Quality of Life and the New 'Baby Doe' Law," *Linacre Quarterly* 52(August, 1985):258–270.

May, William F. "Dealing with Catastrophe," in *Dax's Case: Essays in Medical Ethics and Human Meaning,* ed. Lonnie D. Kliever (Dallas: Southern Methodist University Press, 1989), pp. 131–150.

O'Rourke, Kevin. "The A.M.A. Statement on Tube Feeding: An Ethical Analysis," *America* 155(November 22, 1986):321–323 and 331.

Paris, John J. and McCormick, Richard A. "The Catholic Tradition on the Use of Nutrition and Fluids," *America* 156(May 2, 1987):356–361.

Pius XII. "The Prolongation of Life," *The Pope Speaks* 4(Spring, 1958):393–398.

Ruse, Michael. "Genetics and the Quality of Life," *Social Indicators Research* 7(1980):419–441.

Siegler, Mark and Weisbard, Alan J. "Against the Emerging Stream: Should Fluids and Nutritional Support Be Discontinued?," *Archives of Internal Medicine* 145(January, 1985):129–131.

Walter, James J. "Food & Water: An Ethical Burden," *Commonweal* 113(November 21, 1986):616–619.

PRENATAL DIAGNOSIS
AND ABORTION

10

Who Shall Live?

Leonard J. Weber

In an attempt to explain and analyze the different ways in which life is valued in the questions of abortion and euthanasia, two conflicting approaches are sometimes compared. These two have come to be known as the "sanctity of life ethic" and the "quality of life ethic." The sanctity of life ethic holds that every human life is intrinsically good, that no one life is more valuable than another, that lives not yet fully developed (embryonic and fetal stages) and lives with no great potential (the suffering lives of the terminally ill or the pathetic lives of the severely handicapped) are still sacred. The condition of a life does not reduce its value or justify its termination. The quality of life ethic puts the emphasis on the type of life being lived, not upon the fact of life. Lives are not all of one kind; some lives are of great value to the person himself and to others while others are not. What the life means to someone is what is important. Keeping this in mind, it is not inappropriate to say that some lives are of greater value than others, that the condition or meaning of life does have much to do with the justification for terminating that life.

The sanctity of life ethic defends two propositions:

1. That human life is sacred by the very fact of its existence; its value does not depend upon a certain condition or perfection of that life.
2. That, therefore, all human lives are of equal value; all have the same right to life.

The quality of life ethic finds neither of these two propositions acceptable. Things are valuable when they are of value to someone; life is good when it is meaningful to someone, especially to that person himself. The mere fact of life does not immediately mean that life is good or sacred. Thus, ending one type of human life is not always of the same moral nature as ending another type.

"Who Shall Live?" by Leonard J. Weber in Who Shall Live?: The Dilemma of Severely Handicapped Children and Its Meaning for Other Moral Questions, *1976, pp. 41–52. Reprinted with permission of Paulist Press.*

The sanctity of life ethic has acknowledged that there may be times when it is morally acceptable to directly kill someone. Traditionally, killing has been recognized as legitimate in self-defense against unjust aggression, in participation in a just war (criteria have been developed to help determine which wars are just and which are not), in capital punishment, and —according to some—in tyrannicide (when an illegitimate and unjust ruler can be removed in no other way). In all four of these cases, killing is justified because the one being killed has, by his actions, forfeited his right to life. Killing is not permitted because the lives of some are considered less valuable than the lives of others. Rather, it is permitted only because of the actions taken. This, it is argued, is not a quality of life judgment, but one based on more objective criteria, what the person is doing or has done. When the aggressive actions that forfeit the right to life have not been taken, there is no justification for killing, no matter what the condition of someone's life. Innocent human life may never be directly taken.

Some who are within the sanctity of life tradition think that the tradition may have gone too far in recognizing the legitimacy of killing (as in capital punishment). Others think that the whole emphasis should not be placed on innocence or injustice (as when an innocent fetus threatens the mother's life). But all within the sanctity of life school agree that the killing cannot be justified because someone's life is seen as less valuable on the basis of its condition; killing can only be justified in response to actions which threaten life.

The sanctity of life ethic and the quality of life ethic are not totally exclusive. The sanctity of life ethic is concerned with quality, with the type of life that is being lived. Advocates of this position insist, however, that "if each and every life is not accorded full worth and equality, then the quality of the whole of society will be seriously endangered."[1] The quality of life ethic is not unconcerned with the value of life itself. Advocates of this position maintain, however, that it is impossible to make responsible moral decisions in individual situations if we always place an absolute prohibition on taking innocent life. Placing such absolute value on life is "thoroughly idolatrous"[2] and does not give us the opportunity to give due consideration to other factors. The two positions are not totally exclusive, but their orientations are so different that they disagree on many practical issues.

It is, in fact, precisely these underlying differences in the way life is valued that accounts for much of the disagreement on abortion and euthanasia. Those who emphasize the very fact of life as being the basis for its value (the sanctity school) feel an obligation to respect life totally as soon as it is present. Though life in the early stages of pregnancy is not fully developed, it is life of the human species and, as such, needs to be protected against direct destruction. Its condition does not diminish its value. Those who emphasize the condition and meaning of life (the quality school) feel an obligation to recognize that the woman's life is, at present, of much greater value. She may be justified, therefore, to end the life within in defense of a certain value in her own life. She may also be justified in having an abortion to guard against a life of poor quality for the child who would be born or for other members of the family or society. The obligation to try to bring about a good life for all concerned is more important than the obligation to protect undeveloped human life.

In the case of mercy killing, the sanctity of

life ethic insists that as long as a person is alive, direct killing is always an unjustified attack upon the sacredness of life. This is true even when the killing is requested by the patient himself, because the value of life does not depend upon how much meaning that life has for the individual or for anyone else. It should be noted very carefully, though, that the sanctity of life ethic does *not* insist that everything possible must be done to prolong life in all cases; it is not opposed to the practice of withholding or ceasing treatment at times. That does not directly attack the goodness of life; it recognizes that death is natural and that life is not the only good to be concerned with. But direct killing of an innocent person always violates the goodness of life. The quality of life ethic finds it morally responsible at times to mercy kill because the obligation to avoid a meaningless and severely painful life is greater than the obligation to protect life simply because it is human.

It is something of an oversimplification to suggest that all the ways in which men value human life can be placed in either one of these two categories. This author has elsewhere suggested one way in which the scheme might be refined to include a position that can be called "the sanctity of personal life ethic."[3] This approach argues that all human lives are sacred and of equal value provided they are capable of personal living. The life that is to be considered sacred is not to be identified with biological life of the human species; it is personal life that is sacred. In a sense, then, this position rejects the first but accepts a variation of the second of the sanctity of life propositions.

Some such refinement (and probably others as well) would seem to be necessary to give full justice to the positions that are taken on the value of life. For our purposes here, though, the basic distinction between the sanctity of life and the quality of life positions is sufficient to indicate the fundamental importance of the very way in which persons view life. For many (sanctity), man's obligations are determined by the fact of life and justification for killing has to be based on the objective criteria of actions. For many others (quality) man's obligations are determined by what things mean to persons and justification of killing has to be based on the value that life has for persons. These are two fundamentally different ways of viewing moral obligations. A more careful consideration of these ethical worldviews will help us to understand why people take the moral stands that they do.

Ethical Worldviews

When we get back to one's fundamental ethical orientation we are dealing with the very way in which he sees things as having meaning and value. This is what is being described here as an ethical worldview—one's universe of meaning and value and man's place in that universe.

Recognizing that this involves the same danger of oversimplification as the sanctity of life-quality of life distinction, but recognizing as well that it involves the same usefulness in indicating underlying differences, I would like to describe in the following pages two characteristic ethical worldviews which are behind and shaping the different responses to abortion and euthanasia. It is precisely because they tend toward one or the other of these understandings of man's moral obligations that individuals tend to accept or reject abortion and mercy killing.

Both worldviews have existed side by side

for centuries. One, however, seems to have been the predominant one in the past while the other has been becoming increasingly common in recent times. We can call the first the "classical" or "traditional" worldview and the second the "modern." Both are very much alive today. People are not always able to articulate their own worldviews and they are often not conscious of them, but some such orientation underlies their position-taking.

In the classical worldview, man, both as the race and as the individual, is seen as being a very important part of the universe but he is not at the very center. The world has meaning and value apart from the meaning and value given to it by man. Man's own life, too, has a given meaning and purpose. His moral obligations are to accept, respect, and live in accordance with that meaning and purpose.

To determine what is a morally correct mode of behavior, an individual must attempt to discover the duties and obligations which the given meaning of things imposes upon him. In this classical worldview, the tendency is to stress moral obligations rather than moral rights. The focus is not on the individual, but on the larger context to which the individual must respond. The primary obligation may be expressed in terms of doing the will of God which is largely expressed in the created order of things. Or it may be expressed in terms of one's need to be in tune with nature. Or it may be expressed in terms of responsibility toward fellowmen. But, in any of these expressions, the emphasis is placed on the obligation of the individual to respond. He does not give meaning; he must respect the meaning already present.

For someone of the classical mentality, the starting point of moral analysis is rational reflection. What would the contemplated action involve? What are its implications? Is it in conformity with the obligation to respect the goodness and order of creation? Individual situations and individual differences are not stressed; first it is necessary to understand what any action of this sort involves. By withdrawing slightly from the situation and reflecting upon the larger context, it is possible to draw up guidelines to be followed which indicate one's obligations. To begin the decision-making process by dwelling on the circumstances of an individual case is to court the danger of deciding what is of immediate benefit to the individual rather than deciding what the individual must do to respect a common good. An abortion decision can be made pretty clearly once and for all and does not need to be begun anew in each individual case. A careful analysis of what abortion involves reveals that this is an unjustifiable destruction of human life. Man's obligation is to respect life, to be willing to undergo some suffering in defense of life, and to accept responsibility for his sexual behavior. To resort to the violence of innocent life-taking to solve problems (even serious problems) is contrary to the obligation to protect what is given us to protect. The classical view sees life as a gift, not as a possession.

The ability to decide the morality of questions without focusing on individual cases indicates another characteristic of the classical worldview. Morality is to be understood as a morality of actions rather than (or at least more than) a morality of intentions. Abortion is abortion whether the desire is to avoid a deformity or to not interrupt a career. Abortion is still direct assault upon helpless human life. The intention to abort so that the child will not have to suffer is much more admirable than the intention to abort to avoid an inconvenience, but the intention is not the most important factor. To put too much emphasis on intention is to stress what the action means to the *persons* involved, not how the action affects the right ordering of things that man is bound to respect. Actions have more impact upon the conditions of life than intentions do.

The classical ethical worldview, in summary:

1. The world has meaning apart from the meaning given by man.
2. The individual must *discover* what is the right thing to do.
3. The focus in morality is on the action.
4. The moral obligations of the individual are stressed.
5. The starting point of moral analysis is rational reflection on the nature and implications of actions.
6. Life is a gift.

This leads, in medical ethics, to what has previously been described as the sanctity of life ethic. Human life is good in and of itself; its value does not depend upon what it means to persons.

The relationship between the classical worldview and opposition to mercy killing can be clearly recognized. Because the facts of life are to be accepted and respected, man should accept but not attempt to control death. Because actions are very important morally, there is a sharp moral difference between letting die and killing. Because the emphasis is placed on the general moral obligation and not on individual differences, the suffering of the individual or the hopelessness of the situation is not decisive. Because the end does not justify the means, the fact that the killing is done in mercy does not justify it.

The modern ethical worldview puts much more emphasis on the role of man. Man's role is largely to exercise dominion over the world; man is at or near the center of the universe of meaning and value. Whatever meaning there may be apart from man is not so important as the meaning given by man. Man's moral obligations are not to be defined so much in terms of acceptance and respect as in terms of the need to be compassionate and wise as he exercises control. For the world is what man will make of it, man is what man will make of himself, and the responsibility is to make the world as good a one as possible for humankind.

When an individual is making a moral decision, he should begin by recognizing that there are a variety of options open to him. None of these possibilities should be rejected out of hand. He is free to choose any one of them. Right conduct is not something that is imposed from outside. What is right is to be decided by the individual, who should pick that option which is most likely to meet the needs of the individual and his fellowmen. The focus in morality has to be placed on the "end," the purpose for which an action is undertaken. Man is answerable to himself in morality; he should be expected to do neither more nor less than what, according to his best insight, constitutes an action calculated to do good for persons.

According to the modern worldview, the nature of man and the universe does not impose specific moral obligations. There are no universal moral laws and any guidelines that have been developed are to be used with discrimination. Generally speaking, killing of human persons is wrong. But what about this particular case? Whether killing is right or wrong in this case depends upon the nature of the case, the alternatives, and the probable consequences. Morality must be somewhat individualistic and situational. What is right in one case may not be right in another. Since there is no, objectively speaking, "right" answer to questions of morality, the moral freedom of the individual to decide for himself must be stressed.

As the individual begins his moral analysis, he tends to consult his own experience and perception. What would this action mean for me, in this situation? In an abortion situation, for example, the emphasis is placed on the reasons why an abortion is being considered. It is the best solution to this particular situation that is being sought. Whatever action is chosen is moral as long as it is truly selected as most conducive to the perceived good of those involved.

The modern ethical worldview, in summary:

1. The world is largely meaningless until given meaning by man.
2. The individual must *decide* for himself what is the right thing to do.
3. The focus in morality is on the purpose of the action.
4. The moral freedom and rights of the individual are stressed.
5. The starting point of moral analysis is the experience and perception of individuals.
6. Life is a possession.

The modern worldview involves the attitude that has been discussed as the quality of life ethic. The value of life depends on what it means to someone. Unqualified value cannot be placed upon anything, including human life; it all depends upon the situation.

The modern worldview provides the basis for support of mercy killing. Because it is man's role to exercise dominion over the world, he has a right to exercise control over life and death. Because the morality of an action depends primarily upon the reasons for which it is done, mercy killing is no more evil than withholding treatment in the care of a dying patient. Because individuals are not bound by moral rules, the maxim not to kill an innocent person does not mean that such killing is never justified. Because his moral analysis begins with his individual experience of the situation, he cannot abstract from the suffering and hopelessness of the individual case.

It is possible for both the classical worldview and the modern worldview to be associated with religious faith and with the moral absolute that man must always attempt to do the will of God. But the religious understandings are different. For the classicalist, the moral will of God is identical with his created will. The will of God for man is largely expressed in the natural ordering of creation. Man's obligation is to use his reasoning to come to know what is (what the purpose is) so that he can act out of respect for and in accordance with that created meaning. The modernist sees man's relationship to God and the world somewhat differently. God has created man to exercise dominion over creation. His moral obligation is to use the reason God has given him to fashion a world which is better for man. Creation does not impose moral obligations; it has been given by God as the material with which and the context within which to exercise responsible freedom.

It may be necessary to remind the reader that these two worldviews are artificial constructs. They constitute an attempt on the author's part to help explain some of the underlying differences in orientation that account for the different positions taken on specific issues. A typology of this sort should be used when helpful; no attempt should be made to force the views of individuals into an artificial mold. Most moralists and most citizens, I would suggest, tend toward one or the other of these sets of moral assumptions, though there are probably very few pure types.

Debates on life and death issues in recent years in America have often seen one side accusing the other of a fundamental contradiction. It has been fairly common for support for the American participation in the war in Vietnam to go hand in hand with opposition to abortion. Opponents have been quick to criticize: How can you claim that abortion destroys the sanctity of life while advocating killing in Vietnam? On the other hand, support for abortion has often been accompanied by opposition to the war. This combination has also been criticized as insupportable: How can you say that the war is wrong when you defend the killing of the helpless here at home?

The classical-modern discussion may serve to clarify these positions (without claiming that either is totally consistent). Both become quite understandable when placed in the larger context of how ethical decisions are made.

The anti-war, pro-abortion stand can be related to the modern worldview. The primary focus is not on the actual act of killing, whether the question be war or abortion. The Vietnam war is seen as wrong because it imposed suffering without corresponding benefits and because young men were forced to serve whether they wanted to or not. News coverage of the war made it possible to experience, in a removed but real way, the suffering of the Vietnamese and of the American soldiers. Opposition to the war was thus based upon such goals as the relieving of suffering and the defense of freedom. Support for abortion is often the result of the same motives and

goals. The woman's right to control her own body and the prevention of suffering can both be goals that inspire support for abortion. The fetus' suffering and death in abortion is something that is very hard to identify with, much harder than it is to identify with the suffering of a Vietnamese peasant thousands of miles away. The combination of an anti-war and pro-abortion stand does not strike one as so contradictory when seen as an expression of the modern worldview. If this stand is to be criticized, the criticism probably has to be directed toward the underlying worldview.

The pro-war, anti-abortion stand is sometimes taken by persons who represent the classical worldview. It is innocent human life that may never be directly taken. War can sometimes be justified, especially in defense against aggression. One's moral obligations include the pursuit of individual freedom and relief from suffering, but a more basic obligation is to protect innocent human life, both the lives of human fetuses and the lives of those being unjustly warred upon. Over the centuries, the sanctity of life tradition has recognized that war can sometimes be justified while abortion cannot; the contemporary pro-war, anti-abortion stand reflects this tradition. Some who approach these questions from a classical orientation have found themselves in opposition both to war and to abortion. To them this war was not one of those that could be justified; it is not clear that Americans were defending the innocent against the unjust. But the actual working out of the classical tradition has made it possible for many to support killing in war while opposing abortion. Criticism of the pro-war, anti-abortion stand should probably be directed primarily toward the sanctity of life tradition and its historical development.

The assumptions, attitudes, and values that

11

Implications of Prenatal Diagnosis for the Quality of, and Right to, Human Life: Society as a Standard

Robert S. Morison

My framework will be one of a rather crass pragmatist. I have no expertise, but I once had a fairly close association with public health. And since I was given the topic of talking about amniocentesis from the standpoint of the social standard, I have drawn a little bit on my past public health experience.

Actually, I want to ally myself with that ethical attitude which relies principally on a careful weighing of the probable practical consequences of a given choice of alternatives.

In doing this, I withdraw in horror from the tendency to reduce this utilitarian procedure to a cheap matter of dollars, cents, and simple linear equations. It clearly is a much more complicated matter than that and involves judgment of all kinds of values.

I am also relatively unimpressed with the camel's head argument. I don't think that looking at an ethical viewpoint from the standpoint of—"You do this and inevitably this terrible thing is going to happen later on"—is an acceptable way of going about it.

I have noticed that principles, whatever their logical base, are valid only over a certain limited range; when pushed toward their limit, they tend to conflict with one another or become absurd. Even Oliver Wendell Holmes could not extend the principle of free speech to those who falsely cried "fire" in a crowded theatre. Even the most concerned believers in the sanctity of life do not always equate the life of a four-day-old, yet-to-be-implanted egg with the life of a Mahatma Gandhi.

Again, modern ethical decision-making should be guided by moral policies rather than by principles. Policies are—and indeed usually should be—developed in relation to principles, but they need not be completely bound by them. Policies do not determine decisions

"Implications of Prenatal Diagnosis for the Quality of, and Right to, Human Life: Society as a Standard" by Robert S. Morison in Ethical Issues in Human Genetics, eds. Bruce Hilton, Daniel Callahan, Maureen Harris, Peter Condliffe, and Burton Berkley, 1973, pp. 201–211. Reprinted with permission of Plenum Publishing Corporation.

by themselves. There must always be a decision-maker in the background, or a group of decision-makers.

Fortunately, the decision-makers in the abortion case are already in the process of being identified for us, and we need not spend time on this problem. A steadily-increasing proportion of the developed world is deciding that the principal decision-maker should be the woman carrying the fetus—assisted, perhaps, by her physician. This primacy of the prospective mother cannot be based only or even primarily on the feminist assertion of the woman's right to do what she wants with her own body. As many people have pointed out here, the biological evidence is conclusively that a fetus is something quite different from a right hand or even an eye, which even the Bible urges us to extirpate or pluck out if they are offensive. I realize the Bible is equivocal on this point, and one can quote other passages against self-mutilation. The woman in the case, however much she would like to, cannot help participating as a trustee or guardian of the developing human being. The fact that the fetus is so primitive and so helpless, far from justifying a ruthlessly destructive attitude, should be added reason for compassionate concern.

It seems to me, therefore, that society, in its capacity as protector of the weak and moderator of differences between individuals, should not become indifferent to the welfare of the fetus or to the effect that the continuance or discontinuance of its life will have on the fabric of society as a whole.

The recent worldwide move towards liberalizing the abortion laws should not be construed as reflecting the belief that such laws have no constitutional standing. The change in attitude is so sweeping and so recent, especially in this country, that it is difficult to assess all the reasons that have influenced so many different people to change their minds—including me. But it appears that the majority finally concluded that the old rules were simply not working as acceptable policies.

One way of describing what we have done with our recent legislation is to say we have converted a matter of principle into a series of individual problems in situational ethics. This by no means implies, however, that society should relinquish all interest in the question. In place of the previous formal and legal restraints, it must find informal ways of impressing the decision-makers with the gravity of the situation in which they find themselves.

In reviewing the legislative history of the new arrangements, it appears that principal attention has centered on allowing the mother to base her decision on the effect of another child on her own health, on the welfare of the other children, and on the standard of living of the entire family unit. The particular qualities of the particular fetus to be destroyed were not at issue, in part because they seemed destined to remain unknown.

It may be worthwhile to pause and note that the presumptive unknownness of the individual characteristics of the fetus may have contributed to the lack of concern that some people have felt for the right of the fetus as an individual. As long as it remained in the darkness of the womb, it could be safely dismissed as in limbo, a subhuman entity, a thing rather than a person.

What amniocentesis may have done for us, among other things, is to make it clear that the fetus is an individual with definite, identifiable characteristics. In considering whether or not to abort a fetus because of certain such characteristics we don't happen to like, we recognize her or his individuality in a way we could avoid when we talked simply about the addition of any new member, or an essentially unknown "X," to the family circle.

However much considerations of personal identity will heighten our awareness of what we are doing and increase our sense of what I have called the gravity of the situation, I believe these considerations will not keep us from weighing the finding of amniocentesis in the balance when it comes to deciding on particular abortions.

I will, in fact, argue that society does have substantial interest in both the quantity and quality of the children to be born into its midst, and that it is already expressing this interest in numerous ways. These ways provide a precedent and at least partial justification for expressing an interest in the results of amniocentesis and in the way these findings are used in arriving at individual abortion decisions.

I should explain that I am using the word "society" in a flexible and—you may think—ambiguous way. Part of the time I am thinking of society as what the mathematicians refer to as a "set" or collection of individuals with needs, interests, and rights. More often I include with this notion the formal and informal organizations and institutions through which people express, satisfy, and protect their collective interests and rights.

Any suggestion that society may have some sort of stake in the proceedings may be greeted with the prediction that such ideas lead directly and immediately to the worst abuses of Nazi Germany. Let me say at once, then, that in trying to analyze the interest of society in unborn babies, I am not for a moment suggesting that legislation be passed forcing people to have abortions or to be surgically sterilized. If it turns out that society does have defensible

interests in the number and condition of the infants to be born, it can express these interests in ways that fall far short of totalitarian compulsion.

It can, for example, facilitate or ban abortion. It can develop or not develop genetic counseling and contraceptive services. It may offer bounties or impose taxes on parents for having or not having children. Purists may object to such procedures as invasions of personal liberty, as perhaps they are, but they are the kind of invasions which all societies find necessary for survival.

No modern society could long endure without making it as easy as possible for parents to send children to school. But expressions of interest in individual education do not stop there. Most societies require that children be sent to school for some years under penalty of the law. In most countries the courts have the right to protect children from physical abuse, to order ordinary medical care in opposition to the parent's wishes, and even to remove them entirely from a family environment that appears to be inadequate.

Such protection and fostering of infants and children by the state can be explained wholly in terms of an obligation to protect the child's right to life, liberty, and the pursuit of happiness. But in point of fact, this is not the only consideration. Society is also protecting its own safety and welfare by ensuring that there will be maximal numbers of people capable of protecting the goods and services and composing the songs necessary for a good society. Note that "composing songs." It is not purely a matter of dollars and cents. We want people who are able to contribute at every level. At the same time, society is minimizing the number likely to become public charges or public enemies.

Similarly, the provision of maternal and child clinics and the requiring of vaccination against disease can be explained in part as an expression of society's interest in controlling the spread of disease to third parties, and in part by the desire to ensure that each individual citizen be as healthy as possible. Part of this concern is altruistic, but public health officials can also argue that such preventive measures help society avoid the cost of caring for the incapacitated and handicapped later on.

These social concerns about individual health are not limited to persons already born. They extend back to the period of pregnancy and fetal life. Perhaps one of the earliest legal expressions of society's concern for the unborn infant was the dramatic requirement by the ancient Romans that Cesarean section be performed on all women who died while carrying a viable fetus. Less dramatic perhaps, but far more important quantitatively, are our present procedures for encouraging prospective mothers to eat the right foods, have their blood tested for syphilis and Rh antibodies, and even to give up smoking.

This concern for the unborn extends back into time before the new individual is even conceived. Mothers are urged to check their health and to undergo such procedures as vaccination against German measles before becoming pregnant. Vaccination of young women against German measles is now so fully accepted that we may overlook how sophisticated a procedure it really is. It is not proposed as a protection of the woman, herself, against what is usually a scarcely noticeable illness; its purpose is purely and simply that of protecting an unborn, unknown individual against a small but identifiable probability that it may be born with a congenital defect.

Perhaps the foregoing examples are sufficient to establish the following points:

(1) Society has an interest in the welfare of children and fetuses.
(2) This interest is recognized by the general public as legitimate, and various expressions of it have the sanction of tradition and current practice.
(3) In several important cases, the interest is thought to justify not only the use of educational persuasion, but even the force of law to control or shape the behavior of mothers and prospective mothers.

It is highly probable that different people have different reasons for supporting these policies, and of course there is a minority which has reasons for opposing them. Some will talk of the right of the infant to be born healthy as a part of a more general right to health, which some enthusiasts regard as having been established by the World Health Organization shortly after the close of World War II. Other more utilitarian types will simply point out that the results for both mother and child are usually "better"—and that the cost to society is less.

Still others will maintain that the Christian commandment to love everyone requires society to analyze all the angles in each particular case and that, by and large, love will be maximized if society takes an intelligent interest in the welfare of infants and fetuses.

The important thing to note is not the variety of reasons, but the general agreement on the conclusions. In a pluralistic society one must never lose sight of the fact that it is much more important that people agree on a policy rather than that they agree on the reasons for agreeing.

We must now move from this all too brief discussion of how society is currently expressing its interest in the yet-unborn, to how we can build on this experience to formulate policies to guide mothers and their counselors in adding the facts revealed by amniocentesis to all the other matters in their minds and hearts as they decide whether to continue or interrupt a pregnancy.

In the first place, I will assume that a prospective mother has a right to consider the specific characteristics of a specific fetus as she weighs the probable results of carrying a given pregnancy to term. If so, it follows that a society like ours has an obligation to provide, either through public or private means, facilities for amniocentesis in the same way as it customarily provides diagnostic facilities in other areas of medicine and public health.

So far, everything seems to be in accord with normal public health practice. But as we look a little further we encounter perplexities. The major difficulty is that the facts revealed by amniocentesis do not tell us what to do as clearly as many other laboratory tests do.

When a laboratory test reveals the presence of a streptococcus or a treponema, there is not much doubt in anyone's mind that the thing to do is to get rid of it.

When amniocentesis reveals an hereditary or a congenital defect, the situation is rather different. In the first place, the object to be got rid of is not a bacterium but an incipient human being. In the second place, it is not always immediately clear what the results will be if the defective fetus is allowed to go to term. Who is to say whether a child with Down's syndrome is more or less happy than the child with an IQ of 150 who spends the first 16 years of his life competing with his peers for admission to an Ivy League college? Who is to assess the complex effects on parents of coping with a handicapped child?

Most troublesome is the recognition that the interest of the individuals directly concerned may be more often at variance with those of society than is the case in most public health procedures. For example, most public health officials have little difficulty in urging or even requiring people to be vaccinated, since the risk is very small and the benefits appear to accrue more or less equally to society and to the individual concerned.

The interests of parents and the interests of society in the birth of children, however, may often be quite at odds with one another. In some rapidly growing societies, for example, the birth of additional children of any description may be looked upon with dismay by society as a whole, however much the new citizens may be welcomed by their parents. In societies where the over-all rate of growth is under better control, society may properly still have an interest in maximizing the proportion of new members who can at least take care of themselves, and if possible return some net benefit. Some parents, however, may long for any child to love and to cherish. They may regard any talk of social costs and benefits as shockingly utilitarian.

Even more difficult situations could arise when the prospective child may, himself, be quite normal, a joy to his parents, and a net asset to society—except for the fact that he is a heterozygous carrier of a serious defect who would, as a matter of fact, not have been started at all had the way not been made clear for him by aborting one or more homozygous siblings.

The more one thinks of these problems in abstract, philosophical terms, the more appalled he becomes. I am beginning to suspect, however, that the situation will turn out to be less serious in practice than it is in theory.

In the first place, it seems highly improbable that the wishes of parents and the interests of society will really be at odds in cases of severe defects like Down's syndrome or Tay-Sachs disease. In other words, if the parents' views are such that abortion is an acceptable option on general grounds, they are likely to exercise it for their own reasons in the kinds of cases in which carrying the fetus to term would also be most costly and least beneficial to society. In cases where the option is unacceptable to the individual for religious or similar reasons, society, under existing and generally agreed upon policies, has no business interfering anyway.

At the other end of the spectrum, relatively mild defects which may alter only slightly the subject's chances of becoming a useful citizen, like six fingers, may be safely left to the parents to decide without comment from outside since the social costs of either outcome are likely to be negligible. There may be a number of areas where the net cost to society may be appreciable but hard to quantify and where family attitudes may be quite variable. It would seem unwise to emphasize the possible conflicts between individuals and society in these gray areas until we know a lot more about them.

Particularly troublesome, of course, are those genetic conditions in which the homozygotes suffer a severe disorder while the heterozygotes show little or no deficit. There may come a day when the question of what to do about such heterozygous fetuses may indeed involve ethical problems between the long-run interest of society in its gene pool and the short-run interest of the individual in family life. At present, however, the technical difficulties of identifying heterozygotes in many conditions and especially of evaluating the possibly unusual "fitness" of the latter may excuse us from taking any firm position which might breathe life into a latent conflict between individuals and society.

To point out that the number of potential conflicts is probably not so large as some people have feared is not to say that there is no problem. But the realization may be of some comfort to prudent men as they start to formulate policies.

It is also true that the above analysis depends very largely on the assumption that the general public knows as much about the disorders in question as the representatives of society do and that decisions will be arrived at more or less autonomously. This, of course, is not the case, and we are thus brought to the heart of the problem that worries many moralists and men of good will.

In most instances the facts revealed by amniocentesis must be interpreted to the prospective parents. In advanced countries these interpretative services are likely to be at least partially supported by society. How are we— and perhaps equally important, how is the counselor—to be sure that he is providing the interpretation in the best interests of the patient? Alternatively, how far is he justified in presenting the interests of society, especially if these may appear from some angles to be in conflict with those of the parents? These are indeed difficult questions. But I am not persuaded that they are so difficult as some people think they are.

Some commentators appear to feel that society is making an unjustifiable invasion of personal liberties if it undertakes to persuade an individual to make any decision in the reproductive sphere other than that suggested by his uninstructed instincts. The criticism is particularly severe if the proposed learning experience is coupled with rewards and penalties. It is hard to understand this squeamishness, since societies have been rewarding people from time immemorial for doing things which benefited society and even more enthusiastically penalized its citizens for actions against the public interest.

Even without this background, it is hard to see how offering a man a transistor radio if he refrains from having a child is interfering with his personal freedom. Indeed, one would ordinarily suppose that by increasing the number of options open to him, we increase rather than restrict his freedom. Furthermore, transistor radios may be looked upon primarily as educational devices, a way of making real to a not very sophisticated mind that children impose costs on society—and that society can in turn use its resources to benefit existing individuals if they cooperate in reducing the potential competition.

Again, this increase in understanding should be considered liberating rather than confining.

If society has a definable and legitimate interest in the number of children to be born, then it is clear that it also may have an interest in their quality. This is especially true in a period of sharply reduced birth and death rates. In an earlier day when both were high, normal attrition worked differentially to eliminate the unfit. A much smaller proportion of society's resources was devoted to keeping the unfit alive. Now, when a defective child may cost the society many thousands of dollars a year for a whole lifetime without returning any benefit, it would appear inevitable that society should do what it reasonably can to assure that those children who are born can lead normal and reasonably independent lives. It goes without saying that if the model couple is to be restricted to 2.1 children, it is also more important to them that all their children be normal than it was when an abnormal child was, in effect, diluted by a large number of normal siblings. And the over-all point here again is

that the interests of society and the interests of the family become coincident at this stage, when they both realize that there are a limited number of slots to be filled.

That is really the situation that we are approaching in many countries. There is a limited number of slots that human beings can occupy, and there do seem to be both social and family reasons to see that those increasingly rare slots are occupied by people with the greatest possible potential for themselves and for others.

What then can society reasonably do to work with potential parents to insure as high quality a product as possible? It certainly can encourage and support the development of research in genetics and the physiology of fetal life. It can certainly support, in the same way, work on the technique of amniocentesis. It can make abortion available under appropriate auspices and regulations. Many societies are doing some or all of these things right now.

Our problem, if there is one, centers on what society can and should do in helping the individual mother to use the available information not only in her own best interests, but also in those of the society of which she is a part. And the whole assumption here is that we are not going to require any behavior. We seem to be working toward a position which gives to the mother's physician or genetic counselor the greatest possible influence. Sometimes the two functions may be discharged by the same individual. In either case, the relationship is a professional one, with the individuals giving the advice owing primary responsibility to their patient or client. I think all of us with medical training feel our first obligation in any such situation is to the patient before us.

Just what the amniocentesis counselor will say to a given client is likely to remain a professional matter, biased in favor of the client when her interests and those of society conflict. On the other hand, there seems no good reason to discourage the advisor from pointing out to the client what the interests of society are. Indeed, there seem to be several good reasons for encouraging him to do so.

In the first place it seems proper, even if it is not always precisely true, to assume that the client wishes to be a good citizen as well as a good parent. Thus, it is in some sense an insult to her intelligence and good will to withhold information about social repercussions on the grounds that such advice might curtail her Anglo-Saxon freedom to act ignorantly in her own selfish interest.

It may also be remembered that every professional man is an officer of society—although I realize not everybody agrees with this—as well as an individual counselor. True, most lawyers, clergymen and physicians like to think of themselves as owing a paramount obligation to their patients, clients, and parishioners. But the clergyman has at least a nominal interest in the deity, the lawyer in justice, and the physician in the health of the community.

Fortunately, in medicine at least, the welfare of the patient usually coincides reasonably closely with the welfare of society. But there are well-known cases of conflicts in which the physician is supposed to act in the best interest of society even at some cost to his patients, and sometimes he does.

Thus, the conscientious physician reports his cases of venereal infection and T.B. in order to protect society, even at the risk of embarrassment and inconvenience to his patient. In a similar vein he urges his epileptic patients and those with seriously defective vision not to drive automobiles. These and other examples provide ample precedent for injecting the interests of society into a counseling situation.

I hope it is obvious that when he does so, the counselor will wish to make clear exactly what he is doing and why. It would of course be totally inadmissible for a professional counselor of any kind to deceive his patient or client, in order to gain what he thinks of as a socially desirable end.

We have heard of cases where it may be necessary to deceive a patient for his own good (or what is thought to be his own good), but I don't think any of us would countenance deceiving a patient for society's good.

On the other hand, it would be almost equally reprehensible to conceal the long-term effects on the gene pool of substituting a heterozygous carrier for a homozygote of limited life expectancy, or to fail to mention social dislocations which might follow from a decision to use abortion as a method of sex determination.

In summary, the position I have described is a simple and straightforward one. Many people are likely to feel it is too simple. It is based on the fact that society has placed or is in the process of placing the burden of decision as to whether or not to have an abortion in the hands of the woman carrying the fetus.

It accepts the proposition that in arriving at that decision, she will be allowed to add to a number of already stated considerations, evidence on the probable characteristics of the child.

It does not accept the inference that society no longer has interest in the matter simply because it has released the formal decision-making power.

It suggests that the best way of expressing its

interest is through the counselor-physician, who in effect has a dual responsibility to the individual whom he serves and to the society of which he and she are parts.

Finally, it holds out the hope that instances in which the interests of the individual woman are clearly seen to conflict with the interests of society will be less numerous than might be feared.

In review, I find that I must add one point. Just as I believe there are no simple principles which take precedence over all others, I believe that everything one does affects everything else. We are now all so interdependent that there are no such things as purely private acts.

There is a danger that the present effort to make abortion a crime without a victim will obscure the seriousness of all such decisions.

We will all certainly be diminished as human beings, if not in great moral peril, if we allow ourselves to accept abortion for what are essentially trivial reasons. On the other hand we will, I fear, be in equal danger if we don't accept abortion as one means of ensuring that both the quantity and quality of the human race are kept within reasonable limits.

12

Prenatal Diagnosis
and Selective Abortion

Karen A. Lebacqz

The practice of prenatal diagnosis raises a number of serious ethical dilemmas. I shall focus here on one of these: the selective abortion of defective fetuses. Selective abortion is commonly recognized as the central ethical dilemma in prenatal diagnosis, and it receives new urgency in light of the recent decisions on abortion by the United States Supreme Court.

The questions being raised here are first, what justifications are offered for prenatal diagnosis and selective abortion; and second, what are the implications of the ethical reasoning embodied in these justifications? I shall argue that the current and projected widescale practice of prenatal diagnosis and selective abortion establishes precedents which both violate fundamental principles of justice and threaten the traditional life-preserving orientation of medicine.

I

It may be helpful first to set the entire discussion in the context of two important trends in our changing social ethos. Both these trends have achieved sharp articulation during the time of development of prenatal diagnosis, and both have influenced arguments made on behalf of prenatal diagnosis and selective abortion.

The first trend encompasses a general awareness of "women's rights" and specifically, a movement toward autonomy of women in the reproductive sphere. This trend received significant articulation in the Supreme Court decision in Griswold v. Connecticut (1966), in which a marital right to privacy in reproductive matters was declared to be protected as a constitutional right and its culmination can be

"Prenatal Diagnosis and Selective Abortion" by Karen A. Lebacqz. Reprinted with permission of Linacre Quarterly 40(May, 1973):109–127.

seen in the recent declaration by the Supreme Court that "this right of privacy . . . is broad enough to encompass a woman's decision whether or not to terminate her pregnancy."[1]

Current concern for the effects of rapid population growth and the scarcity of resources has contributed to a second trend which influences this discussion: a movement toward a "quality of life" ethic which, according to an editorial in *California Medicine,* places relative rather than absolute value on human life.[2] This "quality of life" ethic may be seen generally in the trend toward accepting abortion and specifically in arguments that it is better not to be born than to be born unwanted.

Thus prenatal diagnosis has arisen in a general climate of concern for "population growth, women's rights, the consequences of illegal abortions, the number of 'unwanted' children and the discriminatory aspects of current abortion laws."[3] It is within this general framework and its specific articulation in the recent decisions by the Supreme Court that the practice of prenatal diagnosis and selective abortion must be assessed.

Preliminary Observations

Before considering the morality of selective abortion, some preliminary observations are in order. Prenatal diagnosis itself is an information-gathering procedure. Clearly, the information generated can be used in a variety of ways, and not only as the basis for selective abortion. Indeed, practitioners stress the fact that most diagnoses reveal a normal fetus and hence serve to reassure anxious couples[4] and on occasion to prevent a scheduled abortion.[5] Moreover, a few disorders may be treated prenatally or postnatally on the basis of a prenatal diagnosis,[6] and it is hoped that more treatments will be available in the future.[7] Thus prenatal diagnosis is advocated not only to provide for selective abortions, but because it potentially brings these other benefits as well. Nonetheless, a cursory examination reveals the centrality of selective abortion in the practice of prenatal diagnosis, and hence justifies a focus on this one issue.

To begin with, the importance of the "reassurance" rationale can be tested by asking first, whether *any* woman could have an amniocentesis just to make sure that the fetus she carries is normal, and second, whether a woman could get amniocentesis if she had no intention of having an abortion in the event of abnormality. The answer to both these questions is "no." First, not all women are considered eligible for amniocentesis, but only those in "high risk" or "moderate risk" groups.[8] Second, even for those women in high risk groups, amniocentesis will not be performed unless abortion is at least an option,[9] and some practitioners would even say that the woman must be committed to an abortion before diagnosis will be performed.[10] The reason in both cases is simple: the risks associated with the diagnostic procedure are considered sufficiently great so as to preclude the diagnosis in the absence of genuine risk of defect and sufficient benefit —the benefit of reassurance alone does not outweigh the harms of the procedure.[11] No matter how important the reassuring function may be in actual practice, it does not constitute sufficient justification for widescale prenatal diagnosis.

Similarly, the argument that prenatal diagnosis "saves lives" by preventing abortions also depends on the acceptance of selective abortion: the interest here is not in saving the lives of *all* fetuses by preventing *all* abortions, but only in saving the lives of *normal* fetuses by preventing *them* from being aborted. Thus the entire line of reasoning depends on acceptance of the abortion of defective fetuses.

As for treatment, there are currently only a few disorders for which treatments are available and "at the present time, the emphasis is placed on diagnosis of disorders in which there is no treatment."[12] Moreover, even where treatment is available, most practitioners still allow the couple the choice of abortion, and indeed suggest that that is what most parents would prefer.[13] Hence the availability of treatment does not rule out abortion.

Developing Treatments

But even though treatment is not a major possibility now, surely prenatal diagnosis might be justified as a necessary means to gain basic information needed in order to stimulate the development of new treatments.[14] Attractive though this argument might at first seem, however, there are several problems here.

First, if parents would indeed choose abortion over "any but the most trivial treatment,"[15] it is not clear that the impetus to develop treatments will exist.

(But even if future fetuses might indeed benefit from information gained through present diagnoses, there remains a serious question: is it justifiable to subject a fetus to risk in an experiment which carries no hope of benefit to *that* fetus but only to future fetuses? The lack of clear legal and ethical guidelines regarding experimentation on the unborn must not obscure the fact that this is a critical question. Should the fetus be protected, for example, by laws that govern experimentation on minors?

The answer to this question is beyond the scope of this essay; but the question must be recognized.)

Second, whatever hope there may be for future treatments, such future possibilities do not in fact form sufficient justification for the performance of prenatal diagnosis in the eyes of some practitioners. Dancis states that any attempt previously to diagnose defects prior to birth would have met with the response "why bother?" because no intervention was possible.[16] It is "medical intervention of some sort" that justifies the use of prenatal diagnosis. And, as we have seen, intervention "of some sort" usually means abortion.

It is obvious, then, that whatever other benefits may be claimed for prenatal diagnosis, for the present and for the foreseeable future, its "justifying" or "real" purpose is to provide for selective abortion. Ethically, then, the crux of the matter is whether or not selective abortion of defective fetuses is justifiable.

II

Selective abortion is not, of course, a new issue. While it has rarely been a *central* issue in the "abortion debate," it has received at least sporadic attention following rubella epidemics and the thalidomide scare. A "eugenic abortion" clause has appeared in almost every proposed model code for abortion reform, and a number of states have included such a clause in revised abortion statutes within the last few years.[17] Hence, the issue itself is not new.

What is new in selective abortion following prenatal diagnosis is the certainty of the diagnosis. Previously, a decision for selective or "eugenic" abortion had to be based on statistical probability or "risk" figures; now, an "actual diagnosis" can be made.[18] Thus prenatal diagnosis is hailed as a great advance for "taking the gamble out" of pregnancy and genetic counseling.[19]

The advent of prenatal diagnosis therefore *focuses* the question of selective abortion in a new and dramatic way: for the first time, the problem of selective abortion arises not because of accident or mishap, but because of the deliberate intervention of medical technology. For the first time, selective abortion is not an occasional and regrettable act, but the planned outcome of deliberate programs of medical practice.

Nonetheless, most of the ethical issues raised by prenatal diagnosis and selective abortion are issues that have been implicit or explicit in the "abortion debate" over the past few years. Now this debate has raged so long and hard and covered so much territory that one is well advised to exercise caution when entering the fray. Moreover, the recent decisions by the Supreme Court suggest that the wisest course might be to assume that the legal resolution of the issue also resolves the moral dilemmas.

Arguments Examined

However, I suggest that previous debate and present legal framework notwithstanding, there may yet be a little room for clarification of the issues and moral decision-making with regard to selective abortion. Therefore, I shall examine the arguments offered as justification for selective abortion and place those arguments within a logical framework which will help to ascertain what is really at stake in this practice.

The matter is complicated at the outset by the fact that few practitioners present explicit arguments to justify selective abortion. Most advocates simply refer to the legality of abortion or its acceptance within a significant reference group—for example, "therapeutic abortion may be offered where it is legal,"[20] "most people would probably prefer abortion,"[21] "most obstetricians would regard abortion as acceptable,"[22] and so on. Indeed, some practitioners specifically exempt themselves from responsibility for making the ethical decision, on grounds that it is their job to lay the empirical foundations on which legal, ethical, and political decisions will be made by others.[23]

Nonetheless, alongside specific disclaimers and vague references to decision-making groups there emerges from the discussion a constellation of claims for selective abortion.

First, selective abortion is justified on grounds that it procures benefits for individual families: it protects them from the financial and emotional strains associated with bearing and rearing a child with a genetic disease[24] and it minimizes the risks involved in pregnancy. Special pleas are made on behalf of families with a previous history of devastating defect, who may be afraid to "take a chance" with another pregnancy unless they can have prenatal diagnosis.[25]

In addition, there is considerable emphasis on the rights of women and couples and especially on freedom of choice and autonomy in the reproductive sphere. Amniocentesis is seen as a technique which "opens doors"—that is, which expands the options available to women and their spouses, thus enabling them to exercise freedom of choice.[26] It is a cardinal rule in the practice of prenatal diagnosis that the "ultimate" decision for both diagnosis and abortion is to be made by the couple.[27] One practitioner has even suggested that parents have a *right* to healthy children.[28]

First Rationale

Thus the first rationale given for selective abortion is that of the benefits accruing to individual women and their families. As this rationale begins to shade over into questions of women's rights and reproductive freedom, it takes on the character of the first social trend enumerated above, assimilating the trend and contributing to it.

Alongside this concern for the pregnant woman and her family, there emerges another concern: an interest in the impact of genetic disease on society as a whole, and in the public health aspects of prenatal diagnosis. Justification for diagnosis and abortion is therefore also derived from benefits to society gained through wide-scale screening programs.

In the first place, geneticists contend that screening programs could have a eugenic effect in eliminating deleterious genes from the gene pool.[29] In the second place, practitioners argue that screening and abortion would significantly reduce financial burdens to the state, since fewer children would be born needing costly medical or institutional care. Elaborate cost-benefit economic analyses have been made for several disorders.[30] Concern for protection of society at large is thus the second reason given as justification for selective abortion.

Just as arguments regarding benefits to women "shaded over" into arguments about women's rights and procreative freedom, so here the arguments regarding benefits to society shade over into a larger concern, which may be encompassed by the phrase "quality of life." Prenatal diagnosis and selective abortion are justified because they function to preserve a *norm of genetic health* which is a part of the "quality of life."[31]

The concern for a standard of genetic health may be seen to operate, first, in the assumption that prenatal diagnosis and selective abortion function as "preventive medicine." This assumption has been made explicit on several occasions.[32] Moreover, it is implicit in the use of phrases such as "reduce the incidence of disease," "eliminate disease," or "prevent the birth of" rather than "abort." As "preventive medicine," prenatal diagnosis and selective abortion combine to preserve the norm of genetic health which is a part of the quality of life.

Second, concern for the norm of genetic health and the quality of life have been raised explicitly by several advocates. Quality of life questions are most often linked to questions of *quantity,* and it is here that the concern for genetic normalcy becomes most apparent. Prenatal diagnosis is seen as a means of quality control in a quantity-limited system. On the level of the individual family, the quantity-quality link is seen clearly in statements to the effect that with increasing pressure to limit family size, parents will not want to risk any departure from the normal in their offspring.[33] Indeed, under pressures of quantity, quality control becomes a right: "if the size of our families must be limited, surely we are entitled to children who are healthy rather than defective."[34]

Social Needs

The quality problem is seen not only on the individual level, however, but also as a response to societal needs. Thus one practitioner claims: "The world no longer needs all the individuals we are capable of bringing into it," and argues for selective abortion on these grounds.[35] Prenatal diagnosis becomes a tool to ensure that "both the quantity and quality of the human race are kept within reasonable limits."[36] Maintaining the norm of genetic health thus justifies prenatal diagnosis and selective abortion because maintenance of the norm is a necessary step in ensuring quality of life in a time of concern for population growth. The concern here is well summarized by one practitioner reflecting on the work of several pioneers in the field:

> Dr. Gerbie and his associates have helped us take still another step down the long road which we must follow if we are going to *improve the quality of human existence while searching for better methods of controlling population density.*[37]

Finally, the norm of genetic health may also be seen in the argument that the fetus has a right to be "well-born."[38] The argument here is that there is a fundamental right to be born "with normal body and mind" and that if this right is not to be fulfilled, then it is better not to be born at all.[39]

In sum, the importance of genetic health is taken as a *given,* which carries its own justification. It is only necessary to know that there is a choice between health and disease: the obvious choice on the part of all parties—family, society, and the individual concerned—will be for health.[40]

These, then, are the justifications for selective abortion: benefits to the woman and family and to society as a whole, both in terms of specific and measurable emotional and economic factors and in terms of the maintenance or restoration of the norm of genetic health.

III

We can now ask how these justifications fit into the context of the "abortion debate,"

what other assumptions are necessary to explicate them, and what it means to follow out their implications logically.

Several of the justifications offered for selective abortion following prenatal diagnosis are similar to specific arguments used to establish other categories of "indications for abortion."

The concern to protect the woman and family emotionally and financially is not a new concern in the abortion debate, nor is it unique to selective (or eugenic) abortion; rather, it is reminiscent of the "psychiatric" and "socio-economic" indications for abortion. Thus if these arguments are used to justify selective abortion, the justification becomes similar to that used for the psychiatric and socio-economic indications. And indeed, it appears to be the practice in some places to require a psychiatric examination and justify the abortion as "therapeutic" on these grounds.[41]

However, some advocates reject the "psychiatric indications" argument: one practitioner calls it "circuitous" and "ridiculous" to require psychiatric examination of the woman following diagnosis of defect in the fetus.[42] They want the presence of defect alone to be sufficient justification for abortion. This argument, therefore, parallels the traditional arguments for a separate category of "eugenic" abortion which has validity independently of other criteria.

The assertion that there should be an independent category of abortion for "eugenic" indications, in which the very presence of defect justifies abortion, is a logical outcome of reasoning on the basis of a norm of genetic health. Thus a psychiatrist commenting on prenatal diagnosis notes that "for some people, abortion of a defective fetus is less unsavory than abortion of a presumably normal fetus," and he explains this fact on the basis that it is "in line with our medical orientation that makes the extirpation of disease a noble act."[43]

If arguments for selective abortion appear at first glance to coincide with various arguments for "indications" for abortion, however, there is also evidence of affinities between arguments used for selective abortion and the so-called "abortion on demand" arguments.[44] Here, the basic claim is that the woman's freedom is an overriding value which dictates the availability of abortion "without reason" (that is, without public or legislative consensus on the reason proffered). Women may thus choose to have a child or not, to have a defective child or not, as they please.

Clearly, then, it is necessary to examine the arguments for selective abortion both within the general context of "abortion on demand" and within the more specific context of special claims made in the case of defect. It will also be necessary to suggest ways in which the recent Supreme Court decision impinges on the various arguments and sets the context for any future action.

IV

I shall begin by examining very briefly the question of "abortion on demand." (Before doing so, however, a brief note is necessary regarding the relation of abortion on demand to the more specialized arguments for abortion in selected categories. The history of the abortion controversy makes it obvious that it is possible to argue for selected categories of justifiable abortion without also condoning abortion on demand. I would argue that it is also *logically* possible to condone abortion on demand without necessarily condoning eugenic abortion. Logically, one can argue that a woman has the right to determine whether or not she is prepared to accept a pregnancy, but that having made that determination the particular status of the fetus should be irrelevant.)

The abortion on demand argument gives primacy to the freedom of choice of the woman. However, it must also deal with the fact that freedom of choice of one human being does not usually extend to the point of killing another human being; that is, there is a *presumption* that a human being has a right to life and that my freedom does not normally extend to the point where it deprives another of his right to life. Thus if the fetus is considered to be a human being, the woman would not normally have the right to kill that human being. To counter this difficulty, advocates of abortion on demand usually take either of two positions: First, they argue that the fetus is not a human being—or not "fully" human—and hence has no right to life. Second, they argue that although the fetus is human and hence has a right to life, there is something in the unique relationship of the woman and fetus that destroys the "normal" prohibition against killing.

Most advocates have taken the first approach: they assert that the fetus is not (fully) human. Arguments of this sort range from those that assert that the fetus is a mere "tissue" or part of the woman's body[45] to those that recognize the fetus as a "developing" or "potential" human being, but argue that full humanity is not present until a specified time.

Must Set Time

The difficulty with this view is that advocates must then determine a time at which the developing embryo/fetus/neonate is considered to be (fully) human—six weeks? three months? at viability? one year after birth? That is, they are caught in a line-drawing problem: *When* does the individual acquire full human status? The designation of a *time* of attainment of full humanity always presupposes the choice of *criteria* according to which humanity is determined—brain function? lung capacity? personality? speech?

Now these criteria for determining that one has reached full humanity always have to do with functional capacity and personal development. Hence it is always possible to ask whether there would be others besides fetuses who would, logically speaking, be subject to the determination that they are not "fully human" and hence not protectable under the law.

For example, geneticist Joshua Lederberg argues that the moment of conception should not be considered "as the start of human life"; rather, he suggests, "an operationally useful point of divergence of the developing organism would be at approximately the first year of life,"[46] on the basis of development of language and cognitive interaction with others. However, the establishment of this time point on these criteria would obviously allow for the destruction of the newborn child up to one year of age. Logically speaking, Lederberg's criteria would allow for infanticide. At this point, Lederberg draws back from accepting the logical conclusions of his standards and refuses to discuss infanticide, on grounds that our emotional involvement with infants is sufficient to establish "a pragmatically useful dividing line." He then implies that the "tastes" or emotional involvement of "the majority" determines one's status as a human being to be given full protection under the law: "To discuss the fetus during prenatal life as if he were a human

being is merely to reflect the emotional involvement of that observer, according to a set of tastes not now shared by the majority." One must ask, then, whether persons or groups who do not meet the standard of emotional involvement would be considered less than fully human and not protectable—for example, the convicted criminal or any outcast group.[47] Once again, Lederberg draws back from the logical conclusions of his own argument and suggests that the criterion of emotional involvement "should not be confused with any objective biological standard by which we can set up principles of social order."

Lederberg's search for an "objective biological standard" to get him out of the problems he encounters with his own criteria illustrates as well as anything the inherent difficulty in this basic line of approach: any biological point that is chosen will be chosen on the basis of other criteria, and these criteria are all too often the results of our very human weaknesses. (Do we choose "spontaneous lung function" as the determining criterion of humanness because we *really* think it is a decisive criterion, or rather because we would *like* to be able to destroy the fetus prior to viability?) Are we willing to accept the consequences of our choices—what about those who must exist with the help of an iron lung?

Human Standards

In short, there is no "objective biological standard," but only very real *human* standards. To be sure, some choices make more sense than others: Fletcher has suggested, for example, that in order to be consistent with our increasing orientation toward brain activity in defining the *end* of human life, we should also define the *beginning* of human life in terms of brain activity.[48] Certainly, consistency is a desirable trait in both logical thinking and human interaction; indeed, this suggestion makes considerable sense. However, since the presence of brain activity in the fetus has been measured as early as six weeks, considerably before amniocentesis can be performed, Fletcher's criterion would preclude prenatal diagnosis and selective abortion.

In view of the difficulties of drawing a line on the developmental continuum, several advocates of abortion on demand have preferred to take the second route: they argue for abortion on the basis of the special relationship between the woman and the fetus which is deemed to nullify the prohibition against killing. The most intriguing exposition of an argument along this line is that of Judith Jarvis Thomson.[49]

Thomson proposes that we accept, for the sake of argument, the claim that the fetus is human.[50] The question then is, under what circumstances may we justifiably kill a human being? Suppose, says Thomson, that you wake one morning strapped to a famous unconscious violinist who needs your kidneys to survive; "is it morally incumbent on you to accede to this situation? Does the right to life of the violinist require this heroic and self-sacrificing act on the part of another person? Thomson concludes that it does not: "nobody is morally *required* to make large sacrifices, of health, of all other interests and concerns, of all other duties and commitments, for nine years, or even for nine months, in order to keep another person alive." In essence, Thomson's argument rests upon the moral right of the woman to *remove herself* from the violinist—or from the fetus. While separating woman and fetus *in*

fact secures the death of the fetus, Thomson is not arguing that a woman has a right to secure the death of the fetus, but only to remove herself. Presumably, if prenatal adoption or an artificial womb were available, either of the options could be used to preserve the fetus while freeing the woman.

This argument is more than intriguing; it has a certain force in its logic. Nonetheless, I think it also admits of some difficulties. Thomson claims that the woman has a right to remove herself from the fetus; the fact that the fetus then dies is perhaps unfortunate, but not central to the moral issue. Perhaps a different scenario will help elucidate the issues.

If one grants, as Thomson does, that the fetus is human, then the issue is whether one human being may remove herself from another when that other is dependent upon her body functions for survival. Surely the closest parallel to pregnancy, then, is the case of siamese twins, in which separation would cause the death of one twin. The moral question then is: could an adult siamese twin choose to "remove" herself from her twin, knowing full well that the twin would die, but claiming that her freedom was the more important value? (The medical practice of involuntarily separating siamese twins at birth, with the resultant death of one, does not change the *moral* argument regarding the rights of adult siamese twins.) If anything, it could be argued that we should feel *more* sympathy toward the plight of the siamese twin than toward the pregnant woman —the twin's predicament is both involuntary and lifelong. Yet I wonder if we would be willing to accept the twin's argument; would we not be inclined to consider the "removal" of one adult twin with the resultant death of the other to be murder, or wrongful killing? It is not clear to me that we are ready to argue *logi-*

cally that one human being may "remove" himself from another when that removal causes the other's death.

Other Examples

Indeed, to bring the scenario a little "closer to home" for most of us, let us suppose that a man is responsible for the continued care of his elderly and dependent father, who will die if no one is in attendance at his bedside. Surely this man is morally free to leave his father's bedside if there is someone else to sit and watch over his father. But what if there is no one else? Is he then morally free to walk off, leaving his father to die? Or, suppose a young child needs medication every few hours to survive; is not that child's mother morally (and perhaps legally) culpable if she "removes" herself from the child and it dies?

In short, Thomson's distinction between removing oneself from another and securing the death of another becomes problematic when we consider a variety of cases. In cases where our nurturing function could be served by others, we are perhaps willing to argue that we have a right to remove ourselves provided that we have secured someone else to carry on the nurturing. But in cases where there is no one else to carry on that function—i.e., in pregnancy today, and in the case of siamese twins—I suggest that a view that really respects the full humanity of the other will not so readily allow us to argue that we may "remove ourselves," causing thereby the death of the other. (Hence, I suspect that Thomson has not really taken the human status of the fetus seriously, that she has not really overcome her own predisposition "that the fetus is not a person from the moment of conception.")

To accept Thomson's argument means to accept what it logically entails: the right of any human being to remove himself from one who is dependent on him, even if that removal results in the other's death—the elderly father, the child in need of medication, and the adult siamese twin. Once again, the argument allows for the destruction of other human beings. If we are not willing to accept these consequences, then we must reject the premises.

V

Thus far, I have dealt with the general question of abortion under the rubric "abortion on demand," locating two basic ways of approaching this issue and suggesting that there are problems in the extension of logic in either of these approaches. It has not been my intention to resolve the issue of whether or not the fetus is entitled to protection of its life, but only to illustrate the difficulties encountered in a position that denies protection to the fetus.

However, the question of selective abortion introduces a new element to the discussion. As Daniel Callahan suggests, with selective abortion we are dealing not with the problem of an unwanted *pregnancy,* but with the problem of an unwanted *child.*[51] A logical exercise will illustrate what is at stake: Suppose that an artificial womb were available. Then, if the purpose of abortion is to free the woman from an unwanted pregnancy, logically the fetus would be placed in the artificial womb. Would a defective fetus also be thus preserved, or would its genetic status somehow "make a difference" in how it is treated?

Since the purpose of selective abortion is not only to protect the woman but also to protect society and preserve the norm of genetic health, it seems logical to assume that simply moving the fetus from one location to another would not be sufficient to fulfill the purposes of selective abortion. To the extent that selective abortion is oriented toward maintenance of the norm of genetic health or the "quality of life," it requires the destruction of those who do not meet this norm.

Now this illustration of the artificial womb is, of course, a hypothetical situation at present. Nonetheless, there are indications in the current practice that demonstrate the centrality of destruction of defective fetuses in this practice.

Determining Sex

First, prenatal diagnosis is used to determine the sex of the fetus in cases at risk for sex-linked disorders such as hemophilia. In such cases, the male fetus which is aborted has a 50 percent chance of being normal. Thus half of the fetuses which are aborted in sex-linked cases will in fact be normal; this destruction of normal fetuses is allowed in order to ensure destruction of defective fetuses.

Now in the case of sex-linked disorders, one does not know whether a *particular* fetus is defective or normal; hence the abortion is done on the supposition that the fetus *might* be defective. A more complicated case, therefore, would be that of a diagnosis of twins which revealed one normal twin and one defective twin. In such a case, in order to "get rid of" the defective fetus, it would be necessary to destroy the normal fetus as well. Would this destruction of normal fetuses be allowed? To date, prenatal diagnosis has missed the presence of twins, but practitioners agree that par-

ents would be allowed the choice.[52] Thus even a known normal fetus could be aborted in order to abort an abnormal fetus.

Finally, since there is always a possibility of error in diagnosis, we can ask whether advocates prefer a false positive which would result in the abortion of a normal fetus, or a false negative which would result in the birth of an affected child. Practitioners disagree here. One states flatly that the loss of the "rare normal pregnancy" would be "an undefendable catastrophe."[53] Another, however, suggests that it is a "more critical" error if a negative diagnosis is given and the child is born defective than if a positive diagnosis results in abortion of a presumed defective fetus and the defect is not confirmed upon examination of the abortus.[54]

It seems clear that the practice of prenatal diagnosis establishes a distinction between the normal and the defective fetus, and allows for differential treatment of the fetus on this basis. As one concerned practitioner put it: "We are faced with problems of assigning values to individuals with given genetic characteristics and designing programs directed against them."[55]

Serious Problems

What are the implications of adopting this kind of reasoning—of treating fetuses differentially according to their genetic constitution? I suggest that there are a number of serious problems in establishing this kind of precedent, and I shall deal briefly with several of these, illustrating where appropriate with difficulties encountered already in the practice of prenatal diagnosis.[56]

The first problem is that of determining the *categories* of fetuses considered destructible. Where is the line to be drawn on the determination of what constitutes sufficient "quality of life" to enable the fetus to live?

This problem will be encountered in two forms. In the first form, it has to do with the severity of genetic defect. The normative use of prenatal diagnosis is for severe, untreatable disorders (e.g., Tay-Sachs, Down's syndrome). However, even present techniques will diagnose less severe disorders (e.g., XO), and with expanding technology such incidents may be anticipated more frequently. Will abortion be allowed for less severe genetic disorders, or for disorders where treatment is available?

Already this problem is being encountered in the practice of prenatal diagnosis, and advocates appear to be divided in their responses. While some would maintain that "if there is an effective intrauterine treatment, then, of course, it should be applied,"[57] probably most would agree that abortion in the case of a treatable disorder "remains a parental decision based on the informed counsel of their physician."[58]

Second, the determination of destructible fetuses may be extended from clear *genetic* categories to categories of *social desirability* or usefulness. As Kass says, "Once the principle, 'Defectives should not be born,' is established, grounds other than cytological and biochemical may very well be sought."[59] The beginnings of this trend may already be seen in the treatment of fetuses with XYY chromosomes, where the "prognosis" for the child is problematic primarily because of the possibility of socially undesirable behavior. If XYY fetuses are to be aborted, then what about fetuses of women living in undesirable circumstances—for example, women on welfare? Will "quality of life" come to be determined more on the basis of social usefulness than clear genetic disorder? One practitioner has already argued for prenatal diagnosis on grounds that "the world no longer needs all the individuals we are capable of bringing into it—especially those who are unable to compete and are an unhappy burden to others."[60] Surely such criteria as "ability to compete" extend the range of destructible fetuses far beyond the severely genetically handicapped.

Indeed, I would stress the fact that *all* categories chosen depend on some social criteria —even those that are most closely tied to genetic anomaly. For example, most practitioners consider Down's syndrome to be a "clear-cut" case calling for abortion.[61] Certainly the genetic component—a trisomy G— is clear enough; and this genetic component is related to certain clinical symptoms such as mental retardation. But to determine therefore that fetuses with trisomy G should be aborted is to make a *social* judgment about the place of retarded individuals in society. It is possible to judge disability or deviation from a norm medically, but to determine that this deviation constitutes a significant handicap is to make a social judgment.[62]

Drawing a Line

The first point, then, is that it is extremely difficult to "draw a line" with regard to the *categories* of fetuses which will be considered destructible, since all determination of such categories includes a social component and will be subject to the vagaries of social opinion. The phrase "quality of life" defines a continuum from the severely disabled through the socially undesirable to the "optimal" child. Where on this continuum will the line be drawn?

The second "line drawing" problem has to

do with the *time* continuum. As one practitioner asks: "Are we going to be faced with demands to do away with a child with 21-trisomy whose mother was only 34 years old during her pregnancy and therefore was denied the benefits of prenatal diagnosis?[63] Do not the same arguments that justify abortion of a five month old fetus also justify infanticide?

That this question is not just fanciful is borne out by a recently publicized case at Johns Hopkins Hospital in which a newborn child with Down's syndrome was reportedly starved to death because its parents refused surgery necessary to save its life.[64] It seemed clear that had the child been normal, the surgery would have been performed.

Indeed, some physicians now argue explicitly for a different standard of treatment for newborn children with Down's syndrome. One has said: "Parents of mongoloids have the legal (and I believe the moral) responsibility of determining if their child . . . should live or die," and he suggests that this decision may be seen as a "second chance" for abortion.[65]

Thus it seems that infanticide is simply the logical extension of prenatal diagnosis. Indeed, one practitioner comments: "Early abortion based on prenatal diagnosis can be viewed as the modern counterpart of infanticide based on congenital defect."[66] This, then, is the second serious problem implicit in the reasoning behind prenatal diagnosis and selective abortion.

These first two problems have been line-drawing problems—problems of determining the categories of destructible fetuses, and the time of destruction. The third problem is of a somewhat different nature. It involves the *locus of decision-making* and the possible conflict between "women's rights" on the one

hand and the "quality of life" on the other. I suggest that as increasing value is assigned to the "preventive" function of prenatal diagnosis and selective abortion, the concern to eliminate defectives and preserve the "quality of life" may logically be extended to deprive women and families of decision-making power.

Quality of Life

To be sure, at present advocates assume that the concept of "quality of life" embraces both the familial and the social aspects of prenatal diagnosis, and that there will be a concurrence of benefits to individuals and to society. They assume that if women are given freedom of choice, they will choose to abort defective fetuses and hence their choices will serve the best interests of society as well.

However, it is obvious that the interests of individual families and of society at large will not always coincide—even in the decision to abort the defective fetus. For example, it has been calculated that if all male fetuses at risk for hemophilia were aborted and "replaced" by female children, the result would be a dramatic increase in the number of female carriers of hemophilia—a 50 percent increase in the gene frequency in each generation.[67] Hence, decisions made to benefit individual families might have a dysgenic effect on society as a whole.

On the other hand, at times where it would be beneficial financially to society for a fetus to be aborted, the woman or family might prefer not to abort. Would the woman's freedom of choice be restricted here on grounds of benefiting society or preserving the genetic health? One concerned practitioner has raised the problem by suggesting that the uncertainties

> could result in an accentuation of the conflict in our society between personal choice and governmental control, which could possibly come in the form of selected programs of compulsory screening and mandatory abortion for some conditions that are deemed socially intolerable.[68]

Indeed, compulsory abortion has already been proposed.[69]

In a situation where the fetus has no inherent rights and genetic health becomes an overriding value, compulsory amniocentesis and abortion is a logical outcome, as one practitioner rightly anticipates:

> The decision to terminate the life of a fetus has traditionally been denied even to the couple at risk, but the more widespread legal acceptance of abortion, the growing awareness of the impending crisis inherent in the population explosion, and increased concern for the social cost of genetic disease lead me to think that attempts to legislate eugenic programs may not be so untimely or even so far in the future as many of us have expected. Individuals in a society which is willing to allow even normal fetuses to be aborted simply at the request of the parents are not likely to be very tolerant of a known abnormal fetus.[70]

To be sure, several practitioners have expressed their alarm and rejection of compulsory programs at the same time as they raise the question. But the point is that the movement toward compulsory abortion of defective fetuses is a logical outcome of elevating the norm of genetic health to override any rights of the fetus.

Further, once a principle has been established that the genetically unequal may be treated unequally in accordance with their genetic potential, other forms of unequal treatment will be encompassed by this principle. One of the first areas to be affected by the application of this principle will be that of procreation: the suggestion has already been made that reproduction be regulated in accordance with genetic inheritance—that "quality control" have a built-in "quality control" component.[71] A practitioner has even claimed that "most of the women screened should not have been pregnant in the first place. All women who would have genetically high-risk pregnancies should be offered sterilization or an effective method of contraception.[72] Thus the way is opened up for other kinds of restrictive programs as well.

Impact on Medicine

Finally, the acceptance of selective abortion and its principle of unequal treatment of unequals will have profound implications for the practice of medicine. On the one hand, if selective abortion is a woman's right, then the physician is *obligated* to provide for it.[73] As with "abortion on demand," the role of the physician is thus radically changed: "For the first time . . . doctors will be expected to do an operation simply because the patient asks that it be done."[74] The physician, then, becomes a technician performing according to the desires of others.

There is evidence already that this dilemma

is being encountered in the practice of prenatal diagnosis, and that many practitioners are reluctant to give up entirely their traditional decision-making function. Thus, for example, one suggests that amniocentesis should not be done in cases of LSD ingestion because the physician would be obligated to provide for an abortion if chromosome breaks are found;[75] here, the physician retains his power of making a medical judgment. Another practitioner has suggested that the use of prenatal diagnosis simply to determine the sex of the fetus constitutes an "abuse" of prenatal diagnosis and that information on the sex of the fetus should be withheld "unless it is crucial for management of the case."[76] Prenatal diagnosis, in this view, is not to be a tool for the "frivolous" uses of women; yet if abortion is a woman's right, then it must be performed no matter how "cold-blooded and contrived" it seems to the physician.

On the other hand, if selective abortion is justified not as a woman's right but as a means of maintaining the norm of genetic health and promoting "quality of life," the physician is in danger of becoming a technician for society. Theologian Helmut Thielicke declares that the doctor becomes an "engineer, a technician doing manipulations for a productive society."[77] Thus Friedmann suggests that "it is not difficult to imagine the emergence of pressures to set standards for desirability in genetically determined human characteristics" and we must ask whose standards they might be.[78]

Thus in the long run, this practice threatens the basic orientation of medicine: as geneticist Jerome Lejeune puts it, to "capitulate in the face of our ignorance and propose to eliminate those we cannot help" is to reverse the entire course of medicine. Not only do the principles established here have serious implications for human rights in society, but they also challenge the foundations of medical practice.

VI

Now clearly, many of these same problems have arisen in the general debate on abortion, and are not unique to selective abortion. In a sense, one could say that selective abortion gives a prismatic view of the implications of abortion in general—of the problems of extension of logic, the threats to human rights and to medical practice. Both abortion in general and selective abortion in particular involve the assignment of relative rather than absolute value to human life on the basis of some social criteria; hence both establish precedents which violate fundamental principles of justice as we have understood those principles in Western society.

Nonetheless, if the basic logic of selective abortion does not differ from that of abortion in general, it is focused and reinforced here in a way which makes its implications more striking and perhaps more threatening. As Kass suggests, precisely because the *quality* of the fetus is at stake in the decision for selective abortion, this decision undermines the fundamental moral equality of all human beings.[79]

Further, the practice of prenatal diagnosis adds something to this equation: the deliberate institution of medical programs designed to foster selective treatment of human life. Friedmann captures the truth well in his haunting statement that:

Prenatal genetic diagnosis seemed at first no different from most other new diagnostic methods. Now we see that we are faced with problems of assigning values to individuals and designing programs directed against them.[80]

For all these reasons, I submit that the current practice of prenatal diagnosis and selective abortion threatens basic human rights and I urge practitioners to reconsider the implementation of wide-scale programs of diagnosis and abortion. Prenatal diagnosis is indeed a very exciting new technology with many potentially beneficial uses in providing "therapy" for the afflicted fetus and help to anxious parents. These justifiable uses should not be overshadowed by allowing it to become strictly an exercise in selective abortion.

Violate Equality

Even more than abortion on demand, it seems to me, selective abortion embodies principles of unequal treatment which violate the fundamental moral and legal equality of all human beings. In the long run, this violation of fundamental rights of equal treatment is a more serious threat to the "quality of life" of all of us than the birth of numerous children with defects will ever be. I am heartened by the seriousness with which this matter has been taken in general both by parents and by physicians; nonetheless, it is a dangerous move to aid parents by eliminating their children. We must beware of the implications of moving to a "quality of life" ethic in which persons are judged according to their social utility and hence "some are more equal than others."

But perhaps it will be objected that in view of the recent Supreme Court decisions on abortion, physicians really have no choice: Does not the woman now have a right to an abortion, and if so, does the medical practitioner have any choice but to offer prenatal diagnosis and selective abortion?

Admittedly, the Supreme Court's decisions are ambiguous. The Court declares that the "right of privacy" established in the Constitution is "broad enough to encompass a woman's decision whether or not to terminate her pregnancy."[81] At the same time, however, the Court also maintains that "the abortion decision" is "inherently, and primarily, a medical decision," and at all points it appears to give the decision-making power to the physician: "The abortion decision and its effectuation must be left to the medical judgment of the pregnant woman's attending physician."[82] Thus it is not clear that physicians must comply with the demands of the woman; there appears to be room for "medical judgment" in all cases, and especially in cases involving late abortion. Minimally, physicians can choose to make a true "medical judgment" regarding the woman's "life and health" in each case, and not simply to allow the very presence of defect to be considered sufficient justification for abortion without further consideration of the "full setting of the case."[83]

Finally, it seems to me that all of us, physicians and lay persons alike, have a responsibility to women and families to provide the emotional and financial support needed to enable families to care for children born with defects; although I discourage wide-scale prenatal diagnosis and selective abortion because of the serious threats to basic freedoms involved in this practice, I do not think the matter is settled morally by rejecting abortion. The birth of a child with a defect can indeed be a shattering experience for a family; it is the responsibility of all of us to ensure that families are provided with adequate resources. Ironically, as I write this, federal funds for many supportive programs are being curtailed; this we must not allow to happen.

If indeed the strength of a people can be measured by their attitude toward the weak, the defenseless, and the outcast, then selective abortion points to the weaknesses in our society and in ourselves. It seems appropriate, therefore, to close with a word of warning offered by Ralph Potter:

> When a fetus is aborted no one asks for whom the bell tolls. No bell is tolled. But do not feel indifferent and secure. The fetus symbolizes you and me and our tenuous hold upon a future here at the mercy of our fellow men.[84]

Notes

1. *Roe v. Wade,* 41:4213 at 4225. [Reprinted as Chapter 68 of this volume; see p. 408.]
2. *California Medicine,* September 1970.
3. A. Milunsky, J. W. Littlefield, J. N. Kanfer, E. H. Kolodny, V. E. Smith, and L. Atkins, "Prenatal Genetic Diagnosis," in *New England Journal of Medicine* 283: 1370 and 283: 1498, 1970, at 1501.
4. Ibid., at 1503: "It should be emphasized that for the vast majority of women, these prenatal studies will serve as reassurance that their offspring will be chromosomally normal."
5. See, for example, M. Neil MacIntyre, "Prenatal Chromosome Analysis—A Lifesaving Procedure," *Southern Medical Journal* 64, Supplement 1: 85, 1971.
6. See William Cole, "The Right to Be Well-Born," *Today's Health,* January 1971.

7. Henry Nadler argues repeatedly for the possibility of future treatment; see "Antenatal Detection of Hereditary Disorders," *Pediatrics* 42: 912, 1968.
8. Considerable attention is given to delineating categories of women "at risk." See, for example, John W. Littlefield, "The Pregnancy at Risk for a Genetic Disorder," *New England Journal of Medicine* 282: 627, 1970.
9. MacIntyre expresses the common sentiment when he says: "If I am involved in a situation in which the parents decide that they will continue the pregnancy under any circumstances, I will be opposed to undertaking the amniocentesis." In Maureen Harris (ed.), *Early Diagnosis of Human Genetic Defects,* (Washington, D.C.: D.H.E.W.), 1970, p. 143.
10. For example, T. N. Evans declares: "She must first be committed to an indicated abortion before amniocentesis is justified." In Albert B. Gerbie, Henry L. Nadler, Melvin W. Gerbie, "Amniocentesis in Genetic Counseling," *American Journal of Obstetrics-Gynecology* 109: 765, 1971.
11. Thus MacIntyre declares: "In my judgment, it is wrong to subject a pregnant mother and her fetus to even the slight risk of amniocentesis if the information thus derived will have no effect upon the parents' decision." In Harris, *op. cit.,* p. 143.
12. Henry Nadler, "Human Genetics and Intra-Uterine Diagnosis," in Donald J. Stedman (ed.), *Current Issues in Mental Retardation and Human Development* (The President's Committee on Mental Retardation, 1971.)
13. See, for example, Milunsky *et al., op. cit.* at 1378 and 1502.
14. Nadler argues that "despite the moral, legal and ethical questions" involved in selective abortion, prenatal diagnosis is

warranted because it will enable modification of disorders in the future. Nadler, "Antenatal Detection of Hereditary Disorders."

15. A. G. Motulsky, G. R. Fraser, and J. Felsenstein, "Public Health and Long-Term Genetic Implications of Intrauterine Diagnosis and Selective Abortion," in Daniel Bergsma (ed.), *Symposium on Intrauterine Diagnosis* (The National Foundation—March of Dimes, Vol. VII, no. 5, April 1971.)

16. Joseph Dancis, "The Prenatal Detection of Hereditary Defects," *Hospital Practice* 4: 37, 1969.

17. I am indebted to Charles P. Kindregan's excellent discussion, "Eugenic Abortion," *Suffolk University Law Review* 6: 405, 1972.

18. Milunsky *et al., op. cit.,* at 1503. There are, of course, occasional errors in diagnosis: in every publicized instance thus far in which twins were delivered following prenatal diagnosis, the diagnosis failed to reveal this fact.

19. The medical literature is replete with phrases such as "take the gamble out," "reduce the risk," "not take a blind risk," etc.

20. Henry A. Thiede, "Amniocentesis: A New Approach to Some Old Problems in Obstetrics," *Surgery* 67: 383, 1970.

21. Milunsky *et al., op. cit.* at 1504.

22. J. H. Edwards, "Uses of Amniocentesis," *Lancet* 1: 608, 1970.

23. For example, Nadler says: "I do not want to argue the pros and cons of abortion. . . . We are trying to provide a way in which accurate diagnosis can be made in the case of those people with risk factors. Then, *if they wish to,* they can take advantage of that diagnosis." (Nadler, "Human Genetics and Intra-Uterine Diagnosis," emphasis mine.) While Nadler here gives the decision-making power to the individual couple involved, Milunsky *et al.* suggest that it rests with society: "The medical, moral, legal and economic issues, problems and implications that have been raised will require extensive study over time. . . . Moreover, the challenge of these new responsibilities must be shared with society." Milunsky *et al., op. cit.,* at 1503.

24. "The most obvious purpose of such procedures is to reduce or eliminate the occurrence of genetic diseases that impose a devastating emotional burden on the parents. . . ." Theodore Friedmann, "Prenatal Diagnosis of Genetic Disease," *Scientific American* 225: 34, 1971.

25. See, for example, C. O. Carter, "Practical Aspects of Early Diagnosis," in Harris, *op. cit.,* p. 19.

26. See, for example, MacIntyre, "Prenatal Chromosome Analysis—A Lifesaving Procedure.

27. A statement by Milunsky *et al.* is typical: "The decision for amniocentesis and subsequent intervention for an affected fetus will be made primarily by the family. . . ." Milunsky *et al., op. cit.,* at 1502.

28. John W. Littlefield, "Prenatal Diagnosis and Therapeutic Abortion," *New England Journal of Medicine* 280: 722, 1969.

29. The most extensive work on the question of *genetic* impact of prenatal diagnosis is the study by Motulsky *et al., op. cit.;* in describing this study, Friedmann concludes: "The directed elimination of genes by selective abortion after prenatal detection is certainly feasible. . . ." Friedmann, *op. cit.,* p. 40.

30. For example, the following calculation of comparative costs was made for Tay-Sachs disease: "The cost of the whole program—of screening the entire Jewish population of the area and monitoring the at-risk pregnancies—is put at some-

where between $100,000 and $200,000, less than the medical costs incurred in caring for just two Tay-Sachs children during their short lives." "Mass Screen for Tay-Sachs Carriers," *Medical World News,* May 14, 1971.

31. I am indebted to Leon Kass for his helpful analysis of "nature as a standard" in "Implications of Prenatal Diagnosis for the Human Right to Life," presented to the Fogarty International Center Symposium at Airlie House on October 12, 1971.

32. In the early stages of development of prenatal genetic diagnosis, J. H. Edwards declared that it had "opened up the possibility of a new field of preventive medicine." Edwards, "Antenatal Detection of Hereditary Disorders," *Lancet* I: 579, 1956.

33. Milunsky *et al., op. cit.,* at 1502. This view is shared by Robert Morison, who suggests that if the "model couple" is to be restricted to 2.1 children, it becomes more important to *them* that all their children be normal (draft essay: "Implications of Prenatal Diagnosis for the Quality of, and Right to, Human Life," presented to the Fogarty International Center Symposium at Airlie House, October 12, 1971).

34. Littlefield, "Prenatal Diagnosis."

35. *Ibid.*

36. Morison, *op. cit.*

37. Dr. T. N. Evans, responding in Gerbie, Nadler, and Gerbie, *op. cit.* (emphasis mine).

38. Cole, *op. cit.* The strongest argument of this sort is that of Normal John Berrill: "If a human right exists at all, it is the right to be born with a normal body and mind, with the prospect of developing further to fulfillment. If this is to be denied, then life and conscience are mockery and a chance should be made for an-

other throw of the ovarian dice." *The Person in the Womb,* p. 153.

39. This line of reasoning has been consistently rejected by the courts.

40. Thus, for example, Irving I. Gottesman and L. Erlenmeyer-Kimling claim: "We accepted as articles of faith that health was better than illness and that normal intelligence was better than mental retardation. Therefore, it is reasonable to maintain that a fetus should not be brought to term when it is known, by amniocentesis, to be a victim of Down's syndrome (mongolism), Tay-Sachs disease, or any of a host of detectable and catastrophic errors of nature." "A Foundation for Informed Eugenics," *Social Biology,* 24: 54, 1971.

41. Nadler, "Human Genetics and Intra-Uterine Diagnosis."

42. *Ibid.*

43. E. James Lieberman, "Psychosocial Aspects of Selective Abortion," in Bergsma, *op. cit.,* p. 20.

44. The term "abortion on demand" is problematic. While it focuses attention on the woman's claim to have an abortion, it also implies an obligation to comply with the demand in any and all circumstances, and appears to ignore the physician's right to "conscientious objection."

45. This view is not only medically inaccurate, it is antithetical to the practice of prenatal diagnosis; the separateness of the fetus from the woman enables practitioners to call the fetus the "patient." See Nadler, "Human Genetics and Intra-Uterine Diagnosis."

46. Joshua Lederberg, "A Geneticist Looks at Contraception and Abortion," *Annals of Internal Medicine* 67: 25, 1967.

47. While our present movement away from capital punishment may indicate a trend to preserve even the lives of those who are most hated in society, we do have a

history of treating persons who are "different" as less than human (for example, during the second World War, Japanese Americans were interned in concentration camps without due process of law).

48. Joseph Fletcher, "Ethical Aspects of Genetic Controls," *New England Journal of Medicine* 285: 776, 1971.

49. Judith Jarvis Thomson, "A Defense of Abortion," *Philosophy and Public Affairs* 1: 1, 1971. [Reprinted as Chapter 70 of this volume.]

50. She says: "I am inclined to agree . . . that the prospects for 'drawing a line' in the development of the fetus look dim. I am inclined to think also that we shall probably have to agree that the fetus has already become a human person well before birth."

51. Daniel Callahan, *Abortion: Law, Choice, & Morality* (New York: Macmillan, 1970).

52. In one case where a male fetus was detected and the pregnancy terminated, the practitioners comment that "to the surprise of all, non-identical twin male fetuses were delivered." C. J. Epstein, E. L. Schneider, F. A. Conte, and S. Friedman, "Prenatal Detection of Genetic Disorders," *American Journal of Human Genetics* 24: 214, 1972.

53. Michael Kaback in Harris, *op. cit.*, p. 85. The context for this statement is actually not that of assessing false positives versus false negatives, but of concern for possible complications in widescale use of amniocentesis. Thus it is not certain that Kaback would prefer a false negative to a false positive, although he is clearly concerned about the destruction of normal fetuses.

54. Fritz Fuchs, "Amniocentesis: Techniques and Complications," in Harris, *op. cit.*, p. 15.

55. Friedmann, *op. cit.*, p. 42.

56. There are several critical questions which I ignore here. For example, Leon Kass has suggested that a program to eliminate defective fetuses may have serious implications for our treatment of living persons with defects—undetected by diagnostic mechanisms, who are born with defects in spite of all our efforts (see Kass, *op. cit.*). This is indeed a serious problem, but will not be dealt with here.

Another serious problem which I ignore is that of experimentation on fetuses—particularly, experimentation with new genetic technologies such as cloning, in vitro fertilization, and such. Decisions made with regard to prenatal diagnosis will establish precedents for the treatment of fetal life in and outside the womb, before and after abortion.

57. Carter, *op. cit.*, p. 18.

58. Milunsky *et al.*, *op. cit.*, at 1378.

59. Kass, *op. cit.*, p. 13.

60. Littlefield, "Prenatal Diagnosis," p. 723.

61. Lubs says: ". . . we can approach the prenatal diagnosis of this syndrome with confidence. This is the simplest situation in the spectrum of probabilities with which we and the parents must work." Herbert A. Lubs, "Cytogenetic Problems in Antenatal Diagnosis," in Harris, *op. cit.*, p. 71.

62. The distinction between medical determination of disability and social determination of handicap is forcefully drawn by Beatrice Wright in *Physical Disability: A Psychological Approach* (New York: Harper, 1960).

63. Orlando J. Miller, "An Overview of Problems Arising from Prenatal Diagnosis," in Harris, *op. cit.*, p. 29.

64. This case has been widely publicized. See, for example, the report in *Technology Review*, January 1972.

65. Anthony Shaw, " 'Doctor, Do We Have

a Choice?' " *The New York Times Magazine*, January 30, 1972.

66. James V. Neel, "Ethical Issues Resulting from Prenatal Diagnosis," in Harris, *op. cit.*, p. 221.

67. Friedmann, *op. cit.*, p. 40.

68. Ibid., p. 42.

69. In "Human Heredity and Ethical Problems," Bentley Glass asks: "Should not the abortion of a seriously defective fetus be obligatory?" *Perspectives in Biology and Medicine*, 15: 252, 1972.

70. Orlando J. Miller, "An Overview of Problems Arising from Amniocentesis," in Harris, *op. cit.*, p. 28.

71. See William Vukowich, "The Dawning of the Brave New World: Legal, Ethical and Social Issues of Eugenics," 1971 *University of Illinois Law Forum* 189, for an elaborate system of quality regulation in accordance with genetic endowment. A more generalized statement is the following by Ingle: "I believe that since man must limit his numbers, efforts to control conception should be focused on those who for cultural, genetic, or medical reasons are unable to endow children with a reasonable chance to achieve health, happiness, self-sufficiency, and good citizenship." Dwight J. Ingle, "Ethics of Biomedical Interventions," *Perspectives in Biology and Medicine*, Spring 1970.

72. Dr. T. N. Evans, responding to Gerbie *et al.*, *op. cit.* Clearly, Evans's response is not the intent of the current practice of prenatal diagnosis, which can be seen as a means to enable couples at "high risk" to "take a chance" with a pregnancy. Nonetheless, Evans's statement is a logical possibility given acceptance of the basic principle that "some are more equal than others."

73. Nadler and Gerbie state: "The physician who detects a genetic disorder prenatally is committed to providing therapy—if the results indicate an abnormality and the parents wish termination of the pregnancy." Henry Nadler and Albert Gerbie, "Present State of Amniocentesis in Intrauterine Diagnosis of Genetic Defects," *Obstetrics-Gynecology* 38: 789, 1971. Of course, the physician does not have to *perform* the abortion.

74. "A Statement on Abortion by One Hundred Professors of Obstetrics," *American Journal of Obstetrics and Gynecology* 112: 992, 1972.

75. Valenti, in Harris, *op. cit.*, p. 179.

76. "An Abuse of Prenatal Diagnosis," letter to the editor, *JAMA* 221: 408, 1972.

77. Helmut Thielicke, "The Doctor as Judge of Who Shall Live and Who Shall Die," in Kenneth Vaux (ed.), *Who Shall Live?* (Philadelphia: Fortress Press, 1970).

78. Friedmann, *op. cit.*, p. 41.

79. Kass, *op. cit.*

80. Friedmann, *op. cit.*, p. 42.

81. *Roe v. Wade;* 41 *Law Week* 4225.

82. *Ibid.*, 4229.

83. Justice Douglas, concurring opinion in *Doe v. Bolton*, 41 *Law Week* 4244.

84. Ralph B. Potter, "The Abortion Debate," in Donald Cutler (ed.), *Updating Life and Death* (Boston: Beacon Press, 1968).

IMPERILED NEWBORNS

13

Terminating Treatment for Newborns: A Theological Perspective

John J. Paris, S.J.

In a recent issue of the *Hastings Center Report*,[1] Paul and Marilyn Bridge discuss the difficulties and frustrations they encountered with the physicians and hospital concerning a proposal to withhold treatment from their severely defective newborn son, Christopher. Born some three months prematurely, he had signs of viral encephalitis. His long-term outlook was quite dim: he had severe mental retardation, and would possibly suffer from uncontrollable convulsions, deafness, blindness, and quadraplegia. Brain damage was extensive, and was thought to extend to the cortex. While Christopher was not terminally ill nor in any immediate danger of dying, the pediatrician suggested that there would be situations in the future which perhaps ought not be treated, such as infection or the aspiration of food. The family rejected that option, and insisted on treatment until Christopher, on his 75th day of life, suffered cardiac arrest. After three days of ventilator support, the parents agreed to discontinue the "heroic" means supporting their son whom they now believed to be "terminally ill" and approaching brain death.

The purpose of their article was to plead for a better way to make decisions than what they had encountered. Their relations with the pediatrician became strained; they feared the legal implications of passive euthanasia for a newborn; they believed that generally parents were too ill-informed, too emotionally involved to make decisions in the best interest of the child. In their words: "We regard any decision making by concerned physicians and parents behind closed doors of the pediatric unit as a haphazard approach."[2] In so doing, they rejected the well-known proposal of Drs. Duff and Campbell of the Yale-New Haven Hospital that such decisions should be left to the families with only general guidance from the

"Terminating Treatment for Newborns: A Theological Perspective" by John J. Paris, S.J. Reprinted with permission of Law, Medicine and Health Care 10(June, 1982):120–124, & 144, a publication of the American Society of Law and Medicine.

attending physician.[3] Their rejection pinpoints one of the limitations of the Duff and Campbell proposal: it is normless. There are no guidelines, no principles for the physician's recommendations. They are simply ad hoc decisions and, as a result, they can be made quite poorly as easily as quite well.

As the famous Johns Hopkins case makes abundantly clear, parents or physicians may determine not to treat on such slender grounds as "a Down syndrome child with duodenal atresia would be a financial and emotional burden on the rest of the family."[4] That standard is, I believe, too low to be normative. We have to ask ourselves what principles apply to such decisions? What type of ethical decision making fits such cases? The first thing we must have is an adequate factual basis. We simply have to know the facts. Then we must examine the response of the family and, because every response, every decision is a value-laden one, we must try to discern what the values are. We must rank the operative values and then make the decision, looking to the past for guidance, and, more important, to the future for the implications of the decision. What would be the implications of using the standard of the Johns Hopkins case, of saying that whenever children are going to present financial and emotional burdens to the family, that their right to life is truncated? Do we want to make that a general norm or principle? I would say an emphatic "no."

The second question the Bridges raised is: how are we to decide or, rather, who is to make the decision? They wisely discerned that while some lawyers may favor and profit from turning these cases over to courts, the courts are ill-equipped to resolve such difficult issues. Should we doubt this proposition, a survey of some of the cases will put that doubt to rest. A good example is *Maine Medical Center v. Houle*,[5] which involved a profoundly defective newborn suffering from multiple maladies, whom the family and physician had decided not to treat. Some other physicians in that hospital objected, and the case was brought to court. Superior Court Judge David Roberts began his analysis this way: "Though recent decisions may have cast doubt upon the legal rights of an unborn child, at the moment of live birth there does exist a human being entitled to the fullest protection of the law." Then, in words which give a clue to his order, Judge Roberts states: "The most basic right enjoyed by every human being is the right to life itself." In his view, the issue before the court was not the prospective quality of the life to be preserved, but the medical feasibility of the proposed treatment compared with the almost certain risk of death should the treatment (surgical correction of the tracheal esophageal fistula) be withheld. With that premise, the judge then asked only whether there is a medical need, and whether there is a medically feasible response. If these two questions can be answered affirmatively, then, Judge Roberts argued, regardless of the quality of life, the surgery must be performed. The surgery was performed, but the child, nonetheless, died.

A similar ruling occurred in the case of Karen Ann McNulty who was born with congenital rubella.[6] She had cataracts on both eyes, suffered congenital heart failure, a coaxion of the aorta, and respiratory problems; additionally, she was retarded and apparently deaf. The family did not want the cardiac surgery, which, according to the physician, had a 50 to 60 percent mortality rate. The surgeon took the case to court and the judge followed the standards set by the Massachusetts Supreme Judicial Court in *Saikewicz*,[7] i.e., that quality of life was not to be a consideration for such decisions, and ruled: "If there is any life-saving treatment available, it must be undertaken regardless of the quality of life that will result."

Houle and *McNulty* illustrate a stance that is widespread in medicine and society: vitalism. This is premised on the theory that life is the ultimate value, and something that is to be preserved regardless of prognosis, regardless of cost, and regardless of social considerations. The Bridges argue that we should have a more broadly based locus for this decision making process. I think they are right because, as we see in Judge Roberts' opinion, courts do not provide that kind of objective, dispassionate analysis that those who would like to bring cases to courts would have us expect. There is a marvelously insightful example of this difficulty in a little-known case decided by the New York State Supreme Court, *Powell v. Columbia Presbyterian Hospital.*[8]

Mrs. Powell, a Jehovah's Witness who was suffering from massive bleeding following a Caesarian delivery, refused a blood transfusion. The physician, fearing she would bleed to death, took the issue to court. Judge Jacob Markowitz raised a theological issue which illustrates the personal basis of many judicial decisions. He stated:

> I was reminded of *The Fall* by Camus and I knew that no release, no legalistic absolution would absolve me or the court from responsibility if, speaking for the court, I answered "No" to the question "Am I my brother's keeper?" This woman wants to live. I cannot let her die.[9]

If you examine the court's opinion, you see some very interesting theology. As a Jehovah's Witness, Mrs. Powell firmly believed that if she were to "drink" blood, she would be separated everlastingly from the God Jehovah. Judge Jacob Markowitz believed that if he failed to be his brother's keeper he would be eternally damned. What would you do in that case? Judge Markowitz ordered the transfusion. And so, on that great Day of Judgment, he will enter through the pearly gates and be asked: "Were you your sister's keeper?" He'll answer, "Yes," and go to heaven. Mrs. Powell will be asked: "Did you drink blood?" She will answer, "Yes," and go to hell. Such a decision may make good sense for the judge, but does it make equally good sense for the patient? The decision in this case serves as a warning to those who think that courts can provide clear, dispassionate answers to complex moral dilemmas. It also illustrates the fact that courts are like loose cannon on a rolling ship: dangerous, unpredictable and difficult to restrain.

In their article, the Bridges propose a more broadly-based decision making mechanism, some sort of a committee which will consist not only of physicians and professionals, but also of a wide spectrum of people so that we could gain the wisdom of society. Where do we find that wisdom? Alexander Solzhenitzyn in *The Gulag Archipelago* tells us that at one point he had lost his moral compass; he was engaged in things that were wrong. He very discerningly said, "I forgot the lessons I learned from my grandmother as she stood there before the icon." That is, he had lost the religious sentiments which are a coalescence of much wisdom and much understanding of human nature and the human condition. Seymour Glick, in a marvelously insightful article in the *New England Journal of Medicine,* wrote that Western society, having abandoned its religious traditions and substituted the secular values of pragmatism and science, is now adrift in a morass of competing values. If there is any focus, it is on personal gratification and autonomy at the expense of societal interests and general humanitarian concerns.[10]

There is, I would propose, a need for some value structure in our lives, a need which each of us finds and each of us feels. If, as Glick proposes, we have really lost our religious traditions then something else will come to replace those traditions. This is an insight which Dostoyevsky had long ago when writing *The Grand Inquisitor.* He said: "Men and women do not want freedom because that involves responsibility." Responsibility involves living with ambiguity, anxiety, doubt, and guilt. Since we do not want that, we seek something or someone to take that burden from us. Today, with the demise of religious traditions, science and technology remove these burdens. When the difficult questions concerning the appropriate care of defective neonates arise, the easiest solution is simply to do everything technology allows: plug the kid in. That way, one is absolved from having to make difficult anguishing decisions.

Glick is correct when he states that what we need is a re-analysis and a reinvigoration of religious traditions. What in the Judaeo-Christian tradition would equip us for, and help us to resolve, some of the terribly difficult ethical dilemmas that confront parents, physicians, and society with the birth of a severely defective newborn? Before examining that specific question, let us examine some of the general theological themes of the Christian tradition that can provide the understanding and wisdom of what it means to be human. The tradition begins with the belief that God is the creator of life and its preserver, that life is a gift, and that life has value because God is its end and goal. In Gustav Mahler's Second Symphony it is stated: "We have come from God and to Him we must return." We also see that theme in the Gospel: "Unless the grain of wheat die, it shall not have life." Life is not only a gift and a task, it is also a journey. We are on a journey from God back to God, and death is a part of that journey. Death is not the victor, it is the transition state, not a final state. What within the Christian tradition is the significance of life? It is that life is destined for God. Its ultimate goal is the restoration of the fullness of the kingdom. Thus, it is eternal life and not life itself which is the ultimate. For the Christian who believes in the life, death, and resurrection of Jesus, death has been overcome. It is not the final victor, and all those who believe and accept that message likewise have overcome its defeat. They, in the words of John's Gospel "will be raised up on the last day."

Then comes the question, what is the chief role of human activity? It is simply love, the giving and receiving of love which is not a flaccid "niceness" but a love that proves itself in the concrete world of justice, gratitude, forbearance, and charity. If we think theologically about these kinds of questions, then whatever the decision we make, it has to fit into the context of that story: that life is a gift from God, that life is a journey from God back to God. For the believer, this story provides the meaning, the purpose, and the value of personhood, and it tells us the meaning, the purpose, and the value of life's journey. When decision making is separated from this story, it loses its perspective.

An example of that lost perspective can be seen in the famous Brother Fox case.[11] Brother Fox was a believing Christian, and a man who lived his life in the context of that story. At age 83 he went to the hospital for a hernia operation, suffered cardiac failure, was resuscitated, incurred massive anoxia, and ended in a chronic, vegetative condition. When, after two days of neurological examinations that condition was confirmed, his religious superior, Father Eichner, said: "I know the values of Brother Fox. They are that he is on this pilgrimage to God. There is no further benefit to him in this life. His journey has reached its fullness; let him go." But the hospital spokesman replied that the hospital's mission is to do everything possible to maintain life, and that it could never disconnect the respirator. The implication, of course, is that mere respirator-assisted breathing, mere biological continuation, is the ultimate value. While such a view may be in accord with the Hippocratic Oath, the Christian story simply will not support that theory.

It was belief in the Christian story which led Father Eichner to request the discontinuation of Brother Fox's treatment. But, in the secularized world in which the hospital is located, that story is considered pious but meaningless. The values that are honored are autonomy and technology. The result of that value system was the continued treatment of Brother Fox regardless of the costs or grim prognosis. While the legal battle raged on, Brother Fox's heart gave out, but not until he had incurred $87,000 in medical costs and $20,000 in legal fees. It is the elevation of technology to the ultimate value that has created the problems we see today and that has distanced us so far from the kind of wisdom every caring grandmother in this country would know how to apply to these questions.

How, then, does this wisdom apply to the infant Houle or to others in similar circumstances? First, if you believe the story, you know that there is one absolute God, and you understand the meaning of life and the meaning of death. But, with the demise of that story, with the lack of significance of that story in the lives that we live today, those beliefs are frequently lost. If you doubt that this is an age of nonbelief, ask yourself what is the response of all those believing Christians who enter hospitals when the death process begins. When was the last time you heard anyone say: "This patient had a wonderful life; he fought the good fight; he has finished the race. He kept the faith. Now it is time for him to go to his Maker." Rather, is not the call: "He is dying. Do something." The most glaring example of that reality is that today nobody dies in the hospital, they arrest! For the individual whose journey has indeed come to its conclusion, for example, the individual with end-stage liver disease whose heart stops, we do not say: "At last he is at peace." Instead, we shout: "Code Blue." That is the problem.

The problem comes from the idolatry of the modern age: life is not sacred, it is ultimate. Death is not a part of the human condition; it is a failure, a disaster, an absolute, unmitigated evil to be avoided at all costs. I am reminded of a scene in the film *Whose Life Is It Anyway?* where the attending physician, Dr. Emerson, is making rounds and comes upon a recently deceased body. Emerson asks the group of young residents, "Doesn't this make you sick?" One of the group replies, "No. I've seen lots of bodies." Emerson shouts, "Well, it should make you sick. It is evil, it's awful, it's disgusting, it's failure and we can never tolerate it as physicians."

Emerson's view is clear, but it is idolatrous; it is heresy for those who truly believe in the Christian perspective. Death in that context is not an absolute, unmitigated, total, awful evil. It is simply a part of the human condition, a part of the process of what it means to be human, a part of the journey which is the totality of life. For the believer, life is good, but it is not the ultimate good; as such, the duty to preserve it is a limited one. Normally we are obliged only to use so-called ordinary means for its preservation. Ordinary means are those which are not disproportionately costly, burdensome or painful, and—this is the important part—they must also offer substantial hope of benefit to the patient as a person, not simply to his liver, lungs, or heart. What we are to be valued for is our personhood, and if the treatment cannot offer substantial benefit to the person, not just to his or her chemistries, it is extraordinary and need not be applied.

To make these decisions, we must consider the quality of life of our patients. The Massachusetts Supreme Judicial Court, for all its wisdom, is simply wrong when it claims we ought not consider quality of life in making these decisions.[12] Since we cannot avoid that issue, the question becomes: what do we mean by quality? Richard McCormick has suggested that quality of life means to be able to live this life of loving and being loved. If one's potential for that is ended or is so burdened with the mere struggle for survival, then, he argues, it has reached its fullness.[13] When no further benefit can accrue to the person, we have the norm and the guideline for the decision to say: "This is the will of God and I accept." In his article, Father McCormick is reflecting upon the theological analysis found in Teilhard de Chardin's *The Divine Milieu*. Teilhard asserts that there is a real danger in the Christian dispensation of saying at the first sign of difficulty, "This is the will of God" and then giving up. Teilhard suggests that is not the way for a Christian to proceed. God has entrusted to us the responsibility for caring for ourselves, and that responsibility means work, that means effort, that means human action, that means human activity. But is human activity always called for? "No," says Teilhard. "We must discern what is going on." Our task in the face of the forces of diminishment is to struggle with all of our energy, talents, and might to reverse it. If having exhausted those, we still find that the forces of diminishment overcome us, then we can say, "This is the will of God." We can now concede and accept that this is no longer a reversible phenomenon; that it is not defeat, but part of the Divine plan. Teilhard maintains that if one believes this story then one will realize that there comes a time in the life of everyone—the 80 year old with metastatic cancer who has dwindled to the point of death, or the one-day old infant whose potential for future relationships, for loving, and for being loved does not exist or is submerged in the mere struggle to survive—when the journey has reached its end.

This is not to say that those lives have no value; those lives are valued precisely because they are an act of divine love. It is to say that the Author of that act has decreed that the value is to be of this duration, a decision which is not ours but His to make. The guidelines that the Bridges seek, that McCormick would suggest, and with which I agree, involve the potential to benefit from the treatment so as to arrive at a capacity to enter into human relationships. If that potential is exhausted, if that potential is nonexistent—as is true, for instance, in the 5,000 patients we find today in chronic, vegetative conditions—then the best treatment is no treatment. In fact, to treat is to do a disservice to the humanity of the individuals involved. This is not such a surprising standard. In fact, this standard has been suggested in a staff report of the President's Commission for the Study of Ethical Problems in Medicine and Biomedical and Behavioral Research. The report argued that the appropriate care for patients in persistent vegetative states was non-treatment, and that it would be difficult to justify resuscitation of such patients.[14]

There are, of course, those who argue that such non-treatment is euthanasia and a threat to mankind. Yet, I think that the greatest impetus toward active euthanasia in this country is going to come from reaction to the right-to-lifers who insist that life is ultimate and that everything possible must be done to sustain it. They are responsible for creating disastrous coma ward situations in this country which will soon become so abhorrent that there will be a public outcry to stop that madness by actively terminating the lives of such victims of our technology. Likewise, there are some forces that oppose brain-death statutes. The President's Commission last summer proposed a uniform brain-death statute and some of the more radical right-to-lifers opposed it on the grounds that we can never be certain one is dead until there is disintegration of tissues and cells, *i.e.*, until the body putrifies. That argument, I propose, stinks!

The Karen Ann Quinlan case[15] is a prime example of the vitalist mind set and its effect on the treatment of patients in chronic, vegetative conditions. It is a case that is badly misunderstood, and I recommend Joseph Quinlan's book, *Karen Ann,* to all those really interested in what happened.[16] After the Supreme Court of New Jersey authorized the removal of Karen's respirator, the family went to the treating physician and in essence said: "Following the guidelines of the court, and exercising the right of a guardian, we request that the respirator be removed." Dr. Morse refused, stating that he would follow only standard medical protocol, *i.e.*, do everything to preserve life. So, for the next few weeks, Dr. Morse tried to wean Karen off the respirator, and replaced it whenever it seemed that Karen would not make it on her own. When the family asked how long he intended to continue this process, he responded, "For as long as it takes. Forever."[17] Similarly, the family then met with the physicians and the administrators of St. Clare's Hospital, a Catholic hospital in Morristown, New Jersey, to ask to have the respirator removed. The nun who was in charge refused and said: "Speaking on behalf of the Board of Trustees . . . we feel it is morally incorrect." When the family suggested that the local bishop had stated that it was legitimate to remove the respirator, the nun responded, "In this hospital we don't kill people."[18] Finally, six weeks after the Supreme Court ruled on the case (and it could have been six months or six years), Karen Ann Quinlan was weaned from the respirator. Today, six years later, she continues to exist in a calcified, fetal position, as unconscious and unresponsive as ever. [Editor's Note: Karen Ann Quinlan died in June, 1985.]

The ideas that I have expressed are consistent with the Vatican's 1980 *Declaration on Euthanasia.* After reading this statement, it is clear that the Catholic Church has been the great champion of the sacredness of life. The *Declaration* is the Church's official pronouncement that today we have to protect life against the dangers of technological abuse which threaten its sanctity and its Christian understanding. The text concludes that it is appropriate, when there is no hope of benefit to the patient, to withdraw or to withhold treatment. It is interesting to note that the *Declaration* argues that there is more moral warrant for withdrawing a treatment after it has been shown to be non-effective than there is for never having started it. Stated another way, there is more moral justification for stopping a respirator than there is for never having started it. The *Declaration* states:

> It is also permitted, with the patient's consent, to interrupt these means, where results fall short of expectations. But for such a decision to be made, account will have to be taken of the reasonable wishes of the patient's family, as also of the advice of the doctors who are specially competent in the matter.[19]

It is also important to consider what the *Declaration* says about the role and responsibility of the physician: "The latter may in particular judge that the investment in instruments and personnel is disproportionate to the results foreseen. . . ."[20] That is, patients or families may have unreasonable expectations as to what medicine can do, unreasonable in great part because of the idea that physicians are miracle workers who always take high risks and always win. The Vatican's position is that the doctor must exercise prudent professional judgment. It states that the physicians may also judge that the technique imposes on the patient strain or suffering which is out of proportion to the benefit to be gained. One cannot impose an obligation to have recourse to a technique which is already in use but which carries a risk of burdensomeness. Such refusal is not on the patient's part the equivalent of suicide and is not on the physician's part the equivalent of euthanasia. "On the contrary," says the *Declaration*, "it should be considered

as an acceptance of the human condition, or a wish to avoid the application of a medical procedure disproportionate to the results that can be expected, or a desire not to impose excessive expense on the family, or the community." It concludes:

> When inevitable death is imminent in spite of the means used, it is permitted in conscience to take the decision to refuse forms of treatment that would only secure a precarious and burdensome prolongation of life, so long as the normal care due to the sick person in similar cases is not interrupted. In such circumstances the doctor has no reason to reproach himself with failing to help the person in danger.[21]

A failure to exercise such judgment is evidenced by the case of a 27 year old woman who fell off a horse, was decerebrate, quadriplegic, and maintained in the community hospital for some 18 years.[22] The physicians who wrote the report, prescinded from the economics of the case, were proud of the wonderful care the woman received for 18 years, proud of their compassion for the parents who did not want their daughter to die, proud of their fidelity to the principle that where there's life there's hope. They noted that the cost of such care would be astronomical, almost beyond belief. Well, if one calculates at a very low rate of $300 a day, and builds in an inflation factor of 12 percent, 18 years of such care comes to $6,104,590. The Vatican reaffirms the duty of physicians to take such considerations into account. Dr. Samuel Sherman, the chairman of the Judicial Council of the American Medical Association, commented on that case: "The numerous physicians in attendance had no choice but to abide by the parents' decision to maintain life regardless of cost and pessimistic outlook for reversal of coma."[23] If that were true, the physician would be reduced to a mere extension of the family's whim, and I for one would not approve of such a view of the professional judgment of physicians.

In this regard, I am reminded of a speech that I gave to the Maine Medical Society in Portland, Maine. The day before, there had been a blizzard. I asked the physicians, if during that blizzard, one of them had asked the cab driver to take him to Bangor, what would the cab driver say? He'd say, "You're crazy, of course I'm not going to do that. It's madness." I propose physicians ought to rise to that degree of professional judgment exercised by the cab driver.

In all of this, there are certain dangers: the danger of what Dr. Franz Ingelfinger labels "arrogance" on the part of physicians who usurp all of the decision making and the danger of using guidelines as definitive rules which preempt decision making. We must realize that we deal mainly with gray areas in these cases. Some things, however, are very clear. The anacephaleptic child obviously need not be treated; the otherwise healthy child with some degree of mental retardation has a right to continued life. Other decisions are not so obvious. With those decisions we know that mistakes will be made, and there is no avoiding that. That is what it is to be human. Mistakes will be made; risks must be taken. In doing so we should always proceed with humility, with caution, with tentativeness, with a tilt to the side of life; with the understanding there is no such thing as a life without value, that all life is valued as a gift of God and is precious in His eyes and, hence, sacred for us; that whatever decision we make should be in the best interest of the child and not based on functional util-

ity. There is the everpresent danger that we will value people not as gifts of God, but for what they can do for us. And I believe that as a final theological insight we must always realize that the pride of the Judaeo-Christian tradition has been a concern for the neighbor in need—for the weak, the defenseless, the powerless, the unwanted, the defective, the newborn.

Notes

1. Bridge, P., Bridge, M., *The Brief Life and Death of Christopher Bridge,* HASTINGS CENTER REPORT 11(6): 17–19 (December 1981).
2. *Id.* at 19.
3. Duff, R.S., Campbell, A.G.M., *Moral and Ethical Dilemmas in the Special Care Nursery,* NEW ENGLAND JOURNAL OF MEDICINE 289(17): 890–94 (October 25, 1973).
4. For a discussion of the Johns Hopkins case, *see* Gustafson, *Mongolism, Parental Desires, and the Right to Life,* PERSPECTIVES IN BIOLOGY & MEDICINE 16(4): 524, 529–33 (1973).
5. Maine Medical Center v. Houle, No. 74-145 (Superior Ct., Cumberland Cty., Me.) (February 14, 1974).
6. In re McNulty, No. 1960 (Probate Ct., Essex Cty., Mass.) (February 15, 1978).
7. Superintendent of Belchertown State School v. Saikewicz, 370 N.E. 2d 417 (Mass. 1978) [hereinafter cited as *Saikewicz*].
8. Powell v. Columbia Presbyterian Hosp., 267 N.Y.S.2d 450 (Sup. Ct. Spec. Term 1965).
9. *Id.* at 452.
10. Glick, S., *Humanistic Medicine in the Modern Age,* NEW ENGLAND JOURNAL OF

MEDICINE 304(17): 1036–38 (April 23, 1981).

11. Eichner v. Dillon, 426 N.Y.S.2d 517 (App. Div. 1980), *affirmed and modified sub nom.* In re Storar, 438 N.Y.S.2d 266 (N.Y. 1981).

12. *Saikewicz, supra* note 7, at 432.

13. McCormick, R., *To Save or Let Die,* JOURNAL OF THE AMERICAN MEDICAL ASSOCIATION 229(2): 172–76 (July 8, 1974).

14. Staff Draft: Deciding to Forego Life-Sustaining Therapy (prepared for June 10–11, 1982, meeting of President's Commission for the Study of Ethical Problems in Medicine and Biomedical Research, in Washington, D.C.).

15. In re Quinlan, 355 A.2d 647 (N.J. 1976).

16. J. Quinlan, J. Quinlan, P. Battelle. KAREN ANN: THE QUINLANS TELL THEIR STORY (Doubleday, Garden City, N.Y.) (1977) at 279–94.

17. *Id.* at 287.

18. *Id.* at 291–92.

19. SACRED CONGREGATION FOR THE DOCTRINE OF THE FAITH, DECLARATION ON EUTHANASIA (May 5, 1980).

20. *Id.*

21. *Id.*

22. Field, R.E., Romanus, R.J., *A Decerebrate Patient: Eighteen Years of Care,* ILLINOIS JOURNAL OF MEDICINE (February 1977) *reprinted in* CONNECTICUT MEDICINE 45(11): 717–20 (November 1981).

23. Sherman, S.R., *Commentary on a Decerebrate Patient,* CONNECTICUT MEDICINE 45(11): 721 (November 1981).

14

Quality of Life and Defective Newborn Children: An Ethical Analysis

Warren T. Reich

The Ethical Problem: Quality of Life in the Newborn Situation

Introduction

A crucial question in contemporary bioethics is whether some human lives ought to be sustained in an impaired or handicapped condition. This question has frequently arisen in discussions concerning genetically defective fetal life and the terminal patient. Now, increasingly, the question is being asked: What does the situation of the physically and/or mentally defective newborn child require when medical treatment can sustain the patient's life and improve his health, but without appreciably altering the basic defect?

"Quality of life" is seen as a relevant or even determining factor in making decisions concerning the continuation and support of human life. Ultimately, the quality of life question has relevance because one wants to know what actions should be considered ethically permissible and which impermissible, and whether quality of life has a bearing on this normative judgment.

It seems that three normative judgments are possible with regard to the newborn child: (1) to (continue to) treat with maximal available treatment regardless of the consequences; (2) to actively, directly, and intentionally terminate the life of the defective newborn child; and (3) to omit some or all treatment because of justifying circumstances.

"Quality of Life and Defective Newborn Children: An Ethical Analysis" by Warren T. Reich in Decision Making and the Defective Newborn: Proceedings of a Conference on Spina Bifida and Ethics, *ed. Chester A. Swinyard, 1978, pp. 489–511. Reprinted with permission of Charles C. Thomas, Publisher, Springfield, Illinois.*

The author's purpose is to (1) present a normative framework for analyzing the quality-of-life aspects of decision making in the newborn situation; (2) analyze briefly the views of two physicians and two theologians; and (3) explain the claims and justification of the classic "ordinary/extraordinary means" ethic and how it might apply to the newborn situation.

Quality of Life: Normative Implications

The term "quality of life" appears with increasing frequency in the literature dealing with defective newborn children.[1] When the term is used descriptively, for example, in depicting the medical and social fate of the spina bifida child, one receives an impression about the suffering which is usually associated with negative qualities and the satisfaction that can be experienced with the maintenance of good qualities in the child. But medical ethics is not concerned so much with a *descriptive* account of the qualities of human living as it is with such questions as these. (1.) Which qualities of human life are valued, or should be valued? (2.) How does one know that a quality is or should be a value? From some philosophical consideration, or from a religious basis, or perhaps from some combination of both? (3.) How is a valued quality of life used in a normative statement indicating what sort of action is permissible or impermissible? (4.) How is the normative criterion (which is based on a valued quality) applied to an actual situation, particularly when values are in conflict?[2-4]

Two considerations complicate the issue. First, the selection of valued human qualities is a complex task because there are innumerable human qualities: general and universal: particular and measurable: interpersonal: and more abstract and generally immeasurable qualities. Isolating fundamental qualities of humanness (or of "humanhood" or of "personhood") from contingent and variable qualities which contribute to an individual's well-being has become a crucial matter in the determination of the level of treatment to be employed. Second, one's normative ethical system largely influences the choice of criteria for quality of life judgments. One system would judge the normative value of life from the consequences of various courses of action ("consequentialist" ethics), while the other takes as its starting point the inherent and inalienable rights of individuals ("deontological" ethics).[5-7]

For the *consequentialist* method (which is frequently identified with its well-known form of utilitarianism), moral claims concerning value of life are based on predictable qualitative consequences for the individual or for others whose interests are involved in the case. Personalistic utilitarianism justifies actions by the anticipated benefits to the individual; social utilitarianism builds on the maxim "the greatest good for the greatest number" and tends to judge what is good by a calculus of the impact which quantified, predicted consequences or "payoffs" have on a variety of concerned persons and on society.

The principal objections against utilitarianism arise from concerns about justice, viz., that the utilitarian method: (1) can easily lead to withholding protection from those who are weak or "useless" or who create a serious inconvenience for others, while assuring greater safety for the powerful; (2) tends to be dominated by a single value, a somewhat vague goal such as happiness, which is then taken to justify a variety of actions; (3) employs "slippery criteria" in its attempt to quantify nonquantifiable values (such as "happiness" or "meaningful existence"); and (4) is especially vulnerable to making arbitrary decisions on relative grounds, for in establishing the value of life it must determine—necessarily, somewhat arbitrarily—which consequences are relevant to the decision, how predictable and proximate the benefits and harms must be in order to be relevant, and whether future contingencies will in fact produce excessively onerous consequences.

The *deontological* position has as its base line the inherent and inalienable moral rights of individuals. This position holds that there are obligatory limits on what can be done to an individual because of moral claims which are prior to and not dependent on the possible undesirable or beneficial consequences of the human being living out the course of his or her life. A prime example of this in medical ethics is the classic Judeo-Christian position which asserts the inherent worth of every human being, on this basis prohibits the direct and deliberate killing of an innocent patient of any age, and supports the duty to sustain human life, even of the weak, the disadvantaged, and those who are unwanted by society.

The most common objection against a deontological ethic is its absolutism. However, a deontological system is not necessarily absolutistic: It is not unthinkable that some qualifications and exceptions be made, at least as regards certain obligations in some circumstances, in light of undesirable consequences.

The author's ethical position is the classic deontological position which posits a fundamental duty to protect life—by refraining from direct killing and by positively sustaining life—yet which also takes the contingent values of the patient's internal and external circumstances into account in determining that there is no strict moral obligation to use "extraordinary means" to preserve life. The author believes this approach is applicable to the

situation of the defective newborn child, but within well-defined limitations.

Neonatal Euthanasia
Joseph Fletcher and John Freeman

Joseph Fletcher: The Criterion of "Humanhood" in Infancy

Joseph Fletcher attempts to unravel the dilemmas created by severe impairment of the newborn child by appealing to an ethic of social utilitarianism.[9,13] The direct killing of a human is good, Fletcher claims, whenever the purpose or consequence is justified by the highest value (human happiness or well-being), or whenever the desirable consequences outweigh any disvalue in the action, according to a cost-benefit analysis. Thus, neonatal euthanasia is justified whenever death is judged to be a desirable goal representing a proportionate good.

Criteria for judging which children should be terminated hinge on whether the child has a "viable potential" for "typically human behavior." In an attempt to specify what is "typically human," Fletcher[9,13] offers twenty tentative criteria of "humanhood," which include a great variety of personal assets and desirable personality characteristics. Among them only mentation, or a minimal level of intelligence, is the key requirement.

However, the presence of "mentation" does not assure personhood (indeed, personhood remains elusive because of the idealistic nature of the twenty criteria), and even if it did, this would not assure any decisive value of life for the "person" since, in Fletcher's utilitarianism, the value of life is always judged according to humanly desirable needs in the situation. In the case of defective newborn children, what is decisive ethically is not the quality of "person-hood," but whether the foreseeable conse-quences of the child's life will be too onerous for all those who will be affected by the child's defects. In any case, none of the twenty "indi-cators of humanhood" can be verified of a newborn child; hence, they never work consis-tently in favor of, but potentially always against, the protection of the child. For if the newborn infant does not meet the criteria for "personal status," it is "subhuman" and can be terminated without personal offense, for it is only an "object," not a subject, and hence can have no rights.[10,11]

This points to the obvious flaws in Fletcher's utilitarian ethic: The weak have no convincing moral assurance of protection when placed in the balance with social conse-quences; there is no firm, inherent, and abiding grounds for the worth of a human being; highly discriminatory and relative criteria are offered for the normative value of the life of human beings; and the calculus on the future meaningfulness of the life of a child—on which the child's "right" to life depends—is vulnerable to an arbitrary decision.

John Freeman: The "Inhumaneness" of Waiting for Death

John Freeman, a physician writing with compassion, observes that many babies with meningomyelocele who are left untreated do not die quickly, but they do die slowly, over a period of several months or years. Some actu-ally survive, but in a more impaired condition than if they had had early and vigorous treat-ment. Freeman singles out the "inhumane-ness" involved in waiting for the death of the untreated child, with its accompanying suffer-ing, as the principal moral problem. The suffer-ing which he believes should be taken into ac-count is not just the suffering of the child, but

that of the parents and the professional per-sonnel who attend the child, as well.[14,15]

Freeman's response to the problem relies heavily on social utilitarian reasoning. For the most severe cases, the principal ethical crite-rion seems to be the avoidance of the disvalue of suffering. Arguing from consequences, he pleads for the moral permissibility of active eu-thanasia, based not just on what will be in the best interests of the child, but in the *best inter-ests of the parents, the siblings, and society as a whole*. He does not deny that the child has rights, but believes that the rights of these other parties may at times be preferred to the child's right to life.

Freeman's desire to convert from passive to active euthanasia in the case of the most se-verely affected infants is also supported by his conviction that any ethical difference between terminating life and withholding treatment is "fiction." Once the decision is made not to operate—which is the same as condemning the infant to death—the way should be open to resort to active euthanasia. However, Freeman believes that until euthanasia becomes accept-able to society, vigorous treatment should be pursued for virtually every case.

Within the scope of this paper it is impossi-ble to discuss the many crucial issues raised by Freeman, e.g. the moral significance of suffer-ing, the meaning of death, the goals of the med-ical profession, and most importantly, the eth-ical difference between active intervention to bring about death and the withholding of treatment. However, a word must be said about Freeman's opinion that waiting for the death of the untreated baby *ought* to be re-garded as so inhumane as to warrant terminat-ing its life. Here the question is not whether sometimes the decision not to operate is ethi-cally appropriate. The question is, rather, whether the right of the family to be free from serious suffering takes precedence over the afflicted child's right to life.

Great care is needed in the use of the term "rights." No one would doubt that in many cases the child's right to life conflicts with the interests, claims, or needs of the parents; but it can be misleading to refer to every interest or claim as a right, thus giving the impression that the conflict between the child's and parents' interests is between roughly equivalent claims. The author does not believe a sound argument can be made for the claim that everyone has a *right* to be free from all seriously distressing disadvantages and discomforts—a right that must be positively respected by all others in society, even at the price of another's fundamental right to life.[16] This can be argued on the basis of the inherent value of human life which should be a hindrance to direct killing for the sake of the better well-being of others. But even from a consequentialist perspective, there are values (or valued "qualities of life"—social and long-term values) which support a moral policy against involuntary pediatric euthanasia.

First, the prohibition of killing specifies a constraint that members of a community must observe if the community is to be viable at all. Second, far from being opposed to mercy and compassion, the prohibition of killing places humans in a situation that stimulates compassion much more so than a policy that would eliminate the need for compassion by eliminating the sufferer or the one who causes suffering.

Allowing To Die: John Lorber's View

Lorber's Medicoethical Position on "Selectivity"

Dr. John Lorber, who formerly had championed vigorous and comprehensive treatment for all newborn spina bifida children, more recently has assessed the long-term results of treating his patients over a twelve-year period and has concluded that the pendulum has swung too far—from excessive deaths due to lack of expert care to excessive handicaps for those who otherwise would have died. He found that full and vigorous treatment had produced a questionable benefit in terms of survival rate, severe mental and physical disability, and other constant risks to life from complications. He has concluded that greater selectivity in treatment is needed.[18-20]

On close scrutiny, Lorber's thesis on selectivity exhibits three levels of normative qualities of life: (1) the physical criteria which are contraindications to treatment; (2) the future physical, mental, and social qualities of life which make the treatment desirable or undesirable; and (3) those more ultimate qualities of life which account for the unacceptability of some adverse qualities in the patient.

At the first level, Lorber's view on selectivity is that a decision to treat or not to treat should be made on the first day after birth, before any therapeutic procedure is undertaken, on the basis of simple, readily recognizable "objective data"—physical signs which, he believes, are indicative of what the future disability of the infant will be if he or she is treated. He offers five "adverse criteria," emphasizing particularly the long-term prognostic importance of the site of the spinal lesion and the degree of paralysis at birth.

While most attention has been drawn to Lorber's first-day selectivity, he does suggest criteria for the possible interruption of comprehensive treatment at several significant points in the subsequent history of the child, a decision emotionally much more difficult than first-day selection.

In addition to the physical criteria, social

factors which point to a bad prognosis should also be taken into account. For example, Lorber believes that "to treat a badly handicapped, abandoned, illegitimate baby is total disaster for the baby if he survives."[18,19]

Once a decision is made not to treat, Lorber omits all treatment specific to the disorder. Normal, custodial nursing care is provided with ordinary feeding, but without incubators, oxygen, tube feeding, or resuscitation.

At the second level of analysis, Lorber seeks to identify the degree of disability in the survivor which represents an unacceptable quality of life. To take some of the guesswork out of the decision, Lorber attempted to classify in various categories of disability those infants with meningomyelocele who are given to total care, and to show the correlation between the categories of disabilities observed in two groups of treated children with data concerning the "adverse criteria" obtained on the first day of life.

In summarizing the results of the first group, he offered a "composite picture" of the quality of survivors in five somewhat gross categories of physical and mental defects, ranging from no handicap, through moderate and severe, to gross handicaps.[18] Those five categories constitute what would be the desirable and undesirable results of treatment. Since, for Lorber, "gross multiple malformations" represent an unacceptable quality of life which cannot be notably altered by treatment, he advocates treating only those who fall into the categories manifesting no to moderate handicaps. Pointing out how the categories of more serious defects observed in the survivors (as well as their survival rate) tend to correlate with the adverse physical criteria observed at birth, Lorber concludes that it is principally the degree of paralysis, or more specifically, the site of the lesion, which offers an accurate prognosis of future quality of life. Therefore, when the degree of paralysis at birth, together with the head circumference and other physical criteria, singly or in combination, indicate "severe multi-system physical handicaps," there is good reason for not treating the child.

At the second level of analysis then, the two sets of categories of handicaps observed in surviving patients serve as more detailed *descriptive* indications of where Lorber would want to draw the line in terms of the anticipated physical and mental qualities of survivors. The next question is, *why* are only mild or moderate handicaps acceptable qualities of life? Lorber's reasons constitute what may be called the third level of his normative thesis: They are the qualities, both particular and general, which are used in explaining why a certain level of defect is so undesirable as to call for nontreatment.

Lorber's primary reasons pertain to the interests of the patient, but intertwined with these, and with increasing emphasis, he includes social consequences as justifications for omitting treatment. In the first category, a level of handicap is acceptable to the extent that it is consistent with "self-respect, earning capacity, happiness and even marriage," and would be unacceptable to the extent that it portends repeated operations, hospitalization, absence from home and school, less than a full life span, exposure to repeated risk of death, and, generally a severe restriction of opportunities in life.[18,20] In the second category, Lorber speaks about the children's future ability to "earn their own living in competitive employment and be self-supporting with a secure, independent place in society."[19,20] He places emphasis on the impact the child will have on others: on family life and finances, on health care personnel and resources, and on the schools and community. The cost of treatment is mentioned with increasing emphasis as a contraindication to treatment.[19,20]

Commentary on Lorber's "Selectivity"

What seems to be most significant about Lorber's thesis is, first, that it offers specific, observable criteria, backed by medical data, for omitting treatment in severe cases; second, it has had the wide-spread effect of causing a shift in clinical practice toward nontreatment of spina bifida newborn children, with the result that fewer of these infants now survive; and third, he has taken the risk of expressing his value presuppositions, which is so essential if physicians and others are to contribute to a better understanding of the ethical issues and policy questions concerning "to treat or not to treat."

The author is in general agreement with Lorber's position on the permissibility of withholding comprehensive surgical and medical treatment in certain severe cases of meningomyelocele. In saying this, the author is abstracting for the moment from the question of the medical reliability of his prognostic "adverse criteria," as well as from the question as to where to draw the line on severity of impairment.

The author takes this generally favorable view in light of the principles relative to the ethical permissibility of withholding extraordinary therapeutic measures. As the author assesses that ethical tradition, a medical treatment is extraordinary (and hence nonobligatory) if the same treatment which sustains life also has the effect of causing or perpetuating an excessive hardship which the patient cannot sustain or cannot reasonably be expected to sustain, or if the treatment of the patient causes unreasonably excessive hardship for those persons who have the principal responsi-

bility of caring for the patient, or if the treatment does not hold out a reasonable hope of medical benefit to the patient. In this view, the fundamental worth of the person—which accounts for the duty to avoid killing or negligently abandoning a person—does not depend on this (admittedly consequential) assessment of hardship.

In another fundamental respect the author would not be in agreement with Lorber, viz., in his ethical (as distinct from legal) view on euthanasia. Lorber has written that "in expert and conscientious hands (positive euthanasia) could be the most humane way of dealing with such a situation," but that euthanasia should not be legalized, for that would be "a most dangerous weapon in the hands of the State or ignorant or unscrupulous individuals." The author would be opposed to euthanasia on an individual or a policy level, partly because the worth of the person is so important that life should not be subjected even to the knowledgeable and scrupulous exercise of direct power over life.

The author questions, too, whether the use of "adverse criteria," particularly a single physical criteria, is a just standard for protecting the child's interests, namely his right to life. There are four points to be made.

(1) The strict application of Lorber's single symptom or set of symptoms at birth is probably too gross a criterion for judging fairly whether a human life should be preserved, for it casts the net too wide: Many patients who would have only moderate sequelae, as well as some of the more severely impaired infants whose lives need not be without meaning, would be left to die.

(2) The use of specific, isolated physical criteria as sufficient for deciding whether

to treat (except perhaps in the most severe cases where the very humanness of the offspring can be questioned) seems unwarranted on medical grounds: Medical knowledge is constantly progressing and is always open to interpretation; consequently, the static application of specific criteria would become prejudicial to the interests and rights of the patient, for it would tend to exclude the application of new knowledge and variable interpretations to the advantage of the patient.

(3) The use of physical criteria at birth is also insufficient on moral grounds. Such "substantive standards" are important but are not sufficient for indicating the limits of the moral duty to sustain life in the vast majority of cases, for according to the author, the principal indicator of the limits of the duty to preserve life is whether life in that condition or the effort to preserve life would be excessively burdensome to bear—which depends to a considerable extent on moral strength, social support, and other nonmedical factors.

(4) Nonetheless, for the sake of an equitable policy in the newborn situation, general guidelines should be developed indicating the medical, personal, and social factors which provide the presumptive parameters of the duty to sustain life. These factors will ultimately call for *relative* assessments, which consequently resist concrete, substantive formulation.

In analyzing the degree of disability in the survivor that represents an unacceptable quality of life, Lorber draws the line at moderate

handicaps and offers as his reason a mixture of values partly the "best interests of the patient" and partly "the interests of parents and society." If one admits the moral relevance of these two sets of circumstantial factors in limiting the duty to sustain life, one must also acknowledge that it is not easy to know concretely to what extent one can acknowledge these factors without subverting the demands of justice and the individual's fundamental claim to support and protection.

There is the ever-present danger of subverting the worth of the individual to standards of social usefulness in the appeal to "the interests of parents and society." Even the "best interests of the patient," if understood as self-respect and happiness, can be equated with variable and somewhat capricious standards of social acceptability. The author would place far less decisive value on social respect and personal social fulfillment than Lorber, and far more value on the inner life of man in freedom which is the condition for self-realization and which can perdure with meaning in spite of many (though not all) obstacles.

Richard McCormick's View: "Relational Potential"

In an important and widely discussed series of essays, Richard A. McCormick, the Roman Catholic moral theologian, discussed the nature and limits of the duty to sustain the lives of defective newborn children.[21-23] McCormick believes that the duty to preserve the life of a defective newborn child is determined not only by whether the means necessary to preserve life are ordinary or extraordinary, i.e. whether or not they entail grave hardship, but by the quality of the life thus saved.

McCormick states that in the Judeo-Christian tradition, life is not a value to be preserved in and for itself: It is a relative good—a value to be preserved *insofar as* the higher, spiritual purposes of life are attainable. The duty to preserve physical life, as well as the limits of that duty, are based on the possibility of attaining to these higher values. The "higher spiritual goods" are love of God and neighbor, which are inseparable loves. Because God demands to be recognized and loved in others, it can be concluded that the meaning and consummation of life are found in human relationships.[21] Consequently, *"life is a value to be preserved only insofar as it contains some potentiality for human relationships."*[21]

McCormick applies this value theory to defective newborn children: The criterion for deciding which efforts must be made and which efforts need not be made to sustain the child's life is "the potential for human relationships associated with the infant's condition."[21] He understands this as applying in two ways: (1) if this potentiality is totally absent; or (2) if it would be totally undeveloped or utterly subordinated to the mere effort for survival, human life "has achieved its potential," and no treatment is obligatory. The baby may be allowed to die.

McCormick attempts to make his guideline more concrete: It is the task of physicians to provide "concrete categories or presumptive biological symptoms" for the judgment about the baby's relational potential. Between Down's syndrome and anencephaly, there are many other categories with "biological symptoms" by which one can judge whether "grossly deformed and deprived infants" have relational potential. McCormick concludes that "nearly all would very likely agree that the anencephalic infant is without relational potential," while "the same cannot be said of the mongoloid infant."[21]

Much sensitivity for values, and disvalues, characterizes McCormick's treatment of a very delicate problem in bioethics. The author agrees with the general notion that it can be morally responsible to withhold treatment from some excessively defective newborn children, but the principal elements of his ethical method raises some serious problems. Comments here will focus on (1) issues related to justice and (2) his underlying theory on the value of life.

First, the "relational potential" criterion is vague, indeterminate, and relative, and therefore an unjust criterion for protecting the value of life and the claim to the preservation of one's life. "Human relationships" can be found in a vast variety of forms; and it is not at all clear why the patient should be examined for his or her capacities for relationships without taking account of how other persons might enable a meaningful relationship for the disadvantaged person. Furthermore, how does one *measure* in newborn children their capacity for "meaningful" relationships? If one may assume that being mentally handicapped can more certainly be an obstacle to loving relations than physical handicaps and that something more than "vegetative"[22] life is needed to achieve the consummation in love which McCormick requires, what *degree* of mental handicap makes the life not worth preserving? In his attempt to be more specific, McCormick attaches relational potential not to "biological symptoms" but to broad *diagnostic categories*—anencephaly, Down's syndrome, and other categories in between. Such categories, which usually embrace great variations in mental and physical handicaps, represent a misleading quantification of an elusive relational quality.

To use the diagnostic categories as ethical criteria for judging whether the babies should be treated is to unjustly and unjustifiably encourage generalizations that the "x-symptom" baby is worth preserving and the "y-symptom" baby is not. (The anencephalic child is an ambiguous example, for one may question not only its relational potential, but whether it is a person, since, without any brain, it would seem to lack the minimal prerequisites for a body-spirit individual.)*

The first objection against the "relational" standard, therefore is that it is unjust because it lacks equality, which is a fundamental characteristic of justice.[24] According to McCormick's criterion, the fundamental value of life which accounts for even the minimal obligation to sustain human life depends on whether and insofar as the infant has a specific quality —a certain level of relational potential— which is simply not shared by all and which is inherently variable in the way it is found in people, and that is not just. The claim to life-support treatment is not an unlimited one, especially in the face of death and other adverse circumstances, as the authors who have discussed the contingencies of justice and charity to one's neighbor have indicated; but to make the assets of the individual a fundamental and absolute requirement for these values and claims is not only opposed to the tradition of natural rights but to some basic teachings of the Judeo-Christian tradition on the meaning of man.

The second major problem raised by McCormick's theory pertains to the way "value of life" is established. First it should be noted that there is ambiguity in his use of "value of life." While insisting that every human being is of incalculable worth, he nonetheless teaches, on theological grounds, that no human life represents a value worth preserving except on the basis of the spiritual goals it can accomplish. His basic normative method, then, is a form of religious consequentialism or personalistic utilitarianism. It pertains to a utilitarian school of thought, for it holds that (1) life is a *value* worth preserving, (2) there is a *duty* to sustain and care for human life, and (3) *actions* supportive of life are right or wrong, precisely insofar as the assets or qualities of the individual offer the potentiality for achieving a higher single value.*

Contrary to McCormick's assertion on "the Judeo-Christian perspective," this tradition has commonly held that human life is a value worth preserving and that there is a duty to sustain life fundamentally on the basis of what the person is (a deontological perspective), rather than on the basis of what the individual is able to accomplish (McCormick's consequentialism). While McCormick suggests a bilevel view of man in which *physical* life should be sustained only insofar as it has an *instrumental* value for attaining *spiritual* goods, in both Jewish law[25-27] and Christian (referring particularly though not exclusively to Roman Catholic) theology,[28,33] † human life is valued holistically as the body-spirit life of the entire person; in these traditions the basis of the duty

---

* Use of anencephaly as a reference point for discussion is not very useful because nearly all of these are stillborn or survive but a few hours to a day.

---

* McCormick expressed the hope that decisions about defective newborn children not be shaped from utilitarian perspectives. Perhaps, in making this cautionary remark, he was intending to warn against that type of utilitarianism which would judge the value of human life according to standards of crass social utility, i.e. judging from how "useful" the person would be in contemporary society.

† The author is referring not only to the general Christian views on value of life, but particularly as they have been articulated in the literature which discusses "ordinary and extraordinary means."

to sustain human life is not known from one's physical or mental abilities, nor even from an individual's capacities for spiritual activity, but from qualities which are predicated of all humans, principally the notion that all men are created as persons in the image of God. Thus, in traditional Catholic thought, the concept of "personhood," which requires only the unity of body and soul, accounts for the value of human life and the duty to preserve and foster life.[34]

One can also question whether "human relationships" really expresses the total meaning and consummation of life "in Judeo-Christian perspective," as McCormick claims, since there are other ways of viewing the meaning of man in these traditions. Thus, in the Christian tradition, the value of caring for and supporting the life of even the totally disadvantaged person finds its meaning and source "in ways not dependent on our human purposes and strengths": It is the task of humanity to strive to offer supportive care as an act of love even for the handicapped person "who can never understand the very opportunity of love he offers."[35] Again, this is not to argue for an unrestricted duty and a rigid right to treatment, but simply to say that the value of sustaining a handicapped life and the task of caring for the weak are greatly distorted in a Christian context when the fundamental and unconditional requirement for preserving life is the measure of relationships of which they appear capable.*

Yet the qualities of the life of a highly defective newborn child are relevant to the decision to treat or not to treat. In the final section the author attempts a brief outline of an ethical frame of reference which will take contingent qualities into account without denying the fundamental value of the life of every person.

The Limits of Sustaining Life: Hardship

The author's own preference is to work within the framework of the ethic which speaks of ordinary and extraordinary means.[28,33] Although McCormick uses that school of thought as his starting point, he departs notably from that tradition by employing a consequentialist ethic for establishing the value and duty of preserving life, by utilizing criteria of humanhood (the relational assets of the individual upon which a fundamental value of life utterly depends), and by advocating a fundamentally unjust criterion for judging the basic value of a "life to be preserved."

Historically, it is not accurate to suggest that in the "extraordinary means" concept one was speaking of the *means themselves* being extraordinary, whereas now it is the quality of the life of the patient that is spoken of as being extraordinary, hence not requiring treatment. As the author sees it, the "extraordinary means" concept was never concerned about the means themselves, but about whether the *qualitative* aspects (pain, hardship, futility of treatment, the extremely adverse condition of the survivor) of the *use* of some medical or other life-support effort might in a given *situation* diminish the obligation to treat. Hence the question is not whether "quality of life" is relevant, since it is unquestionably relevant for anyone who does not adopt an absolutely vitalistic position, but *what normative system* one uses in employing "quality of life" considerations in measuring or limiting the duty to care for others.

---

* Thus, the author would not agree with the accuracy of the qualifications made by McCormick in his statement that "It is the pride of Judeo-Christian tradition that the weak and defenseless . . . —that is, those *whose potential is real but reduced*—are cherished and protected as our neighbors in greatest need."

The author's normative position would be stated this way: There is a "deontological" moral duty not to directly and deliberately kill an innocent patient, whether through acts of commission or omission; there is a fundamental prima facie obligation to sustain human life; and the practical limitations on the duty to offer life-supporting efforts are indicated by consequences or qualitative concerns (called "extraordinary" circumstances) in conflict situations.

In the classic Catholic tradition (in which the "extraordinary means" doctrine developed), the basis of this twofold duty was seen in the value and dignity which every human has from being created as a person in the image of God; from the notion that, since man's life and dignity come from God, man has stewardship but not absolute mastery over life; and from a natural law theory which builds on a rational insight into the inclination to self-preservation as a fundamental good.

However, when one speaks of the positive duty to sustain life—which could be accomplished through a variety of possible actions, some beneficial, some futile, some extremely adverse—there are reasonable limits to one's obligation, as there are to all positive obligations arising from the requirements of justice or love. When circumstances indicate the overriding reasons for restricting or terminating treatment, the life of that person continues to be a value, precisely a "value to be preserved," and that is why it is such a profound conflict.

More specifically, the duty to sustain a human life is limited principally by what would be judged an excessive hardship; that is, when the very means or effort to sustain a human life inseparably involves a truly grave hardship, one may discontinue those efforts. An additional contributory factor is when the available means of treatment do not hold out a reasonable hope of success. When one speaks of something being *unreasonably* burdensome or nonbeneficial, it becomes difficult but still necessary to make such an approximation on behalf of an incompetent person such as a newborn child; yet it would seem that for a person who has not yet had the opportunity for life and who is totally dependent on others, one should be more than customarily skeptical about what is truly "extraordinary." Furthermore, it might be noted that it is not just the isolated procedure which may be an extraordinary or nonobligatory therapeutic means, but the entire course of comprehensive care.

Life-sustaining efforts can become "extraordinary" in three ways, all applicable to newborn children, depending on the way in which negative qualities are caused by or associated with the treatment.

WHEN EXCESSIVELY BURDENSOME QUALITIES ARE DIRECTLY ASSOCIATED WITH THE MEANS USED. For example, a standard medical treatment more obviously carries with it the assumption of being obligatory, whereas procedures which are not established or proven may not be obligatory. For example, shunting of the meningomyelocele patient has been and still could be "extraordinary" in some circumstances today. Similarly, the excessive pain (physical or psychological) directly associated with the course of the treatment might create a situation which a "reasonable person" would find morally impossible to accept. Also, the nonavailability of resources, due to excessive expense and other problems in the distribution of life-supporting resources, could make the treatment "virtually impossible" or so associated with negative results as to make the continued therapy unreasonable.

WHEN EXCESSIVELY BURDENSOME QUALITIES ARE CAUSED BY THE LIFE-SUSTAINING TREATMENT. For example, the maimed condition following an amputation, particularly when no prosthetic devices and very little human support are available, may be at least subjectively a proportionate reason for not accepting treatment. Similarly, a terminally ill patient, in need of specialized intensive care available only in a hospital and realizing that that course of treatment will have the negative effect of depersonalizing his final days, decides to go home to be with his loved ones, even though this indirectly entails a shortening of his life. Here, the treatment is not obligatory, not simply because "that kind of life is not worth preserving," but because, during the patient's important final days, the treatment would be an unreasonable obstacle to achieving what in the circumstances is valued higher than a small extension of life, namely, being surrounded by his loved ones in relative peace. In contrast to McCormick, the author does not imply that life is a "value to be preserved" *only if* higher goods like friendship, peace, and love are possible, but simply that in a conflict case when both cannot be achieved and when the effort to sustain life effectively blocks out the higher values associated with a personalized environment, human life—while *still* being a "value to be preserved"—need not be sustained with all efforts in *those* conflicting circumstances.

WHEN EXCESSIVELY BURDENSOME QUALITIES ARE PERPETUATED BY LIFE-SUSTAINING TREATMENT. This category is similar to the previous case and would include some infants afflicted with meningomyelocele and other newborn anomalies. As regards those infants who can be

expected to experience at least a minimal self-consciousness and freedom of will and who therefore will be striving to achieve moral (or moral-religious) self-realization, the duty to preserve life may be limited by the excessive hardship that would foreseeably be experienced by the patient if his entire striving to discover moral meaning in life were to be totally submerged in or utterly strained by the mere effort to survive and by the suffering that accompanies that effort.*

This obviously calls for a "subjective" judgment about the reasonable limits of hardship; but so do the majority of judgments of "extraordinary means"—whether in the "old" medical ethics or the ethics of the "new medicine." The real question here is whether anyone is entitled to make a proxy judgment relative to the treatment of another incompetent person (for such a judgment always entails a value component). The author believes such a judgment can and must be made and that abuses will only be avoided or minimized by a complex set of considerations, including a totally serious commitment to the general rule of sustaining human life and to the reasons (human dignity and human fidelity) that underly it, the refusal to subordinate adverse medical criteria to utilitarian or merely consequentialist considerations, and a dedication to alleviating suffering coupled with the conviction that a life with handicap and suffering can be meaningful. This framework for medical decision making cannot easily be codified—certainly no more so than the formulas for any value-laden art of human behavior. Yet this

---

* In this restricted "hardship" sense, and abstracting from the concept of "relationship," the author would agree with an important insight offered by McCormick.

approach is preferable to a medicoethical system that would categorically and systematically exclude as beneficiaries of a duty to sustain human life those infants or groups of infants who lack some specific asset or some relative endowment.

Conclusion

The foregoing categories, and indeed this entire paper, do little more than offer ethical reflections on ways in which "quality-of-life" factors ought or ought not shape decisions affecting the lives of newborn children. Particularly for those who judge what is permissible only by measurable effects, there is little significance in the distinction between the decision to kill and the decision not to offer life-sustaining treatment; but for those who judge these moral actions according to the bond that exists among inherently valued humans, the arduous work of knowing "where to draw the line" between treatment and nontreatment will remain crucial. The "extraordinary means" axiom suggests an individualized manner of ethical decision making which respects the limitations placed by adverse quality-of-life factors, but without abandoning the normative, deontological role of the more profound and universal qualities of human personhood.

References

1. Duff, R. S. and Campbell, A. G. M.: Moral and ethical dilemmas in the special-care nursery. *N Engl J Med, 289:* 890–894, 1973.
2. Gustafson, J. M.: Genetic engineering and the normative view of the human. In Williams, P. N. (Ed.): *Ethical Issues in Biology and Medicine.* Cambridge, Massachusetts, Schenkman, 1972, pp. 46–58.
3. Gustafson, J. M.: Genetic counseling and the uses of genetic knowledge—an ethical overview. In Hilton, B. et al. (Ed.): *Ethical Issues in Human Genetics.* New York, Plenum Pr, 1973, pp. 101–119.
4. Gustafson, J. M.: What is the normatively human? *The American Ecclesiastical Review, 165:*192–207, 1971.
5. Brandt, R. B.: *Ethical Theory,* Englewood Cliffs, P-H, 1959.
6. Franken, W. K.: *Ethics.* Englewood Cliffs, P-H, 1963.
7. Broad, C. D.: *Five Types of Ethical Theory.* London, Kegal Paul, 1930.
8. Ethics of selective treatment of spina bifida: Report by a working party. *Lancet, 7898:*85–88, 1975.
9. Fletcher, Joseph: Ethics and euthanasia. *Am J Nurs, 73:*670–675, 1973.
10. Fletcher, Joseph: The right to die: A theologian comments. *The Atlantic Monthly, 221:*62–64, 1968.
11. Fletcher, Joseph: Medicine and the nature of man. In Veatch, R. M., Gaylin, W., and Morgan, C. (Eds.): *The Teaching of Medical Ethics.* Hastings-on-Hudson, New York, Institute of Society, Ethics and the Life Sciences, 1973, pp. 47–58.
12. Fletcher, Joseph: Four indicators of humanhood: the enquiry matures. *Hastings Center Report, 4:*4–7, 1974.
13. Fletcher, Joseph: *The Ethics of Genetic Control.* Garden City, New York, Anch. Doubleday, 1974.
14. Freeman, J. M.: Is there a right to die—quickly? *J Pediatr, 80:*904–905, 1972.
15. Freeman, J. M.: To treat or not to treat: Ethical dilemmas of treating the infant with a myelomeningocele. *Clin Neurosurg, 20:*143–144, 1973.
16. Cooke, R. E.: Whose suffering? *J Pediatr, 80:*906, 1972.
17. Dyck, A. J.: An alternative to the ethic of

euthanasia. In Williams, R. H. (Ed.): *To Live and To Die: When, Why and How.* New York, Springer, 1973, pp. 98–112.

18. Lorber, J.: Results of treatment of myelomeningocele: An analysis of 524 unselected cases, with special reference to possible selection for treatment. *Dev Med Child Neurol, 13*:279–303, 1971.

19. Lorber, J.: Spina bifida cystica: Results of treatment of 270 consecutive cases with criteria for selection for the future. *Arch Dis Child, 47*:854–873, 1972.

20. Lorber, J.: Early results of selective treatment of spina bifida cystica. *Br Med J, 4*:201–204, 1973.

21. McCormick, R. A.: To save or let die. *JAMA, 229*:172–176, 1974.

22. McCormick, R. A.: Discussion: To save or let die. *America, 131*:169–173, 1974.

23. McCormick, R. A.: Notes on moral theology: April-September 1974. *Theological Studies, 36*:121–123, 1975.

24. Vlastos, G.: Justice and equality. In Melden, A. I. (Ed.): *Human Rights.* Belmont, California, Wadsworth Pub, 1970, pp. 76–95. Reprinted with some changes from Brandt, R. B. (Ed.): *Social Justice.* Englewood Cliffs, P-H, 1962, pp. 31–72.

25. Jakobovits, I.: *Jewish Medical Ethics,* 2nd ed. New York, Bloch, 1959, pp. 45–58, 123–125.

26. Jakobovits, I.: Euthanasia. *Encyclopedia Judaica.* Jerusalem, Keter Publishing House, Ltd., and New York, Macmillan, 1971, Vol. VI, cols. 978–979.

27. Bosker, B. Z.: Life and death. *Encyclopedia Judaica.* Jerusalem, Keter Publishing House, Ltd., and New York, Macmillan, 1971, vol II, cols, 235–237.

28. Kelly, G.: *Medico-Moral Problems.* St. Louis, The Catholic Hospital Association of the United States and Canada, 1957.

29. Healy, E. F.: *Medical Ethics.* Chicago, Loyola U Pr, 1956.

30. O'Donnell, T.: *Morals in Medicine.* Westminster, Maryland, The Newman Press, 1957.

31. Nolan, K.: The problem of care for the dying. In Curran, C. E. (Ed.): *Absolutes in Moral Theology?* Washington and Cleveland, Corpus Books, 1968, pp. 249–260.

32. Häring, B.: *Medical Ethics.* Notre Dame, Fides, 1973.

33. Ramsey, P.: *The Patient as Person.* New Haven and London, Yale U Pr, 1970, pp. 113–164.

34. Welty, E.: The Structure of the Social Order, Vol. II. In *A Handbook of Christian Social Ethics.* New York, Herder & Herder, 1973, p. 116.

35. Hauerwas, S.: *Vision and Virtue: Essays in Christian Ethical Reflection.* Notre Dame, Fides, 1974, pp. 187–194.

15

Projected Quality of the Patient's Life—A Critique

Richard C. Sparks, C.S.P.

Every live-born issue from a woman's womb, however "normal" or severely handicapped, is to be valued by the sheer fact of being human and being alive. Each newborn is inherently a person and therefore has the right to have his/her life protected and developmental potential fostered. Regardless of the infant's inability at birth to be a moral agent, s/he is to be treated as a potential subject or an end in oneself, never solely as an object or a utilitarian means to further others' ends. Whether rooted in religious convictions about creation, stewardship, and the image of God, or philosophically derived from some humanistic sense of intrinsic dignity, these fundamental presuppositions ground both the quality of life position as well as the ordinary/extraordinary means tradition.

At the same time, adoption of the principle of Totality, holistically interpreted, nuances the above prima facie presumption toward treatment. The best interest of a living human patient is never served by an over-emphasis on vital signs in themselves. Within time and space, one's "life" in its physiological aspects is oriented toward one's more holistic best interest. The Totality principle rightly asserts that the meaning or teleological end for which life in the physical sense exists is one's fuller human flourishing in time and space and eternal life or union with God hereafter. The principle of Totality recognizes this in medical decision making by subordinating the mandate to prolong "life" to concern for one's psychological, social and eternal well-being. One's best interest is neither reduced to vitalistic life-prolongation nor expanded to subjugate the patient to social utilitarian concerns. Rather, "projected quality of the patient's life" proponents are to be commended for their balanced anthropology and patient-centered presuppositions. Burden-to-benefit determinations are holistically-viewed, with "sheer life" rightly yielding to determinations concerning "good

"Projected Quality of the Patient's Life—A Critique" by *Richard C. Sparks, C.S.P. in* To Treat or Not To Treat?: Bioethics and the Handicapped Newborn, *1988, pp. 192–208 and 222–225. Reprinted with permission of Paulist Press.*

life" and even these being subordinate to one's interest in "eternal life."

As a criterion or standard for deciding when to forego potentially life-sustaining treatment, the projected quality of patient's life approach expands and builds upon the core components of the ordinary/extraordinary tradition. It might even be asserted that the two approaches, at least as exemplified by Richard McCormick and Warren Reich respectively, differ primarily in language, but vary little in actual content. Both approaches can be said to be "means related" in that any decision for "nontreatment" by definition is focused on whether or not to inaugurate or continue the use of some proposed means, whether life-saving or merely life-prolonging. By the same token both types are in actuality "quality of the patient's life" standards in that the Totality-rooted decision for or against treatment focuses on the kind or "quality" of life that the handicapped patient will have with versus without the proposed procedure. In those cases in which the quality of the patient's life is judged already excessively burdened and the life-sustaining devices or proposed therapies serve only "to perpetuate" such a tragic quality of the patient's life, it seems to be more a debate over semantics than of content whether one labels the standard ordinary/extraordinary means with a means restriction or openly admits that it is a projected quality of the patient's life decision.

If medical means contribute to or actually cause an excessive burden to the patient, both standards exempt the patient from using these "extraordinary means." However, if the means neither enhance nor inhibit a life quality that is already deemed extraordinarily burdensome, or perhaps experientially "meaningless," from the patient's perspective, then it seems that the phrase "projected quality of the patient's life"

better captures the reason for nontreatment. The concept of "means related" seems to be superfluous. If the question is treatment versus nontreatment, obviously a treatment or a proposed means is on the floor for consideration. If used or foregone the decision may or may not hinge on the benefit/burden of that drug, piece of equipment, or proposed surgery. On the other hand, it will always depend on the projected quality of the patient's life and the benefit/burden such a state in life is to and for the patient, holistically considered. Therefore, with all due respect for the concern contemporary ordinary/extraordinary means proponents have against the possible linkage of quality of life decisions for nontreatment with subsequent decisions for direct infanticide [see negative cautions to follow], it would seem that on the level of treatment/nontreatment decisions, THE morally determinative component is the projected quality of life for the patient, irrespective of means causation.

For that reason, McCormick, Paris, Johnson, et al. are to be commended for opening up the ordinary/extraordinary tradition with regard to nontreatment decisions and for declaring such decisions fundamentally and primarily to be quality of life determinations. The primary advantage of a "quality of life" schema is that it puts the emphasis squarely on the kind of life the patient lives or can live, rather than implying that the focus is dependent on means in any essential sense. It links together under one rationale decisions to withhold treatment in the cases of imminently dying patients with the cases of non-dying patients extraordinarily burdened by the means with those borderline cases in which the excessive burden is due to the amalgam of "diseases" or handicaps irrespective of means.

Ramsey's "curious exceptions" of permanently non-sapient and intractably pained patients as well as Reich and Weber's inordinately burdened cases perpetuated but not caused by means can thereby be incorporated together under this projected quality of the patient's life criterion. If imminently dying, the brevity of time left and one's desires for how to live while dying usually outweigh any minimal biological benefit derivable from interim therapies or cumbersome artificial life-support systems. It is the kind or quality of life one will live while dying that determines the course of treatment/nontreatment. If non-dying, and if the proposed physiologically beneficial means will cause a life qualitatively overburdened by pain, by financial or psychic cost, or by inconvenience, such means are optional. Why? No one is obliged to cause an excessively burdened quality of life for oneself or others just to prolong vital signs, presuming that these harsh burdens inhibit or negate one's broader best interest. Finally, if one is not dying, but lives a life already intractably pained, inordinately costly, excessively inconvenienced, or permanently "unaware" (non-sapient and non-relational), then, like the previous example, no treatment, however life-sustaining, is in this patient's personal, qualitative best interest.

Finally, in the area of positive aspects, "projected quality of the patient's life" proponents, compassionately aware of the Home and Society factors championed by Shaw, defend the inalienable right of those handicapped patients whose lives are saved and sustained to the necessary long-term financial, medical, emotional, and educational aid to make the most of their "defective" potential.[1] To mandate that severely handicapped infants must be treated, as Reagan's "Baby Doe" rulings have done, while simultaneously slashing budgetary funds from social programs designed to meet their postsurgical "care" needs, is a species of dualism

and injustice. Paul Johnson goes so far as to suggest that the converse may be true. "The less often means of increasing life quality are made available, the more choices not to maintain life may be justified." While he notes that ethical and/or medical decisions ought not simply reflect current structures of social justice, neither ought they be made without any reference to them. Recognizing that financial and personnel resources are not unlimited, allocation decisions must be made and consequences faced honestly.[2]

After that basic endorsement of the underlying principles and synthetic methodology of the projected quality of the patient's life standard it would seem that the next step would be to adopt either the more restrictive or the broader interpretation of what qualities are essential to declare a given newborn's life worth treating and below which one could forego further efforts as presumably not in his/her best interests. However, adopting a nontreatment standard based on some measurable quality of life below which "life" is not worth sustaining or prolonging is a tricky proposition, open to honest, prudential debate, as well as possible abuse. The potential in one direction for an over-protective minimalism, or in the opposite direction for a naively high expectation of near-normalcy, can hardly be denied. Sadly, both extremes are exemplified in the projected quality of the patient's life options surveyed here.

Duff, Lorber, Campbell, and Shaw, who adopt a "broader interpretation" of what qualities are essential to declare a handicapped infant's life worth living and sustaining, seem to set the minimum standard required for treatment too high. These physicians tend toward equating one's interest in life prolongation with one's functional ability to participate fully or "well" in personal goods and human experiences. While one's future capacity to be socially independent, to hold a competitive job, and to be able to marry, as Lorber suggests, are indeed kinds or qualities of life hoped for by and for all human beings, are such ideal life potentials essential for a life to have "meaning" and "worth" to a given patient? Surely handicapped rights groups would protest. Being blind, deaf, retarded, quadriplegic, paraplegic, impotent, or handicapped in some other way may inhibit one's potential for these experiential ideals. Yet, dependence on fellow human beings for one's livelihood, joblessness or sheltered workshop employment, and celibacy ought not in themselves constitute a life "worthless," "meaningless," or not worth sustaining.

I suggest that a human life with some minimal functional ability to process one's environmental input—mirrored in apparent enjoyment of food, reaction to pain, discomfort over dirty diapers, some degree of responsiveness to cuddling (cooing, rooting, smiling, muscle relaxation), and some basic "awareness" of significant others (primary care nurse, mother)—can be said to have sufficient meaning for the patient to presume the prima facie mandate to treat. Paralleling the relational potential standard of restrictive quality of the patient's life proponents, this definition of a life of minimally meaningful quality to the patient stands in sharp contrast to the fairly sophisticated functions deemed necessary by Shaw, Lorber, et al. For example, Duff and Campbell suggest that Joseph Fletcher's fifteen humanhood traits might be helpful for determining whether one's own life has enough potential for the patient to be worth saving. Accordingly, anyone with an I.Q. below 40 (a category which includes many happy, albeit handicapped Trisomy 21 citizens) or anyone lacking the mental sophistication to balance feelings

with rationality or anyone unable "to communicate" in some intelligible way thereby could be categorically excluded from treatment. Presumably such patients are excessively burdened by their very mental deficiencies and would prefer non-life (or eternal life) to their present impaired existence.

The access-to-treatment of all mentally handicapped persons on the functional scale between this broader standard espoused by Duff and Campbell and the more restrictive one espoused by McCormick, Paris, et al. are threatened by this broad, near-normalcy interpretation of a quality of life worth saving. Better to err on the side of life, presuming that relatively pain-free life with mild to moderately severe retardation is a life with some potential for mental and relational participation, than to assume, based on some potentially biased middle class expectations, that such life is so devoid of experiential "good vibrations" as to be meaningless. Thus, while allowing some leeway for honest debate as to how much functional ability is essential to declare a mentally handicapped newborn relational, experientially capable of participating in embodied human life at all, it seems discriminatory and biased to set that standard so high that obviously relational retardates would be excluded from further participation, albeit limited, in life's "higher goods."

On the other hand, while espousing, with the more restrictive interpreters, that any newborn with the barest minimal potential to relate and positively experience his/her environment has an interest in life prolongation and a claim on treatment, I am reluctant to interpret the subsequent determination of potential burden in as individualistic a manner as Arras, Veatch, and, to some extent, McCormick and Paris tend to. In their admirable effort to avoid a socially-weighted bias against a patient's own experience of burden vis-à-vis benefit, I believe the more restrictive quality of life proponents have construed the determination of excessive burden too narrowly. The ultimate decision as to whether treatment is in a given patient's total best interest ought to incorporate not only medical or individualistic (i.e., experiential) burden factors, but also broader social factors, viewed from the patient's existentially-contexted vantage point. On this level, the broader interpreters of the quality of the patient's life echo the best of the ordinary/extraordinary means tradition in their insistence that the cost, psychic strain, and degree of inconvenience borne by others, a non-competent's social network, ought rightly to be factored in as part of the patient's burden, holistically considered.

Arras' assertion that such inclusion of social factors is "the rankest kind of discrimination" reflects a tendency by the more restrictive quality of life proponents to isolate the neonate, detaching him/her from the realities of social context and circumstances. His conclusion that treatment decisions must be based "solely on the extent of medical disabilities" truncates the patient's interests, bordering on the medical indications policy.[3] McCormick, Paris, and Arras seem to allow the patient's social nature to impact only to the extent that s/he has physiologically-based potential to relate with others (determining one's minimal capacity to derive benefit from treatment), but to reject communality when it comes to the impact the patient's condition has on one's family or society (burden in the fullest sense). In an effort to forestall the slippery slope to a selfish social utilitarianism on the part of burdened others, the more restrictive quality of life proponents tend to exclude social burdens altogether. Rather, would it not be truer to the wisdom of

the ordinary/extraordinary means tradition and fairer to the patient viewed as a social as well as a personal being to allow familial and even societal burden into the calculus concerning a handicapped patient's best interests?

In his defense of the use of non-competent subjects in non-therapeutic medical research, McCormick eloquently argues for an assumed "solidarity and Christian concern for others" on the part of the non-competent.[4] "Sharing in sociality," infants are in some sense "volunteer-able" to help the common good, provided their own individual well-being is not thereby appreciably burdened. Why, then, do he and Paris seem to exclude similar social solidarity and familial concerns from the calculus of the patient's best interest in treatment decisions related to non-competents? First, one might argue that if familial or other social factors are allowed to overrule a relationally able infant's presumed interest in therapy, the subsequent nontreatment would indeed harm the patient left untreated. Death or a more burdened quality of life seems inevitable. Therefore, contrary to the pain-free experimentation premise, incorporation of social factors in these cases cannot help but harm the patient, at least if nontreatment and foreseen death are considered not in this infant's best interest. Second, it is not clear whether McCormick and Paris absolutely exclude all social burden factors. In their joint *America* article they assert that familial factors ought not dictate an infant's access to treatment, since behind one's nuclear family there is a second line of social support or defense, the society. They decline to speculate whether the cost of handicapped care ever exceeds a society's (finite) resources or the demands in justice for its equitable distribution.

While it is questionable whether social burdens in and of themselves ought ever to so dominate a newborn's best interest as to negate a reasonably good prognosis if one is treated, it seems to be an over-reaction and a potential injustice to the patient to categorically exclude familial and/or wider social concerns altogether. It is possible that the exorbitant emotional and financial drain on a family and society, for an infant with only the barest minimal relational potential (e.g., severe brain damage due to prolonged asphyxia or Trisomy 13), is an extraordinary and optional burden given the extremely minimal benefit of such a practically non-sapient life condition for the patient. One might rightly project that s/he would not only not want to be sustained at such a personally futile quality of life, but would, as a "sharer in solidarity," also not want to so burden one's family and society for so little personal experience and benefit. As a corroborative, potentially scale-tipping element in a patient-centered benefit/burden calculus already heavily leaning toward non-treatment, factors related to one's inherent social nature and impact on others seem morally licit and admissible.

Like traversing a mine field one must tread lightly to avoid both extremes—the over-protective, physiologically-based, somewhat individualistic boundary of the restrictive interpreters as well as any glib incorporation of social concerns that might be deemed trivial, easily bearable, and more symptomatic of a selfish family or society than of a patient actually being over-burdened. To avoid potential bias against the patient, social burden factors ought to always be corroborative of existing patient burden or non-benefit, not set over against obvious benefit and minimal patient burden. With the exception of the means-related proviso, such decisions parallel the benefit/burden calculus of patient-centered factors adopted by the ordinary/extraordinary means standard, which traditionally included burden to one's family and community as an extension of the patient's own total best interests.

More work needs to be done by projected quality of the patient's life proponents across the spectrum to better hone, refine, and nuance both functionally and socially the generic boundaries of a life excessively burdened or without further experiential potential. Presently, D'Youville College professor Paul R. Johnson best exemplifies the middle ground between the restrictive and broader interpreters. From the former he adopts a relational potential, brain-related approach to the functional ability essential for embodied human flourishing and proceeds to clarify more specifically than McCormick et al. have as yet done who populates this category. However, he hovers closer to the so-called broader end of the spectrum in arguing that social or family considerations may over-ride the presumption for treatment in some few instances of relationally able infants. Lest this be seen as a socially-weighted calculus of contrary interests or rights, Johnson suggests integrating family or societal resource limitations into a broader concept of the best interest of the patient. If familial and societal limitations in fact do "affect the actualization of the infant's life quality potential," then they are rightful elements in the benefit/burden calculus concerning that unique patient's total best interests.[5]

At this point two cautions need to be raised concerning the adoption of any projected quality of the patient's life as the basis on which treatment or nontreatment hinges. Note first that a "caution," even if found telling, is not synonymous with an argument against the ethical validity of the quality of the patient's life approach to decision making. However, in the realm of public policy, such cautions may lend themselves to the adoption of a tighter legal boundary than ethics, other things being equal, would sanction.

1. The most practical, case-related caution with regard to any quality of life medical ethic concerns the difficulty of translating what Andre Hellegers called religiously-rooted criterion into "biological criteria like signs, symptoms, IQs or lab results."[6] If one accepts relational potential as the measure of a life minimally worth prolonging from the patient's best interest perspective, as Varga, Childress, Beauchamp, Keyserlingk, McCormick, Paris, Nelson, Dedek, Zachary, E. Mahoney, Jonsen, and Garland tend to do, what anatomical standard will be used to declare a patient devoid of such potential? Surely, as Johnson and Arras define relationality in functional terms, it is intimately connected to the mental activity of one's brain, particularly of the midbrain (gray matter) and frontal lobes (neocortex). What neurological tests and devices are available to measure brain activity and, even more importantly, what level of neuronal function is essential for a child to have the minimal ability to relate with one's environment, especially with significant human others?

First of all, it must be acknowledged that medicine is a scientific art, not pure technology. As "applied" science, its diagnoses and prognoses are at best guesstimates, imprecise determinations of what probably is and projections of what might be in the future. To project the mental capacities essential to sustain relational potential in any patient suffering brain damage or dysfunction is extremely risky and "if" laden, particularly in early infancy. According to the President's Commission much of the difficulty in these cases arises from factual uncertainty. For many premature infants and for some of those with serious congenital defects, the only certainty is that without intensive care they are unlikely to survive. Little is known about how each individual will fare with treatment. "Neonatology is too new a field to allow accurate predictions of which babies will survive and of the complications, handicaps, and potentials that the survivors might have."[7]

In a 1979 article dealing with medical measurement of brain functions, physician Barbara Manroe noted that presently "we cannot measure cognitive functions in the newborn period because we have no techniques for doing so." She suggested that we can only make predictions based on "the correlation of perinatal insults and functioning at later follow-up."[8] For example, a maturationally slow or premature infant may appropriately have an intermittently flat EEG or exhibit no elicitable reflexes, which in an older patient might be diagnostic indicators of cortical death. So also, cerebral "insults" prior to or shortly after birth (hemorrhages, infarctions) may preclude future, as yet inoperative cognitional abilities, rather than causing immediately discernible functional loss. If Manroe's data is still accurate this input makes physiologically-based determination of one's brain capacity and future relational potential difficult to project in the neonatal period. Newborns in general are not "very" animated, responsive, or cognitively dynamic, despite parental pride and assertions to the contrary.[9] Symptomatic determinations, at birth or shortly thereafter, of an infant's mental potential for self-awareness or relationality are tentative at best. Therefore, the possibility of predicting whether a given neonate is or will be capable of human interaction is a guesstimate at best.

Still, relational potential, however vague, refers to the embodied ability of a given patient to ingest sensory input. Simple behavioral observation, confirmed by neurological and behavioral testing over the first weeks or months of life, should be able to discern at least if "no" potential at all exists—anencephaly, exencephaly, severe collateral brain damage, severe Trisomy 13 or 18, severe asphyxia-related or hemorrhage-related brain insult, or a "permanent vegetative state." The cases of patients with greater possibility for brain development should, on the level of functional potential alone, be given the benefit of the doubt. Barring the presence of severe irremediable pain, the prognosis for an extraordinarily burdensome course of treatment, and inordinate social burden for their families or society, treatment should be given to these patients. In the case of premature infants even more time is required for an accurate prognosis because most neurological tests cannot be successfully administered until at least four to six weeks following a normal 38 to 40 week gestation period. Jonsen and Garland rightly suggest that the decision to terminate care for an infant requires "sufficient time for observation, mature assessment, and parental involvement in the decision."[10] They assert that it is more ethical, although perhaps more agonizing, to terminate care after a period of time than to withhold resuscitative measures at the moment of birth. Decisions for nontreatment in many cases may emerge only after a number of months, when the infant's mental prognosis becomes more calculable and increasingly more apparent.

Projected quality of the patient's life proponents, especially those labeled restrictive interpreters, are not unmindful of these cautions when they adopt certain minimal functional abilities as the earmark of an experientially meaningful life and then seek physiologically-based confirmations. Conscious both of the potential fallibility of medical diagnosis/prognosis and also of difficulties in measuring a neonate's mental (i.e., relational) capacities with much accuracy, the authors labeled restrictive interpreters of a patient's quality of life call for "prudent and discerning judgment" in the patient's behalf.[11] When in doubt, presume relational potential! Still, their willingness to forge ahead, making some decisions for nontreatment on the basis of careful, conservative, prudential estimates of mental dysfunction and correlative lack of relational potential is founded on the assumption that failure to do so will lead to greater abuse in terms of well-intentioned vitalistic mandates for over-treatment.

2. It is interesting to note that Duff, Campbell, Shaw, Jonsen, Garland, Veatch, and Weir all allow, at least in theory, for the direct killing of neonatal patients selected for nontreatment, particularly if the nontreatment decision consigns them to a slow, painful, "inhumane" dying process. If intractably pained or permanently unconscious or excessively burdened by one's quality of life itself, merciful infanticide is set forth as a more humane next step as opposed to continued nursing care, possibly accompanied by the licit "desire" (not necessarily a moral intention) for an earlier death. Does the adoption of a projected quality of the patient's life standard, unrestricted by means causation, necessarily lend itself to a pro-euthanasia posture? Broader interpreter John Lorber and more restrictive proponent Richard McCormick think not.

Dr. Lorber, who is accused of practicing subtle, barely veiled, "indirect infanticide" through his removal of nutritional support from those spina bifida infants selected out for nontreatment, rejects direct infanticide based on the wedge or slippery slope argument. If legalized, active euthanasia could become "a dangerous weapon in the hands of the State or ignorant or unscrupulous individuals."[12] Presumably then, if active infanticide were practiced only by wise, scrupulous caretakers, it would not be categorically immoral. Only the utilitarian potential for misuse and abuse seems to lead Lorber to exclude it from the nontreatment arsenal.

Richard McCormick likewise rejects direct infanticide, though his rationale for this "practically absolute" prohibition is not altogether clear.[13] If the obligation to sustain life rests ultimately on that life's experiential meaning and relational potential for the patient, it could be suggested to McCormick that once such meaning or potential ceases, there would be no essential reason to differentiate between nontreatment and direct dispatch. In fact, the latter might be preferable out of respect for the lingering person's eternal destiny and to save the patient's family futile expense and mental anguish.

Fellow Jesuit John Mahoney suggests that this is the potential danger inherent in a quality of life standard based so heavily on relational potential, rather than a sanctity of life standard that sees the obligation to treat grounded in essential personhood, irrespective of functional ability or potential. He asserts that regardless of one's experiential ability to relate with others, that patient remains a child of God, of one's family and society, and therefore a person with the rights to life and equitable treatment. Mahoney concludes, "Only if there is more to man than human relationship potential can one use that potential to justify letting die without also justifying killing."[14]

I suggest that both the contemporary ordinary/extraordinary means proponents as well as quality of the patient's life advocates like McCormick do espouse an inherent right to life and to treatment for each and every newborn, irrespective of handicaps. However, the introduction of the principle of Totality implies that such a prima facie interest in treatment may be waived if the experiential, relational, and spiritual purposes for which one is alive have ceased or are irremediably short-circuited by pain or suffering. To forego treatment based on the lack of relational potential, as an expression of inordinate burden or of "the flame not being worth the candle," is not contingent upon a denial of essential personhood as Mahoney presumes.

Assuming then that a severely handicapped newborn, even one intractably pained or with no measurable relational potential, is still a rights-bearing person, one might still categorically defend his/her life right from directly intended assaults, either by acts of commission or omission, without necessarily mandating aggressive therapy to prolong life at such a burdened or minimal level. Thus, contemporary ordinary/extraordinary means supporters allow patients to die via nontreatment, while categorically condemning direct euthanasia. It would seem that McCormick is appropriating this same rationale, though his adoption of a proportionalist approach to the discussion of direct killing makes the distinction between direct and indirect "means" less airtight, in some sense less compelling.[15]

It is this researcher's belief that the tenacity with which contemporary ordinary/extraordinary means proponents like Warren Reich and Leonard Weber hold to the language of "means related," even in the cases in which the use of life-saving or life-sustaining means serve only to perpetuate an already inordinately burdened life, bespeaks their subtle, perhaps subconscious realization that with the open admission that the extraordinary burden may be one's quality of life itself, direct infanticide becomes at least arguably a humane action to relieve the nontreated non-terminal patient who lingers on. By linking the decision to the use of proposed means, even when such means neither cause nor increase one's already tragically burdened quality of life, at least one can claim to be dealing only with the nontreatment option vis-à-vis the means being contemplated.

A logical case can be made, based on acceptance of the principle of Totality, that in a few, rare cases of excessively burdened non-dying patients, direct infanticide would seem to be more humane, more patient-centered than merely ceasing treatment, allowing the patient to linger in such a hopeless or pathetic condition. Boston College ethicist Lisa Sowle Cahill develops this cautious pro-euthanasia rationale in two separate *Linacre Quarterly* articles, in which she argues that Pius XII's absolute deontological prohibition of euthanasia is inconsistent with his strong concern for the principle of Totality.[16] Short of social utilitarian or consequentialistic fears of societal abuse, Cahill suggests that one would be hard pressed to categorically reject some rare, perhaps even theoretical allowance of active infanticide, once one accepts quality of life determinations based on the principle of Totality.

The caution raised here concerning a quality of life approach to decisions to forego treatment is that the same projected qualities or lack thereof, which allow for withholding or withdrawing treatment, can likewise be argued as grounds to move from nontreatment to directly intended killing. The subsequent question is whether such active killing is always and everywhere wrong. Granting the long-range potential for abuse, is the active taking of an inordinately pained or mentally "meaningless" life intrinsically immoral?

In summary, a projected quality of the patient's life approach to treatment/nontreatment decision making seems to best synthesize the logic underlying all patient-centered benefit/burden calculus. If the patient remains the quasi-exclusive focus of these decisions, what quality of the patient's life constitutes an existence so excessively burdened that the total best interests of the patient would be better served by nontreatment? Beware familial selfishness and a bourgeois bias against valid stewardship responsibilities. Beware mandating treatment on a patient solely on the basis of one's functional potential, as if s/he is not affected both by other physiological and psychological burdens as well as by the fortunes and foibles of one's family and society. Lastly, beware of premature medical prognoses. Contrary to the old cliché, time does not heal all wounds . . . or handicaps. But time does allow for fuller medical diagnoses and more accurate prognoses of the patient's personal potential. When in doubt as to the level of burden or of a newborn's potential, better to err on the side of continued life and time. Nontreatment decisions can be made beyond the neonatal period too. There is no need to rush to a precipitous judgment. Projecting the functional and social quality of a patient's life requires careful, self-effacing, prudential, patient-centered determinations.

Notes

1. President's Commission, *Deciding to Forego Life-Sustaining Treatment* (Washington, D.C.: U.S. Government Printing Office, 1983), pp. 7, 205, 228–229; Paul Johnson, "Selective Nontreatment of Defective Newborns," *Linacre Quarterly*

47 (February 1980), pp. 42, 46–47; Albert Jonsen and Michael Garland, "A Moral Policy for Life/Death Decisions in the Intensive Care Nursery," in *Ethics of Newborn Intensive Care* (Berkeley: University of California Institute of Governmental Studies, 1976), p. 155; Albert Jonsen et al., "Critical Issues in Newborn Intensive Care," *Pediatrics* 53 (1975), pp. 756, 764; Philip R. Lee and Diane Dooley, "Social Services for the Disabled Child," in *Ethics of Newborn Intensive*, eds. Jonsen and Garland, pp. 64–74; Philip R. Lee, Albert R. Jonsen, and Diane Dooley, "Social and Economic Factors Affecting Public Policy and Decision Making in the Care of the Defective Newborn," in *Decision-making and the Defective Newborn*, ed. Chester A. Swinyard, pp. 315–331; Eunice K. Shriver, "The Challenge of the Mentally Retarded," in *Medical Moral Problems*, ed. Robert Heyer (New York: Paulist Press, 1976), pp. 1–5.

2. Johnson, "Selective Nontreatment of Defective Newborns," p. 47.

3. John Arras, "Toward an Ethic of Ambiguity" *Hastings Center Report* 14(April 1984), p. 28.

4. McCormick, "Proxy Consent in the Experimentation Situation," in *How Brave a New World?* p. 63; McCormick, "Sharing in Sociality: Children and Experimentation," in *How Brave a New World?* pp. 87–98.

5. Johnson, "Selective Nontreatment and Spina Bifida," pp. 94, 103–105.

6. Andre Hellegers, "Letting Deformed Newborns Die — McCormick's Approach," Unpublished Paper, Kennedy Institute File 20-5.2 (May 1974), pp. 3–4.

7. President's Commission, *Deciding to Forego,* p. 220.

8. Barbara L. Manroe, "Ethical and Legal Considerations In Decision-Making For Newborns," *Perkins School of Theology Journal* 32 (Summer 1979), p. 5.

9. Interview with Dr. Anne Fletcher, Director NICU, Children's Hospital National Medical Center, Washington, D.C., 16 January 1984.

10. Jonsen and Garland, "A Moral Policy," p. 154; Jonsen et al., "Critical Issues in Newborn Intensive Care," p. 764.

11. President's Commission, *Deciding to Forego,* p. 223; see also McCormick, "To Save or Let Die—A Rejoinder," *America* 131 (October 5, 1974), p. 171.

12. John Lorber, "Early Results of Selective Treatment of Spina Bifida Cystica," *British Medical Journal* 277 (1973), p. 204; see also John Lorber, "Selective Treatment of Myelomeningocele," *Pediatrics* 53 (1974), p. 308; John Lorber, "Ethical Problems in the Management of Myelomeningocele and Hydrocephalus," *Journal of the Royal College of Physicians* 10 (October 1975), pp. 57–58.

13. Richard A. McCormick, "Notes on Moral Theology: 1972," *Theological Studies* 34 (March 1973), pp. 70–74; appears in 1981 compilation, pp. 440–444. In 1973, McCormick rebutted Daniel Maguire's pro-euthanasia stance with a then consequentialistic form of his proportionalism methodology. He asserted that conventional wisdom defends the "convergence of probabilities" that in the practical order the basic human value of life would be threatened or compromised by allowing direct euthanasia of permanently comatose or intractably pained infants and others.

14. John Mahoney, S.J. "McCormick on Medical Ethics," *Month* 14 (December 1981), pp. 410–411.

15. Lisa Sowle Cahill, "Within Shouting Distance: Paul Ramsey and Richard McCormick on Method," *Journal of Medicine and Philosophy* 4 (1979), pp. 398–417,

esp. 412–413: It is Cahill's conviction that McCormick's "practically absolute" prohibition of all direct euthanasia rests on shaky ground once long-term consequences (i.e., slippery slope fears) give way to proportionate validating reasons in the best interests of the suffering or mindless infant. If an infant's pain cannot be held at bay or if s/he is fundamentally incapable of relating with others, might not death, which is not an absolute evil in itself, be welcomed or even caused in the patient's total best interest? As Cahill states her challenge to McCormick, "If proportion justifies killing as a nonmoral evil, then an absolute prohibition against direct euthanasia is possible only if the reason specified (relief of suffering) *never* justifies killing" (p. 413). If embodied life is a relative value, then Cahill finds it difficult to argue that an "intrinsic disproportion" always exists between life and all other goods of the patient.

16. Lisa Sowle Cahill, "A 'Natural Law' Reconsideration of Euthanasia" *Linacre Quarterly* 44 (February 1977), pp. 47–63; Lisa Sowle Cahill, "Comments on Euthanasia," *Linacre Quarterly* 44 (November 1977), pp. 299–300; Lisa Sowle Cahill, "Euthanasia: Continuing the Conversation," *Linacre Quarterly* 48 (August 1981), pp. 243–245.

THE PERMANENTLY
UNCONSCIOUS PATIENT

16

Position of the American Academy of Neurology on Certain Aspects of the Care and Management of the Persistent Vegetative State Patient

American Academy of Neurology

I. The persistent vegetative state is a form of eyes-open permanent unconsciousness in which the patient has periods of wakefulness and physiological sleep/wake cycles, but at no time is the patient aware of him- or herself or the environment. Neurologically, being awake but unaware is the result of a functioning brainstem and the total loss of cerebral cortical functioning.

A. No voluntary action or behavior of any kind is present. Primitive reflexes and vegetative functions that may be present are either controlled by the brainstem or are so elemental that they require no brain regulation at all.

Although the persistent vegetative state patient is generally able to breathe spontaneously because of the intact brainstem, the capacity to chew and swallow in a normal manner is lost because these functions are voluntary, requiring intact cerebral hemispheres.

B. The primary basis for the diagnosis of persistent vegetative state is the careful and extended clinical observation of the patient, supported by laboratory studies. Persistent vegetative state patients will show no behavioral response whatsoever over an extended period of time. The diagnosis of permanent unconsciousness can usually be made with a high degree of medical certainty in cases of hypoxic-ischemic encephalopathy after a period of 1 to 3 months.

C. Patients in a persistent vegetative state

"Position of the American Academy of Neurology on Certain Aspects of the Care and Management of the Persistent Vegetative State Patient" by the American Academy of Neurology in Neurology 39(January, 1989):125–126. Reprinted with permission of the Executive Office of the American Academy of Neurology and the Editor in Chief of Neurology.

may continue to survive for a prolonged period of time ("prolonged survival") as long as the artificial provision of nutrition and fluids is continued. These patients are not "terminally ill."

D. Persistent vegetative state patients do not have the capacity to experience pain or suffering. Pain and suffering are attributes of consciousness requiring cerebral cortical functioning, and patients who are permanently and completely unconscious cannot experience these symptoms.

There are several independent bases for the neurological conclusion that persistent vegetative state patients do not experience pain or suffering.

First, direct clinical experience with these patients demonstrates that there is no behavioral indication of any awareness of pain or suffering.

Second, in all persistent vegetative state patients studied to date, postmortem examination reveals overwhelming bilateral damage to the cerebral hemispheres to a degree incompatible with consciousness or the capacity to experience pain or suffering.

Third, recent data utilizing positron emission tomography indicates that the metabolic rate for glucose in the cerebral cortex is greatly reduced in persistent vegetative state patients, to a degree incompatible with consciousness.

II. The artificial provision of nutrition and hydration is a form of medical treatment and may be discontinued in accordance with the principles and practices governing the withholding and withdrawal of other forms of medical treatment.

A. The Academy recognizes that the decision to discontinue the artificial provision of fluid and nutrition may have special symbolic and emotional significance for the parties in-

volved and for society. Nevertheless, the decision to discontinue this type of treatment should be made in the same manner as other medical decisions, ie, based on a careful evaluation of the patient's diagnosis and prognosis, the prospective benefits and burdens of the treatment, and the stated preferences of the patient and family.

B. The artificial provision of nutrition and hydration is analogous to other forms of life-sustaining treatment, such as the use of the respirator. When a patient is unconscious, both a respirator and an artificial feeding device serve to support or replace normal bodily functions that are compromised as a result of the patient's illness.

C. The administration of fluids and nutrition by medical means, such as a G-tube, is a medical procedure, rather than a nursing procedure, for several reasons.

1. First, the choice of this method of providing fluid and nutrients requires a careful medical judgment as to the relative advantages and disadvantages of this treatment. Second, the use of a G-tube is possible only by the creation of a stoma in the abdominal wall, which is unquestionably a medical or surgical procedure. Third, once the G-tube is in place, it must be carefully monitored by physicians, or other health care personnel working under the direction of physicians, to insure that complications do not arise. Fourth, a physician's judgment is necessary to monitor the patient's tolerance of any response to the nutrients that are provided by means of the G-tube.

2. The fact that the placement of nutrients into the tube is itself a relatively simple process, and that the feeding does not require sophisticated mechanical equipment, does not mean that the provision of fluids and nutrition in this manner is a nursing rather than a medical procedure. Indeed, many forms of medical

treatment, including, for example, chemotherapy or insulin treatments, involve a simple self-administration of prescription drugs by the patient. Yet such treatments are clearly medical and their initiation and monitoring require careful medical attention.

D. In caring for hopelessly ill and dying patients, physicians must often assess the level of medical treatment appropriate to the specific circumstances of each case.

1. The recognition of a patient's right to self-determination is central to the medical, ethical, and legal principles relevant to medical treatment decisions.

2. In conjunction with respecting a patient's right to self-determination, a physician must also attempt to promote the patient's well-being, either by relieving suffering or addressing or reversing a pathological process. Where medical treatment fails to promote a patient's well-being, there is no longer an ethical obligation to provide it.

3. Treatments that provide no benefit to the patient or the family may be discontinued. Medical treatment that offers some hope for recovery should be distinguished from treatment that merely prolongs or suspends the dying process without providing any possible cure. Medical treatment, including the medical provision of artificial nutrition and hydration, provides no benefit to patients in a persistent vegetative state, once the diagnosis has been established to a high degree of medical certainty.

III. When a patient has been reliably diagnosed as being in a persistent vegetative state, and when it is clear that the patient would not want further medical treatment, and the family agrees with the patient, all further medical treatment, including the artificial provision of nutrition and hydration, may be forgone.

A. The Academy believes that this standard is consistent with prevailing medical, ethical, and legal principles, and more specifically with the formal resolution passed on March 15, 1986 by the Council on Ethical and Judicial Affairs of the American Medical Association, entitled "Withholding or Withdrawing Life-Prolonging Medical Treatment."

B. This position is consistent with the medical community's clear support for the principle that persistent vegetative state patients need not be sustained indefinitely by means of medical treatment.

While the moral and ethical views of health care providers deserve recognition, they are in general secondary to the patient's and family's continuing right to grant or to refuse consent for life-sustaining treatment.

C. When the attending physician disagrees with the decision to withhold all further medical treatment, such as artificial nutrition and hydration, and feels that such a course of action is morally objectionable, the physician, under normal circumstances, should not be forced to act against his or her conscience or perceived understanding of prevailing medical standards.

In such situations, every attempt to reconcile differences should be made, including adequate communication among all principal parties and referral to an ethics committee where applicable.

If no consensus can be reached and there appear to be irreconcilable differences, the health care provider has an obligation to bring to the attention of the family the fact that the patient may be transferred to the care of another physician in the same facility or to a different facility where treatment may be discontinued.

D. The Academy encourages health care providers to establish internal consultative procedures, such as ethics committees or other means, to offer guidance in cases of apparent irreconcilable differences. In May 1985, the Academy formally endorsed the voluntary formation of multidisciplinary institutional ethics committees to function as educational, policy-making, and advisory bodies to address ethical dilemmas arising within health care institutions.

IV. It is good medical practice to initiate the artificial provision of fluids and nutrition when the patient's prognosis is uncertain, and to allow for the termination of treatment at a later date when the patient's condition becomes hopeless.

A. A certain amount of time is required before the diagnosis of persistent vegetative state can be made with a high degree of medical certainty. It is not until the patient's complete unconsciousness has lasted a prolonged period —usually 1 to 3 months—that the condition can be reliably considered permanent. During the initial period of assessment and evaluation, it is usually appropriate to provide aggressive medical treatment to sustain the patient.

Even after it may be clear to the medical professionals that a patient will not regain con-

sciousness, it may still take a period of time before the family is able to accept the patient's prognosis. Once the family has had sufficient time to accept the permanence of the patient's condition, the family may then be ready to terminate whatever life-sustaining treatments are being provided.

B. The view that there is a major medical or ethical distinction between the withholding and withdrawal of medical treatment belies common sense and good medical practice, and is inconsistent with prevailing medical, ethical, and legal principles.

C. Given the importance of an adequate trial period of observation and therapy for unconscious patients a family member must retain the ability to withdraw consent for continued artificial feedings well after initial consent has been provided. Otherwise, consent will have been sought for a permanent course of treatment before the hopelessness of the patient's condition has been determined by the attending physician and is fully appreciated by the family.

Adopted by the Executive Board,
American Academy of Neurology,
April 21, 1988, Cincinnati, Ohio.

17

Feeding and Hydrating the Permanently Unconscious and Other Vulnerable Persons

William E. May, Robert Barry, O.P.,
Msgr. Orville Griese, Germain Grisez,
Brian Johnstone, C.Ss.R.,
Thomas J. Marzen,
Bishop James T. McHugh, S.J.D.,
Gilbert Meilaender, Mark Siegler,
and Msgr. William Smith

Recent court cases (such as those involving Claire Conroy, Paul Brophy, and Nancy Ellen Jobes) have called attention to the moral and legal questions concerning the provision by tube of food and fluids to the permanently unconscious (e.g., those diagnosed as being in a "persistent vegetative state") and other seriously debilitated but nondying persons. Is it ever morally right to withhold or withdraw such nutrition and hydration? If so, on what grounds? And what should be the role of law?

Before answering these questions, we think it necessary to state several crucially important presuppositions and principles relevant to the subject and also to reject a rationale offered by some ethicists—and apparently accepted by most courts—for withholding or withdrawing food and fluids provided by tubes from the

"Feeding and Hydrating the Permanently Unconscious and Other Vulnerable Persons" by William E. May et al. Reprinted by permission of the publisher Issues in Law & Medicine, Vol. 3 No. 3, Winter, 1987, pp. 203–211. Copyright © 1987 by the National Legal Center for the Medically Dependent & the Disabled, Inc.

permanently unconscious and other seriously
debilitated but nondying persons.

Presuppositions and Principles

1. Human bodily life is a great good. Such
   life is personal, not subpersonal. It is a
   good *of* the person, not merely *for* the
   person. Such life is inherently good, not
   merely instrumental to other goods.
2. It is never morally right to deliberately
   kill innocent human beings—that is, to
   adopt by choice and carry out a proposal to end their lives. (We here set
   aside questions about killing those who
   are not "innocent," i.e., those convicted of capital crimes, engaged in unjust military actions, or otherwise unjustly attacking others.)
3. It is possible to kill innocent persons by
   acts of omission as well as by acts of
   commission. Whenever the failure to
   provide adequate food and fluids carries out a proposal, adopted by choice,
   to end life, the omission of nutrition
   and hydration is an act of killing by
   omission.
4. The deliberate killing of the innocent,
   even if motivated by an anguished or
   merciful wish to terminate painful and
   burdened life—deliberate killing that
   will henceforth be called "euthanasia"
   —is not morally justified by that
   motive.
5. Like other killing of the innocent, euthanasia can be carried out by acts of
   omission ("passive euthanasia") as well
   as by acts of commission ("active euthanasia"). The distinction makes no
   moral difference.
6. Euthanasia can be voluntary (of a person who gives informed consent to being killed), nonvoluntary (of a person
   incapable of giving informed consent),
   or involuntary (of a person capable of
   giving informed consent who does not
   give it).
7. Morally, for a person who consents to
   be killed, voluntary euthanasia is a
   method of suicide. Nonvoluntary and
   involuntary euthanasia violate not only
   the dignity of innocent human life but
   also the right of the person who is killed
   not to be killed. The law of homicide
   should continue to apply to all forms
   and methods of euthanasia; none
   should be legalized. The law of homicide, in particular, must protect innocent human beings from being killed for
   reasons of mercy.
8. While competent persons have the
   moral and legal right to refuse any useless or excessively burdensome treatment, they must exercise great care in
   reaching the judgment that a treatment
   is useless or excessively burdensome.
   This is necessary both in order to avoid
   any intention to end life on the grounds
   that it is devoid of intrinsic worth and in
   order to fulfill properly the responsibility to respect human life.
9. Likewise, those who have the moral
   duty to make decisions for noncompetent persons (such as infants or the permanently unconscious) have a moral
   right to refuse any useless or excessively
   burdensome treatment for them. This
   right must, however, be exercised with
   great care in order to avoid the temptation, unfortunately not uncommon in
   our society, to devalue the lives of the

noncompetent or to regard such persons chiefly in terms of the utilitarian values they may represent. Too often, unfortunately, the judgment that a treatment is useless or excessively burdensome does not reflect serious consideration of the objectively discernible features of the treatment, but is an expression of attitudes toward the life being treated. Moreover, a sound public policy to protect the rights and interests of noncompetent persons and to promote the common good may require regulation by law of the scope of treatment decisions made by families and other proxies (*cf.* the federal "Child Abuse Amendments of 1984").

10. Human life can be burdened in many ways. But no matter how burdened it may be, human life remains inherently a good of the person. Thus, remaining alive is never rightly regarded as a burden, and deliberately killing innocent human life is never rightly regarded as rendering a benefit.

Contemporary Threats to the Dignity of Innocent Human Life

Some today morally approve and seek the legalization of euthanasia, both active and passive, voluntary and nonvoluntary. (At present, public advocacy of involuntary euthanasia is rare.)

One argument for euthanasia is based on the claim that competent persons have a right to be killed mercifully—a "right to die"—when they think that they would be better off dead than alive.

Another argument for euthanasia is based

on the claim that competent persons can refuse all treatment and may choose to do so precisely in order to end their own lives. Assuming or claiming that it is justifiable to refuse treatment on this basis, some proponents of euthanasia argue that ending life with another's help through "active" euthanasia often would be quicker and easier than choosing death through "passive" euthanasia.

Some proponents of euthanasia employ dehumanizing language to support their proposal that noncompetent persons should be killed when their lives are judged by others to be valueless or excessively burdensome. Those to be killed often are defined as nonpersons or are called "vegetables." Some in poor but stable and nonterminal conditions are reclassified as "terminal." Others are defined as "brain dead," even though some spontaneous functioning of the brain persists and the strict clinical criteria for declaring brain death are not verified.

Certain people claim to oppose euthanasia and do not advocate killing by acts of commission, but nevertheless support the view that treatment may rightly be withheld or withdrawn from noncompetent, nonterminal persons simply because their lives are thought by others to be valueless or excessively burdensome. Adopting this rationale, and accepting the assumption that life itself can be useless or an excessive burden, some American ethicists, physicians, and courts have judged that food and fluids may rightly be withheld or withdrawn from persons who are not terminally ill because they are permanently unconscious or otherwise seriously debilitated.

However, withholding or withdrawing food and fluids *on this rationale* is morally wrong because it is euthanasia by omission. The withholding or withdrawing of food and fluids carries out the proposal, adopted by choice, to end someone's life because that life itself is judged by others to be valueless or excessively burdensome. Moreover, the withholding or withdrawing of food and fluids *on this rationale* should be judged to violate fundamental principles of American law and equity, since it explicitly sanctions status-based discrimination—i.e., discrimination based on the debilitated physical or mental condition of the person. Such discrimination becomes a new basis for deliberate killing by omission—killing that is not justified by the plain language of applicable statutory or constitutional law.

It is cause for very great alarm that some influential physicians, ethicists, and courts have adopted this rationale for withholding or withdrawing food and fluids—and other means of preserving life—from some persons. For in adopting this rationale, they approve and legally sanction euthanasia by omission—deliberate killing—in these cases. In order to prevent the sanctioning, even if unintended, of killing the innocent, everyone with relevant competence—especially ethicists, religious teachers, lawyers, jurists, physicians, and other health care personnel—must repudiate the withholding or withdrawal of food and fluids on this rationale.

If it becomes entrenched practice to kill by omission certain sorts of persons whose condition is very poor and whose lives are judged by others no longer to be worth living, then this method of killing surely will be extended to many other persons. Most of the cases that have attracted attention thus far have involved the very severely brain damaged—those who are permanently unconscious, severely damaged by strokes, in advanced stages of dementia due to Alzheimer's or another disease, and

so on. But the various sorts of damage, defect, debility, and handicap that burden human lives occur in myriad degrees, so that there are always more and less severe cases differing from one another only by degree. Unfortunately, it is not difficult to imagine a future America in which human life may itself be judged excessively burdensome for all persons who cannot care for themselves and have no one willing and able to care for them. Since dying of thirst and starvation can often be slow, very painful, and disfiguring, the demand will inevitably follow that death be hastened by lethal overdose or injection. Thus, ironically, the purportedly "dignified death" of those who die from dehydration and malnutrition would occasion demands for deliberate killing by commission because of the indignity involved in such a death.

The Use of Tubes to Provide Food and Hydration for the Permanently Unconscious and Other Seriously Ill Persons

Providing food and fluids to noncompetent individuals such as infants and the unconscious is, except under extraordinary circumstances, a grave duty. The Second Vatican Council invoked a longstanding tradition of the Church Fathers when it urged individuals and governments: "Feed the man dying of hunger, because if you do not feed him you have killed him" (*Gaudium et spes,* n. 69). Deliberately to deny food and water to such innocent human beings in order to bring about their deaths is homicide, for it is the adoption by choice of a proposal to kill them by starvation and dehydration. Such killing can never be morally right and ought never to be legalized. It follows that it is never right and ought never to be legally permitted to withhold food and fluids from the permanently unconscious or from others who are seriously debilitated (e.g., with strokes, Alzheimer's disease, Lou Gehrig's disease, organic brain syndrome, or AIDS dementia) as a means of securing their deaths.

However, when specific objective conditions are met, the withholding and withdrawing of various forms of treatment, including the provision of food and fluids by artificial means, do not necessarily carry out a proposal to end life. One may rightly choose to withhold or withdraw a means of preserving life if the means employed is judged either useless or excessively burdensome. It is most necessary to note that the judgment made here is *not* that the person's *life* is useless or excessively burdensome; rather, the judgment made is that the *means used to preserve life* is useless or excessively burdensome.

Traditionally, a treatment has been judged useless or relatively useless if the benefits it provides to a person are nil (useless in a strict sense) or are insignificant in comparison to the burdens it imposes (useless in a wider sense). Traditionally, a treatment has been judged excessively burdensome when whatever benefits it offers are not worth pursuing for one or more of several reasons: it is too painful, too damaging to the patient's bodily self and functioning, too psychologically repugnant to the patient, too restrictive of the patient's liberty and preferred activities, too suppressive of the patient's mental life, or too expensive.

An exhaustive examination of each of these factors is beyond the scope of this statement.

We stress, however, that moral certainty of excessive burdensomeness is required to justify foregoing nutrition or hydration. It is necessary, especially in the formulation of law and public policy, to identify with precision the circumstances in which nutrition and hydration may be legitimately foregone.

In judging whether treatment of a noncompetent person is excessively burdensome, one must be fair. Great care should be taken not to employ a double standard, by which consciously or unconsciously one attributes greater weight to burdens imposed by the treatment and less to benefits provided by it because the patient is cognitively impaired or physically debilitated. The logic of such a standard would lead to rationalizing the discriminatory withholding or withdrawing of care from anyone whose condition fails to meet some arbitrary norm for adequate quality of life.

Yet the damaged or debilitated condition of the patient has been the key factor taken into consideration in virtually all the recent court cases that have focused attention on the moral and legal questions concerning the provision by tube of food and fluids to permanently unconscious or other severely debilitated but nondying individuals. Decisions have been made to withdraw food and fluids not because continuing to provide them would be in itself excessively burdensome, but because sustaining life was judged to be no benefit to a person in such poor condition. These decisions have been unjust and, as noted above, they set a dangerous precedent for more extensive passive or even active euthanasia.

Nonetheless, *if it is really useless or excessively burdensome* to provide someone with nutrition and hydration, then these means may rightly be withheld or withdrawn, *provided* that this omission does not carry out a proposal to end the person's life, but rather is chosen to avoid the useless effort or the excessive burden of continuing to provide the food and fluids.

Plainly, when a person is imminently dying, a time often comes when it is really useless or excessively burdensome to continue hydration and nutrition, whether by tube or otherwise. But the question that concerns us is not about patients who are judged to be imminently dying, but rather about persons who are not.

In our judgment, feeding such patients and providing them with fluids by means of tubes is *not* useless in the strict sense because it does bring to these patients a great benefit, namely, the preservation of their lives and the prevention of their death through malnutrition and dehydration. We grant that provision of food and fluids by tubes or other means to such persons could become useless or futile if (a) the person in question is imminently dying, so that any effort to sustain life is futile, or (b) the person is no longer able to assimilate the nourishment or fluids thus provided. But unless these conditions are verified, it is unjust to claim that the provision of food and fluids is useless.

We recognize that provision of food and fluids by IVs and nasogastric tubes can have side-effects (e.g., irritation of the nasal passages, sore throats, collapsing of veins, etc.) that might become serious enough in particular cases to render their use excessively burdensome. But the experience of many physicians and nurses suggests that these side-effects are often transitory and capable of being ameliorated. Moreover, use of gastric tubes does not ordinarily cause the patient grave discomfort. There may be gas pains, diarrhea, or

nose and throat irritation, but ordinarily such discomforts are of passing nature and can be ameliorated. We thus judge that providing food and fluids to the permanently unconscious and other categories of seriously debilitated but nondying persons (e.g., those with strokes or Alzheimer's disease) does not ordinarily impose excessive burdens by reason of pain or damage to bodily self and functioning. Psychological repugnance, restrictions on physical liberty and preferred activities, or harm to the person's mental life are not relevant considerations in the cases with which we are concerned.

The question remains whether providing food and water in this way to these patients is excessively burdensome because of its cost. At the outset we make two critical points. First, the cost of providing food and fluids by enteral tubes is not, in itself, excessive. Such feeding is generally no more costly than other forms of ordinary nursing care (such as cleaning or spoonfeeding a patient) or ordinary maintenance care (such as the maintenance of room temperature through heating or air conditioning). Second, one must also take into account the benefits that such care may provide both to the patient and to the caregivers.

It must be acknowledged that the care of persons in very poor but nonterminal condition, sometimes over a long time, can be quite costly when taken as a whole. For instance, the care of anyone who cannot eat and drink in a normal way requires not only tubal nutrition and hydration, but also a room, which must be supplied appropriately with heat and utilities, and regular nursing care to keep the patient clean, prevent bed sores, and so on. But these forms of care and maintenance are provided to many other classes of persons (e.g., those with severe mental illnesses or retardation, with other long-term disabilities, etc.). The "burdens" involved in each of these instances are similar to those involved in caring for nondying persons who cannot feed themselves.

Some of these patients (e.g., those suffering from strokes) might be cared for at home rather than in an institution; the regular provision of food and fluids by tube is usually not too difficult or complicated to be done by people without professional training if they are properly instructed and supervised. This is not to say that care of such patients, when feasible, is not costly in time and energy. Like care for a baby, it must be carried on constantly; and it may be more difficult in some cases because of the larger size of an adult body.

But such care is not without its benefits. Since it is necessary to sustain life, such care benefits the nondying patient by serving this fundamental personal good—human life itself —which, as we have explained, remains good in itself no matter how burdened it may become due to the patient's poor condition.

Moreover, caring for others expresses recognition of their personhood and responds appropriately to it. For example, care for a baby is the form parental love naturally takes; care for a helpless adult—family member, neighbor, or stranger—expresses compassion and humane appreciation of his or her dignity. It also offers the possibility to the caregiver of nurturing such noble qualities as mercy and compassion.

It is possible to imagine situations in which a society might reasonably consider it too burdensome to continue to care for its helpless members. For example, in some very harsh environments, natural disasters, and war situations, the more able can be forced to make hard choices between caring for themselves (and their children) and providing life-sustaining care for those who are gravely disabled and helpless. However, our society is by no means in such straitened circumstances—in the aftermath of nuclear destruction we may face such a situation, but we are surely not facing one now.

Some Americans might prefer to abandon to death those who require long term care at public or private expense. But comparing the costs of care with its benefits, only one who sets aside the Golden Rule will consider excessively burdensome the provision by our society of life-sustaining care to all its members who require it and can benefit from it. As the Catholic church stated in its 1981 Document for the International Year of Disabled Persons: "The respect, the dedication, the time and means required for the care of handicapped persons, even of those whose mental faculties are gravely affected, is the price that a society should generously pay in order to remain truly human." To withhold or withdraw from those in poor condition the elemental care they need to survive would be to decide that our society no longer values its members insofar as they are persons with dignity—that is, with inherent value independent of what they can do and contribute—but only insofar as they are useful, or so long as their lives have sufficient "quality."

We thus conclude that, in the ordinary circumstances of life in our society today, it is not morally right, nor ought it to be legally permissible, to withhold or withdraw nutrition and hydration provided by artificial means to the permanently unconscious or other categories of seriously debilitated but nonterminal persons. Rather, food and fluids are universally

18

The PVS Patient and the Forgoing/Withdrawing of Medical Nutrition and Hydration

Thomas A. Shannon
James J. Walter

Over the last several decades modern medicine has progressed at a rate that has astonished even its practitioners. Developments in drugs, vaccines, and various technologies have given physicians an incredible amount of success over disease and morbidity, as well as allowing them to make dramatic interventions into the body to repair or replace a problematic system or organ. Yet there are limits we are coming to recognize slowly and only reluctantly. For even many of our best technologies are only halfway technologies, i.e. the technology or intervention compensates for a function but cannot cure the underlying pathology or correct the damaged organ. The respirator is probably the most frequently encountered example of this phenomenon.

Another intervention is our capacity to pro-

vide nutrition and hydration to those in a persistent vegetative state (PVS). For long-term feeding of such individuals, a gastrostomy tube is inserted directly into the stomach and the liquid protein diet is delivered in a controlled fashion by a pump. If the individual is reasonably healthy and other reflexes are intact, the life expectancy may be several decades.[1] The PVS will not be cured, and the liquid protein serves to maintain the status quo. The question of how to treat these patients medically is now heavily debated nationally and internationally.

In this essay we will examine the issue in several ways: (1) report on a survey of the U.S. hierarchy on bioethics committees in general and on forgoing or withdrawing nutrition and hydration in particular; (2) propose a struc-

"The PVS Patient and the Forgoing/Withdrawing of Medical Nutrition and Hydration" by Thomas A. Shannon and James J. Walter. Reprinted with permission of Theological Studies 49(December, 1988):623–647.

tured argument which includes a reconceptualization of "quality of life" judgments; and (3)
offer suggestions for the future conduct of this
debate.

A Survey of the U.S. Hierarchy

General Analysis

In January of 1988 one of the authors (TAS)
developed a brief questionnaire which sought
information on two broad areas: (1) Were
there diocesan bioethics committees and, if so,
what was their composition etc.? (2) Did dioceses have specific policies on the issue of nutrition and hydration?[2]

One hundred and sixty-seven questionnaires
were sent to the ordinaries of the U.S. dioceses. Seventy-eight ordinaries responded. Of
these, 62 indicated that there was no diocesan
bioethics committee; 16 indicated the existence of such a committee, and of these, 7 sent
in detailed information which will be evaluated separately below.

Of those indicating no diocesan committee,
8 said that there were committees at local
Catholic hospitals. Another 8 identified a specific individual within the diocese to whom
the ordinary turned for assistance. Another 3
indicated the formation of such a committee,
either on a diocesan or on a state level. One
respondent stated there was an inoperative
committee.

The survey then asked for a description of
the membership of the committee, frequency
of meetings, its role, whether or not there were
guidelines, and how it functioned within the
diocese. Committee size ranged from 9 to 23
members, which allowed for a good representa-
tion of professions, typically including hospital
administrators, physicians, nurses, chaplains,

ethicists, lawyers, and other theologians. Six of
the committees met monthly, 2 bimonthly,
and 1 as needed. Three respondents said their
role was to set policy, 2 were to be advisory,
and 1 was to be primarily educational. Two
respondents had no guidelines, and 9 indicated
some form of guidelines ranging from church
teachings on medical issues to specific pro-
nouncements of the hierarchy over the past
decade.

Part 2 of the survey focused specifically on
the moral evaluation of feeding tubes. Of the
78 answering, 17 made no comment on Part 2,
37 made some comments, and 22 respondents
reported no cases of PVS patients in their
diocese.

Nine respondents reported knowledge of
PVS patients within their dioceses. Of those 9,
8 reported figures ranging from 1 to 4–5 per
year, and 1 respondent indicated 10 cases in
the past year. Eight committees were asked to
consider cases and 11 had not been asked. Additionally, 4 respondents reported that they
have specific guidelines they follow in such instances and 8 indicated that they have none.

The survey asked if the committee considered feeding tubes to be a medical technology.
Six said yes, 4 said no, 8 gave no answer, and 1
said "it depends." The respondents were then
asked if they considered the use of such feeding tubes to be routine care. Six said yes, 4 said
no, 8 gave no answer, and 1 said "it depends."
The next question was whether the removal of
a feeding tube from a PVS patient was ordinary
or extraordinary, or if they had no position.
Four responded that the care was ordinary, 4
that it was extraordinary, 1 had no position, 9
gave no answer, and 9 said "it depends." The
final question asked whether removal was an
act of involuntary euthanasia which is direct
and forbidden, or indirect and permitted, or
no position. Four responded that removal was

direct, 5 that it was indirect, 2 had no position, 4 said "it depends," and 8 had no answer.

Before turning to an analysis of the seven detailed responses (Documents A–G), we would like to make a few general observations about the data so far.

Given the seriousness of contemporary bioethical questions and their pervasiveness within society, it is surprising that so few dioceses have these committees or that so few local Catholic hospitals were indicated as having one. While neither seeking to bureaucratize all life nor to reject appropriate patient and family autonomy, nonetheless such committees on a diocesan or state level serve a useful function, minimally by providing workshops or other resources to hospitals or other groups in the diocese. Of those that are in place, the composition is well represented from a disciplinary perspective, and the committees meet with appropriate regularity. The committees appear to be accessible and, while maintaining patient privacy and confidentiality, there is some degree of openness in the committees.

Part 2 of the questionnaire provides more interesting data. Nine committees had cases brought to them; taken together, they had a moderately large number of cases, about 45. Six committees considered feeding tubes to be a medical technology and also routine care, 4 thought they were not a medical technology, and 1 did not consider them routine care. One committee was uncertain in each case. Yet of these committees, only 4 thought that feeding tubes were ordinary means whose removal constituted active euthanasia.

Four committees considered the technology ordinary and 4 judged it to be extraordinary. Four thought their removal to be direct euthanasia, while 5 considered it passive euthanasia. But even more interesting is that 9 committees thought that the placing of the technology into the ordinary/extraordinary categories depended on the individual circumstances of the case, and 8 thought the same thing about the determination of active or passive euthanasia. This suggests substantial ambiguity about the moral status of feeding technologies for PVS patients.

First, there is a difference over whether the procedure is a medical technology. If a technology, its moral evaluation fits conceptually more easily into the traditional format of ordinary/extraordinary means. If not, one might have to structure the argument differently. Most interesting are the differences in perception between whether the therapy is considered ordinary or extraordinary means, on the one hand, and whether its forgoing/withdrawal is morally evaluated as direct or indirect euthanasia, on the other. This interest is compounded when combined with the additional judgment—on the part of 9 and 8 respondents respectively—that such a determination "depends" on the circumstances. Such evaluations suggest room for various analyses of the problem and the possible moral acceptability of several resolutions.

Analysis of Specific Guidelines

Seven respondents sent more detailed information about committee make-up and the by-laws governing these committees. We will discuss each document in some detail, but, to maintain a promised confidentiality, we will simply refer to these documents as A–G.

Document A suggests that the primary locus for decision-making is the local hospital, with the diocesan or proposed state-wide committee serving as a resource. Yet part of the task of the proposed state-wide committee will be to develop guidelines for the local committee. At present, discussions are ongoing among committees but no consensus has been reached.

Document A affirms a presumption in favor of the use of feeding tubes but states that each case must be examined on its own merits. On the other hand, in very exceptional and extraordinary cases the withdrawal of feeding tubes might be passive and therefore permissible euthanasia. Thus, while removal of these tubes is exceptional, their removal is not prohibited. As the document states it, "each case must be considered on its own merits."

Document B represents the responses from three diocesan hospitals, since this diocese has no diocesan committee. B1 indicated that, while there have been cases, the committee did not meet as a committee on them. Rather, individual members of the committee served as resources to the medical staff and the families. This document stated that there is no consensus within the hospital about the issue, and so each case is to be examined on its own merits. The committee understands the practice as passive euthanasia and thus permissible, but also recognizes that there is no consistent position in the hospital.

We detect a problematic area in this document. B1 argues that feeding tubes might be withdrawn on the basis "that continued treatment *will result* in prolonged total dependence, persistent pain, or discomfort, or in a *persistent vegetative state*" (emphasis added). However, one wonders how the withdrawal of feeding tubes causes PVS. This technology is used to *support* patients in this condition; its administration does not *result* in PVS.

Document B2 states that their consultation has been on the placement of such technologies rather than on their withdrawal. Since it has no fixed policy, each case must be dealt with individually. Additionally, this committee considers tube feeding to be a medical technol-

ogy and can become an extraordinary means in specific cases "which must be individually assessed and reassessed." The decisions are to be considered in "light of the effect of this nutrition and/or the burden to the patient which would be experienced." Again, these decisions cannot be based on a broad application of a policy but must be made according to "case-specific evaluations."

Document B3 comes from an ethicist at a medical center which has no committee. The respondent indicates that conversations about this problem show that many individuals at the medical center have concerns about the issue. Tube feeding, in this individual's judgment, is a technology, but its moral significance resides in "its function in the ongoing treatment of the patient." Thus the central issue is: Does the treatment contribute to restoring life and health, or does it prolong the patient's dying? "If the former, I think it [is] routinely required. If the latter, I judge it foregoable, permissibly not obligatorily foregoable. . . . Tube feeding in some cases is proportionate, hence required, in others, disproportionate, hence not required."

Two other relevant comments were made by this hospital ethicist. First, can feeding tubes ever be withdrawn? If one can

admit that sometimes tubal feeding need not be *instituted*, then you are already describing conditions which might eventuate *within a case* which justify discontinuing tubal feeding. Put another way, a patient on tubal feeding might become the sort of patient you don't want to begin on tubal feeding. Since you need not start the intervention on the latter patient, why must you stay with it for the former one? (Emphasis in the original.)

Second, never starting or, once begun, removing the tubes is not an intending of death; rather, these decisions indicate that families "recognize and consent to (accept) a dying process which is judged irreversible and imminent."

The two common themes in these three documents from diocesan hospitals are a recognition of the ambiguities in the issue and a strong affirmation of a case-by-case evaluation. The more crucial moral elements are case-specific and determining the usefulness of the technology in relation to the condition of the patient. In addition, the suggestion to use the same criteria for not instituting the therapy and for withdrawing it is a helpful one and could aid in resolving several problems.

Document C is testimony to a state legislature on a natural-death act. At issue is the inclusion of a proviso for withholding feeding tubes in a living will. After a strong affirmation of the dignity, sanctity, and value of all human life, this document states: "The concern to affirm life, however, does not require the maintenance of physiological life by all means. It is recognized that aggressive overtreatment is as ethically unacceptable as is undertreatment. Both lack respect for the dignity and welfare of each person."

This testimony makes four points that lay out several issues very clearly.

1. A clear presumption in favor of life should be established. People who are able to eat, but only with assistance, cannot be discriminated against or be refused appropriate treatment.

2. The law should recognize the right of individuals to be allowed to die in circumstances where medical treatments, including nutrition and hydration, are ineffective or too burdensome for the patient.

3. The law must carefully define useless or ineffective treatment to clearly identify those treatments that offer no benefit of recovery or no relief of pain. The burdens associated with continued medical treatment should be defined in terms of the burdens that an individual experiences in pursuing the goals or ends of life and not defined by a level of invasiveness that may or may not be associated with forced feeding.

4. The clinical setting distinguishes between nutrition and hydration. Although both terms are used as though they are identical, it should be recognized that individuals may not require forced nutrition while still requiring hydration to alleviate thirst, provide comfort, relieve pain, or provide an open channel for IV medications.

Document C is very nuanced and makes careful distinctions. In particular, the document emphasizes the distinction between basic nutrition and hydration that requires time and effort on the part of medical personnel to feed the patient orally and the medical procedures that require total parenteral nutritional support (TPN) or invasive medical techniques to provide nutrition and hydration, e.g. insertion of gastrostomy tubes.

Document D comes from a research center whose writings and contributions were mentioned by many respondents as a source of guidance for their committees. Two major points are made. First, forgoing or withdrawing foods and fluids on the rationale of the "assumption that life itself can be useless or an excessive burden" is morally wrong because it is euthanasia by omission. This carries out the "proposal, adopted by choice, to end someone's life because that life itself is judged by others to be valueless or excessively burdensome." The crucial issues here are the moral intention of those who would withdraw the means of providing nutrition, on the one hand, and the justification for the argument adduced to support such a withdrawal, on the other. For this document, the intention is to end life, and the justification for so acting is that the life is burdensome or useless. This constitutes direct euthanasia.

Second, the forgoing/withdrawing of medically provided nutrition and hydration "do not necessarily carry out a proposal to end life." When certain conditions are met—"if the means employed is judged either useless or excessively burdensome"—one may forgo or withdraw treatment.

> Nonetheless, *if it is really useless or excessively burdensome* to provide someone with nutrition and hydration, then these means may rightly be withheld or withdrawn, *provided* that this omission does not carry out a proposal to end the person's life, but rather is chosen to avoid the useless effort or the excessive burden of continuing to provide the food and fluids. (Emphasis in the original.)

Two applications follow. If death is imminent, nutrition may become useless and burdensome, whether administered by tube or otherwise. On the other hand, if the patients are not dying, feeding provides a great benefit: "the preservation of their lives and the prevention of their death through malnutrition and dehydration." Yet even in this instance this treatment could become useless or futile: "(a)

if the person in question is imminently dying, so that any effort to sustain life is futile, or (b) the person is no longer able to assimilate the nourishment or fluids thus provided."

On the basis of this analysis, Document D concludes:

> We thus conclude that, in the ordinary circumstances of life in our society today, it is not morally right, nor ought it to be legally permissible, to withhold or withdraw nutrition and hydration provided by artificial means to the permanently unconscious or other categories of seriously debilitated but nonterminal persons. Food and fluids are universally needed for the preservation of life, and can generally be provided without the burdens and expense of more aggressive means of supporting life.

This document makes a strong argument in favor of such feeding based on the value of human life, the fact that such feeding can provide benefits to the patient and is not generally burdensome, and that the withdrawal of such technology many times includes the intention to end a person's life. Only when the individual is actually dying and/or cannot assimilate nourishment could the feeding be considered an extraordinary means.

Document E represents an advisory opinion of an archdiocese. This opinion bases its position on Pius XII's teaching on ordinary and extraordinary means, the *Declaration on Euthanasia* of the Congregation for the Doctrine of the Faith, and documents from the Committee for Pro-Life Activities of the National Conference of Catholic Bishops. Document E uses the standards of reasonable hope of success and a determination of excessive burdens as the criteria for decision-making. In addition, it recognizes and accepts the presumption of the use of medically providing nutrition and hydration for individuals.

The advisory opinion makes two statements of importance. The first concerns the decision to forgo or withdraw.

> It can hardly be denied that in certain circumstances artificial hydration and nutrition can be just as burdensome and useless as other means and under these circumstances would not be obligatory. A Catholic in good conscience can come to the conclusion that in a particular set of circumstances such treatment need not be initiated or continued, because it holds no hope that it will be successful in prolonging life or is unduly burdensome for oneself or another.

The second point concerns the intention involved in ending treatment. Document E argues that "even though the omission may shorten life, the intention is not to bring on death but to spare the patient a very burdensome treatment." These actions could constitute direct euthanasia if the intention is to end the life; but if omitted because they are too burdensome or useless in preserving life, "they do not constitute killing any more than any other such omission."

Document E uses the categories of ordinary and extraordinary means and then draws the conclusions that a decision to forgo or withdraw nutrition can be made in good conscience and that people should not be prevented from doing what is morally permissible. While the document does not encourage forgoing or withdrawal, neither does it prohibit such actions.

Document F supports the removal of nutrition and hydration within the context of the Catholic moral tradition that permits withdrawal of all medical technologies either on the basis that a patient has entered the dying phase or that the technologies are nonbeneficial or burdensome. These evaluations are moral as well as medical: "not what will the treatment do . . . , but will the treatment promote human activities and values."

> Merely maintaining biological life is not evaluated as being in and of itself humanly beneficial. Life is something more than biological existence. Life is a conditional value which couples biological existence with social, spiritual and human activities such as loving, praying, remembering, forgiving and experiencing. Life is all these things.

Consequently, when these activities can no longer be realized, there is no moral obligation to continue medical treatment, unless to relieve suffering. The conclusion that treatment can stop "does not mean that the person is worthless, but that the person has activated all human potential." Thus there is "no moral requirement to administer artificial nutrition and hydration. In fact it might be violating the person. . . ." Document F concludes on the interesting note that "people feel intuitively that it is wrong and want to find ways to escape imprisonment by technology."

Finally, Document G discusses this issue within the context of policies of life-sustaining treatment. The general context for thinking about this issue is:

> Prolonging physiological function by itself is not of value if it seems all potential for cognitive functions—mental creativity, the capacity to know and to love—if all that is irreversibly destroyed. Respect for life is at the heart of medicine, and a person in such a condition must not be put to death, but may be allowed to die.

The document then considers various forms of supportive care following the decision to allow to die. First, when medical procedures that prolong life are to be withheld or withdrawn, other medical procedures not directed to supportive care may also be omitted. These include, e.g., lab work, diagnostic procedures, dialysis, nutritional support by mouth or vein, or transfer to an ICU. Measures not to be omitted are "basic nursing care, including patient hygiene, adequate analgesia, oxygen for comfort, positioning, intake for comfort including intravenous hydration, and nutritional support as tolerated." The document then notes that there may be exceptions to hydration and nutritional support.

> Exceptions to the last two care elements do exist, especially when they offer no benefit or comfort to the patient. Intravenous hydration may not be appropriate when it prolongs or increases discomfort. With careful deliberation, nutritional support may be withheld when all three of the following conditions are present, namely: (1) The patient has a terminal condition that is irreversible in the final stages. (2) The patient is comatose and shows no clinical evidence of experiencing hunger or thirst. (3) The patient (or substitute decision-maker) has requested no further treatment. Other situations not meeting the above criteria for withdrawal of nutritional support care will be decided on a case-by-case basis.

Document G concludes that any treatments during this time of dying should aim at maintaining the dignity of the individual and providing compassion and comfort. The guidelines wisely state that the dying are more in need of comfort and company than treatment and diagnostic procedures.

These documents represent a range of opinions, arguments, and conclusions. All are carefully stated, clearly argued, and located squarely within the Catholic tradition. Yet different conclusions are drawn from this common heritage—which indicates that the debate is far from finished. There is strong preference for a case-by-case consideration of the issues and a reluctance to have fixed rules to decide cases. On the other hand, there is a recognition that some consensus needs to be developed. Finally, there is no enthusiasm or joy about the conclusion that forgoing or withdrawing is morally permissible. While the arguments are sound, the conclusion is reached with sadness and reluctance.

In the second part of this paper we turn to our own contribution to the development of a moral consensus by arguing for the permissibility of forgoing or withdrawing medical procedures that provide nutrition and hydration to PVS patients.

Argument in Support of Forgoing or Withdrawing[3]

The Medical Situation

An important fact about a PVS patient is that he or she is not dying. In these patients the brain stem is intact, with the major damage to the brain occurring in the neocortex and cortex. Thus these patients breathe spontaneously, have their eyes open, have a sleep-wake cycle, their pupils respond to light, and they typically have a normal gag and cough reflex.[4]

With respect to the diagnosis of PVS patients, there is "no set of specific medical criteria with as much clinical detail and certainty as the brain-death criteria. Furthermore, even the generally accepted criteria, when properly applied, are not infallible."[5] Furthermore, "It is not uncommon for patients to survive in this condition for five, ten, and twenty years."[6] Survival is contingent on age, economic, familial, and institutional factors, the natural resistance of the body to disease and infection, and changing moral and social views of this condition.

Of critical importance is knowing whether these patients experience pain and/or suffering. Cranford, following the *amicus curiae* brief of the American Academy of Neurology in the Paul Brophy case, argues that PVS patients "may 'react' to painful and other noxious stimuli, but they do not 'feel' (experience) pain in the sense of conscious discomfort . . . ,"[7] because the centers of the brain required for these experiences are too compromised to be functional. Thus PVS patients are not clinically dying and, if they are otherwise in good health and receive appropriate care, they can have a rather long life-expectancy. We obviously have the medical capacity to provide nutrition and hydration for these individuals, but the ethical difficulty, of course, is whether we must do everything we can to sustain their existence in this clinical condition.

The Value of Life

Clearly the preservation of life is an important goal of the human community in general and of the profession of medicine in particular. Intuitively we know life is valuable and sacred; for were it not, then nothing else would be. Yet, when all is said and done, especially in the Christian framework, life—even human life—is not of ultimate value. Philosophically and politically, we affirm a variety of values that transcend human life: justice, freedom, charity, the good of the neighbor, etc. On the basis of these values or for their sake, we can qualify

our protection of individual human lives. Theologically, only God is of ultimate value; all else, no matter how good or valuable, must take second place. Though heresy trials are one, perhaps unfortunate, example of this priority, we also have the celebrated examples of martyrdom and individual self-sacrifice.

This perspective reminds us, particularly in the health-care context, that while preserving life is a good—and even a great good—biological life is neither the highest value nor a value that holds ultimate claim on us. To make biological life the ultimate value is to forget our real priorities and to create an idol by making a lesser good our ultimate reality.

The Quality of Life

The meaning and validity of quality of life judgments have been debated in the literature for quite some time.[8] One example in recent decades is Joseph Fletcher's criteria of humanhood.[9] Although his criteria establish standards for being human, they also implicitly argued that life without a certain level of rationality was not human and consequently not worth living. Most recently Robert Jay Lifton's examination of Nazi doctors emphasized the role of the concept of *lebenunwertes Leben*: life unworthy of life.[10] Such unworthiness consisted primarily in being Jewish, but also extended to mental illness and retardation, as well as to severe physical handicaps.[11]

Quality of life judgments can serve as a code for a life judged to be worthless or useless. This orientation comes partially from our consumerist society, in which quality is linked with individuals' norms of excellence and is limited only by the horizons of their imagination and desires.[12] This perspective realizes one's worst fears about quality of life judgments, because the removal of any transcendent significance or value to human lives gives the state, institutions, or individuals final control over a person's fate.

The two most crucial levels in the quality of life debate are the evaluative and the normative. At the evaluative level three points need to be made. First, it is necessary to distinguish clearly and consistently between physical or biological life and personal life (personhood). When this important distinction is not made, quality of life judgments can equivocate between the value of biological life and the value of personhood.[13] This possibility must be removed. Second, physical life is indeed a value that is not conditioned on any property or characteristic of the person. Here we disagree with Documents F and G, which appear to imply such a conditional value of physical life, e.g. its rationality.[14] In our view physical life is a *bonum onticum,* a true and real value, though created and therefore limited. By arguing that physical life as such is a *bonum onticum* and not a conditional value, i.e. a *bonum utile,* we can affirm that all physical lives are of equal ontic value and that all persons are of equal moral worth. Third, the issue of the evaluative status of physical life may be misplaced from the start. The word "quality" does not and should not refer to a property or attribute of *life.* Rather, the quality that is at issue is the quality of the *relationship* which exists between the medical condition of the patient, on the one hand, and the patient's ability to pursue life's goals and purposes, understood as the values that transcend physical life, on the other.[15] We maintain that this reconceptualization of quality of life judgments is entirely congruent with the substance of the Catholic tradition.

Normatively, those who oppose quality of life judgments fear that life-and-death decisions will be made solely on the presence or absence of certain qualities or properties that a patient's life possesses. This erodes our duties to protect innocent lives, especially of those most vulnerable in our society.

If one contends that our duties to preserve life are based on a prior judgment of whether a specific quality or property of physical life will result in benefits or good consequences to the patient (personal consequentialism) or to society (social consequentialism), then in our judgment those duties to preserve life are improperly grounded in what the patient earns through social accomplishments or potentialities that his/her life might possess. We reject such a normative position because it denies, at least implicitly, the equal ontic value of all physical lives.

We argue that one derives the prima facie duty to preserve physical life from the ontic value of life and the actual moral obligation to preserve life from a teleological, but not consequentialist, assessment of the relationship between the patient's overall condition and his/her ability to pursue life's goals and purposes. The structure of the actual moral obligation is teleological in that the patient's condition is always viewed in relation to the pursuit of life's purposes, and the grounding of the obligation always involves an evaluative assessment of the qualitative relation which exists between these two components. Because physical life is not an absolute value, even those arguing for the sanctity of life position recognize definite limits to the obligation to support life.[16] We should not reject quality of life judgments, but we should rightly reject any normative derivation of our moral duties from the presence of certain properties of physical or personal life.

Quality of life judgments, which are judgments strictly circumscribed by an assessment of the benefits and burdens of medical treatment considered in itself and/or of those benefits and burdens that will accrue to the patient as a result of treatment, function appropriately as ways of qualifying our duties to preserve life. Thus, as long as the value of both physical life and personhood is assured at the evaluative and normative levels, we not only support the role of quality of life judgments in medicine but also judge them to be indispensable in proper decision-making. In our view, then, quality of life judgments properly supplement and enhance the Christian emphasis on the sanctity of life.[17]

The Technological Imperative

We cannot discuss this debate without including a reference to the technological imperative—"if we can do it, we should (or must) do it"—which infers a moral obligation either from a capacity or from the mere existence of a technology.

In the context of high-tech medicine, such an imperative, even if not explicitly subscribed to, is difficult to resist. The same is true even for low-tech or simple technologies. Some medical technologies that administer nutrition and hydration are relatively simple, e.g. parenteral methods of delivering nutrients. Other methods are more invasive, e.g. gastrostomy tubes, and they carry with them potential iatrogenic dangers, such as infection resulting from the surgical creation of the stoma. Yet they are much less invasive than other procedures and are more risk-free if properly cared for. Furthermore, their use provides a clear and demonstrable benefit: the prolongation of physical life. Indeed, feeding tubes may be unique among all medical technologies in that they almost exceptionlessly deliver on their claims. The technological imperative is augmented by simplicity and predictability of outcome and consequently presents an apparently unassailable case for use. But this very simplicity, ease of use, and ready availability disguises the moral dimension of the technology's use.

One must consider the use with respect to outcome. The outcome, of course, is the preservation of physical life. Prima facie such an outcome is valuable, but it must be considered with respect to other values and/or goods, for physical life is not the only or absolute good. Thus other goods, such as human dignity, ought to be considered. Our point is that, in and of itself, the presence of a technology and the capacity to utilize it constitute at most a prima facie case for its use. One cannot automatically or necessarily infer an actual moral obligation from the mere existence or presence of a technology.[18]

The Ordinary/Extraordinary Means Distinction

This well-used distinction can be dated as early as the 17th century and has been used by popes and theologians in arguments to determine one's moral obligation to preserve human life.[19] Some maintain that the key element in the traditional use of the distinction is the *classification* of technologies, medicines, or procedures. Consequently they are considered apart from the patient on whom they are used. Once classified, the moral question is then essentially resolved. In the feeding-tube example, the late John Connery, S.J., argued that since nutrition and hydration kept individuals

alive, the technology fitted the classic definition of ordinary treatment and therefore was
morally mandatory.[20]

If one shifts the perspective from an abstract
classification of technologies to a *patient-centered* approach[21] which gives moral weight to
the autonomy of the patient and looks to the
impact of these technologies on the patient's
medical and nonmedical condition as a whole,
one can establish a different moral argument.
Here the expressed wishes of the patient have
a legitimate moral claim based on our valuing
the dignity of the individual and on our respecting the sacredness of his or her conscience. Second, it is the proportionality or
disproportionality of benefits and burdens *to
the patient* that makes any medical treatment
or procedure, including the medical provision
of nutrition and hydration, obligatory or optional. Because the technology can neither
ameliorate a PVS patient's general clinical condition nor restore this individual to any state
of health where the patient might pursue the
values of life, the means are extraordinary and
not morally required. Therefore ordinary and
extraordinary are determined not by classifying the technology but by considering its impact on the patient and his/her overall condition. Additionally, and following directly from
the above, the distinction must adopt a patient-centered perspective to avoid the technological imperative.

The Burdensomeness of Life

The specific issue here is whether the burdensomeness of the life preserved by the offering of nutrition/hydration can or should be
part of the overall assessment of burden in the
determination of ordinary/extraordinary as
we have just outlined it. Considered only in
itself, the medical provision of nutrition and

hydration would most often be considered ordinary. Thus for some people any considerations beyond the technology itself would lead
to an improper questioning of the value of the
patient's life.

We think the concepts of burden and quality of life should be linked. Burden can accrue
to the patient precisely through the administration of modern technology and can be a consequence of a life lived merely at the biological
level with no hope of restoration or further
pursuit of temporal or even eternal goals. In
this sense the burden is iatrogenic. For the PVS
patient, medicine has reached its limit in bringing this individual to any level of health and
wholeness. Again, this patient-centered approach focuses on the conditions under which
this valued life is to be lived and seeks to identify what interests of the patient can be
achieved. Thus we argue that burden is to be
assessed not only from the perspective of the
burdensome effects of the technology itself
but, like Document C, also from the perspective "of the burdens that an individual experiences in pursuing the goals or ends of life" as a
result of the intervention of the medical technology. Although it is doubtful that the PVS
patient would experience this burden personally, the burden is real, even if experienced
secondhand by the family and/or by those professionals who must care for the patient.[22]

Fear of Being Trapped

The expected benefit of tube feeding is the
preservation of life posttrauma or posttreat-
ment so that other important work can go on,
e.g. treatment or diagnosis. But there comes a
time—sometimes sooner, sometimes later—
when one knows that all has been tried and
cure is not possible. What was formerly appropriate to do, viz. trying to cure, is now inappro-

priate, and our efforts must shift to accompanying the patient on his/her final journey.

We agree with Document F that it is precisely here that a family may feel or actually be trapped. Having appropriately initiated medical feeding to preserve life while other tests, procedures, and medications were tried, the family may now be frustrated in its desire to remove the feeding tube. Though such feeding only preserves biological life, attempts to withdraw the feeding may be challenged by medical personnel or by others.

Our fear is that individuals or families may inappropriately refuse to initiate medical procedures for delivering nutrients because of the fear of not being able to withdraw these procedures when that becomes appropriate. Thus individuals who may genuinely benefit from this type of procedure could be deprived of its goods. Such a situation would be tragic beyond belief. But because of the technological imperative, our near absolutizing of biological life, and the fear of taking personal responsibility in medical decision-making, this outcome is almost guaranteed. However, recognizing patient autonomy and shifting to a patient-centered calculation of benefits and burdens in the fashion we have described will counter this unfortunate situation.

Summary

In our judgment, the cumulative effect of our arguments supports the legitimate forgoing or withdrawing of nutrition and hydration to PVS patients. This judgment can properly be reached without supporting any efforts or claims for euthanasia and without making any improper judgments about the worth of a particular life. After carefully considering both the patient's known wishes and the qualitative relation between the patient's medical condition and the pursuit of life's purposes, one may appropriately judge that such a therapy is disproportionate and morally optional. This conclusion seems to be very close to, if not the same as, the judgment contained in Document E.

Suggestions for Future Discussion

Having reviewed the results of the survey, the points raised in the various documents submitted to us, and identified several ethical arguments supporting the removal of medical feeding tubes, we wish to make some suggestions for the future conduct of this debate.

Nomenclature

Here three issues. First, the misuse of "euthanasia" in the debate. In our survey, ordinaries were asked whether the diocesan committee considered the removal of feeding tubes from PVS patients to be an act of involuntary euthanasia. The responses are very interesting. Most answered that they considered the withdrawal of these tubes to be "passive or indirect and therefore permitted." A significant number responded that "it depends," and only four respondents answered that this action was "active or direct and therefore forbidden."

The response from the research center, Document D, states that the withdrawal of feeding tubes from PVS patients, except in very limited cases, is an act of "euthanasia by omission," and in most cases anyone who does this has the moral intention to end a life which is considered valueless or excessively burdensome. Two assumptions, frequently cited among those who consider such actions as euthanasia, seem to underlie this conclusion. The first is that the medical provision of nutrients offers a benefit by preserving the life of the patient. The second is that this nourishment should be considered as ordinary *care*, similar to all other types of care.

The moral characterization of the intention of the one authorizing withdrawal as "ending a life" forces this discussion into the context of euthanasia. In its brief to the New Jersey Supreme Court on the Nancy Ellen Jobes case, the New Jersey Catholic Conference argued that the withdrawal of feeding tubes is "intentional euthanasia."[23] Because we disagree both with the two basic assumptions which underlie this argument and with the description of the moral intention of these acts of withdrawal as killing, we argue that the use of the term "euthanasia" should be avoided in the debate.

A moral analysis of euthanasia necessarily involves an assessment of the intention. Though they may be motivated by humane reasons, morally all acts of euthanasia intend the death of the patient either by commission or by omission, and thus by definition these acts constitute the unjustified killing of a patient. However, we argue that in withdrawing nutrition and hydration the intent is either to end a procedure that no longer benefits the patient or to prevent the person from being entrapped in technology. The patient's death, while foreseen, results from the justified discontinuance of a technology that itself can neither correct the underlying fatal pathology, i.e. the permanent inability to ingest food and fluids orally, nor offer the patient any reasonable hope for what we have defined as quality of life. In our judgment, then, it is inappropriate to characterize the withdrawal of medical nutrition and hydration from PVS patients as euthanasia.

Second, we suggest that in future discussion

of this issue the word "forgo" should be used rather than "withhold." The reason is that "withhold" connotes that something is denied to someone who has some entitlement to it. When family members appropriately decide that a medical treatment will not truly benefit the PVS patient, their decision is to refrain from pursuing what is not useful to the loved one, not to deny something for which the patient has a need or a right. Our intent is twofold: to avoid a begging of the question and to suggest a terminology which allows the argument to come forward and be evaluated on its own merits. The terminology of forgoing and withdrawing, we think, will prevent the argument from becoming confused linguistically and prejudged methodologically.

Third, how describe *nutrition and hydration?* What to call the nourishment administered to a patient introduces a variety of problems, descriptive as well as symbolic. The terms "food and water" conjure up, among other things, a variety of images depending on taste and ethnic background. They also connote a meal in which one actively participates or, if with others, shares. The symbolism associated with food and water is deep, and rightly so. For they symbolize membership and participation in a community, and to deny these common but significant realities to someone is more than depriving that individual of nourishment; it is cutting him/her off from the community.

The symbolic level of food and water is what inclines several individuals to argue against the removal of nourishment from the PVS patient.[24] The forgoing or the removal of nutrition says that the individual has been marked and put outside the community, outside society. This further signifies the valuelessness of the person and his/her uselessness to the community. Therefore one must continue to provide this nourishment precisely as a symbol of inclusion.

However, one must also recognize the limits of this symbolism, particularly in the case of PVS patients. To begin with, we have a situation in which the patient is fed and does not eat; the experience is entirely passive. Orderlies or nurses do not deny trays of food to patients nor do they forcibly remove these from the hands of patients. Nutrition and hydration are administered to the patient and the body absorbs them; the feeding process is completely involuntary. Second, the symbolism of the meal is utterly absent, even if others are there. There is no meal, only a medical feeding. Though nourishing, it is difficult to consider such a liquid protein diet as food. For food, in addition to having a certain biological reality, is also a human construct and is more than the sum of its nutritional value. It is the color, texture, aroma, taste, and company in which it is shared. For the PVS patient, all of this is absent. To call this nourishment food is to invest it with more meaning than the reality of the situation can bear.

Also, these patients do not consciously hunger or thirst. But even if these states were experienced, medical procedures for supplying nutrition and hydration might not relieve the feelings.[25] "Medical nutrition and hydration" seems an appropriate phrase for this form of nourishment, because it captures in a nonjudgmental fashion the medical provision of the nourishment as well as the passivity of the experience. The patient is fed and consequently the body is nourished, but he/she certainly does not participate in a meal and clearly does not share table fellowship. This terminology also describes the procedure without begging the moral question of whether one ought to

provide it, and it avoids the intrusion of inappropriate symbolism. This terminology will keep us from making more of the situation than is there, but it will also keep us from making less of it.

Ordinary and Extraordinary Treatment

Here are three considerations. First, as noted above, there is a difference in how these traditional terms can be used. For some, the terms are the basis on which the procedure or technology is classified. Once classified, the correct action is relatively clear. If ordinary, the procedure or technology is morally obligatory; if extraordinary, it is morally optional. This schema encounters significant problems when the pace of technological change increases. In addition, the term "ordinary" in its moral or normative sense has been used to declare a certain technology routine or customary in a medical or descriptive sense. The descriptive use of "ordinary" generally refers to what is usually done, but this involves little or no moral analysis of what ought to be done.

These equivocations have precipitated a rethinking of the terminology that now aims at the evaluation of the benefit-burden ratio for the patient.[26] Consequently a procedure is judged ordinary in a normative sense if its effects on the patient provide proportionately more benefits than burdens. On the other hand, a treatment is extraordinary in a moral sense if the evaluation produces the contrary conclusion. Thus these terms are now seen as the conclusion of a process of evaluation rather than as a classification of a procedure. It is not unusual that a Jehovah's Witness would judge a clinically routine blood transfusion morally extraordinary because of the disproportionate consequences for his or her eternal salvation. Similarly, a person on long-term dialysis might conclude in some circumstances that use of this technology is extraordinary because of its impact on diet and life style.

Understanding ordinary and extraordinary as conclusions of an evaluative process rather than as a classification schema permits a much more appropriate use of the terms in the practice of contemporary medicine. Furthermore, the danger of equivocation is now removed and the meaning of the terms is moral, not descriptive.

Second, autonomy. Though the concept has undergone some criticism in the last few years because it has been taken to an extreme by functioning independently of or to the exclusion of other values, nonetheless we might do well to remember the old adage that abuse does not take away use. Autonomy is an important value, and the proper starting point for these discussions is the expressed wishes of the competent patient. To begin at this point is to respect the dignity of patients and their conscientious decisions. Statements that individuals make about their death or the circumstances of their dying are extremely important. Minimally, they form the foundation of any and all discussion about the initiation or withdrawal of therapy. These statements, which need to be discussed and evaluated in light of the clinical situation and other relevant moral values, always constitute a core element in the final decision about treatment.

Third, quality of life considerations and the goal of medicine. As we have noted, quality of life judgments should not be construed as judgments about the worth of either physical or personal life. They are not concerned with assessing qualities or properties that, when present, make life itself valuable. Rather, these judgments are evaluative and normative claims or assessments about the relation between the patient's overall condition and his/her ability to pursue material, moral, and spiritual values which transcend physical life but do not give that life its very meaning and worth. Consequently quality of life judgments help specify concretely the meaning of the terms "benefits," "burdens," and "best interests" of a patient, as well as the limits of medical interventions within a given historical and cultural situation.

Whereas all physical life is of equal ontic worth and all personal life is of equal moral value, the quality of the relation between these lives and the pursuit of values is not equal. Due to multiple factors, some of which have to do with individual genetic endowment and the ways in which we live our lives and some of which are dependent on the nurturing and accessibility of values in a given culture, a large portion of the population is fortunate enough to attain a high quality of life. Other individuals, regrettably, are not as fortunate, and they must live most of their lives pursuing life's purposes at a less than optimal level. But some have no discernible or such a minimal qualitative relation between their overall condition and the pursuit of values that we would argue that those in this last category have no moral obligation to prolong their physical lives. In these cases all treatment can be withdrawn from them. Not long ago all PVS patients' lives would have been mercifully ended by their inability to ingest food orally, but the intervention of modern technology today has not been as merciful.

No doubt, one of the principal factors that has provoked this debate has been the ambiguity about the central goal of medicine itself.

Medicine rightfully seeks to prevent death, especially an untimely death, to alleviate pain and physical suffering, and to promote health as far as possible. Indeed, these are important goals. However, we argue that all these goals are really subordinate to the more encompassing goal of serving the purposefulness of personal existence.[27] In other words, the central and overarching goal of clinical medicine is to enhance the qualitative relation between the patient's condition and the pursuit of life's goods. Thus, other things being equal, when medicine can intervene to ameliorate the quality of the relation between the patient's condition and the pursuit of life's goals, then such an intervention can be considered a benefit to the patient and is in his/her best interests. On the other hand, because of the overall condition of the patient, when a proposed intervention cannot offer the patient any reasonable hope of pursuing life's purposes at all or can only offer the patient a condition where the pursuit of life's purposes will be filled with profound frustration or with utter neglect of these purposes because of the energy needed merely to sustain physical life, then any medical intervention (1) can only offer burden to the life treated, (2) is contrary to the best interests of the patient, (3) can cause iatrogenic harm or the risk of such harm, and (4) has reached its limit based on medicine's own principal reason for existence, and thus treatment should not be given except to palliate or to comfort.[28]

Responsibility in Decision-Making

When the biotechnological revolution began in earnest and humans discovered new powers and capacities, one of the first slogans to describe this new state of affairs was "playing God." This phrase denoted the power humans now wielded over previously untamed and uncontrolled natural realities. But we detect a shift emerging. Rather than humans "playing God," it is now technology that is "playing God." Our machines seem to have developed a life and power of their own. How, for example, does someone with an artificial heart die? How does someone on a respirator stop breathing? How does someone with a feeding tube refuse to be nourished? Very often, once in place, there seems to be no way, short of a cosmic power failure, to end the domination of the machine. We are, clearly, much better about removing machines now than we were initially, but many are still very reluctant to intervene in the activities of the machinery. Often enough, court intervention is the only recourse the family or guardian has to stop a machine.[29]

Have we surrendered our decision-making powers to machines? Do they "play God" by exercising their untiring, endless vigilance over us and our loved ones? We have not improved our situation much if indeed we have turned our appropriate decision-making responsibilities over to machines. Although such decisions are dangerous and difficult at times, humans have a legitimate level of responsibility for deciding about the forgoing or withdrawing of treatment. Surrendering that responsibility because a machine is in place is truly the worship of a false god.

The family typically plays an important role in these decisions, because often the individual most affected by a decision cannot participate directly. Such involvement is proper, because generally the family has a relationship with the patient and knows his/her wishes. The family is normally in the best position to discern the patient's wishes or desires. Thus it can either relate what the patient actually wanted or, failing that, relate its best judgment of what the patient would have wanted. If the family has no direct knowledge of the patient's wishes, it is still the appropriate decision-maker. The family has a socially recognized relation to the patient and can be presumed to have the best interests of the patient in mind.

Should conflicts arise which simply cannot be resolved at the local level with the assistance of the physicians, an ethics committee, a patient's rights advocate, the clergy, or other resources, then—and only then in our judgment—is it appropriate to think of turning to the courts for a resolution of the issue.

Conclusion

On both practical and theoretical levels, the question of forgoing or withdrawing medical nutrition and hydration from PVS patients appears to have reached no clear consensus inside or outside the Catholic community, although our sense is that many, if not most, people are uncomfortable with continuing this technology when there is no reasonable hope of an improvement in the patient's prognosis. This is not to say that there is an atmosphere of joy about the situation or a zeal to begin a withdrawal procedure. Rather, there is a sense of reluctance, a very great sense of caution and care, and a most careful focusing on the moral arguments.

Finally, we wish to highlight two aspects of the debate that we think are particularly crucial. First, the moral intention to forgo or withdraw medical nutrition and hydration is not identical with the intention in euthanasia. This conclusion is confirmed by our own work and in most of the literature. People who ad-

vocate the forgoing or the withdrawal of feeding tubes are not advocating any kind of euthanasia policy. The clear intent is to end a procedure that is not proportionately benefiting the person or to release the person from entrapment in technology. Thus, while forgoing or withdrawing feeding tubes is not "medical killing," maintaining them may well produce "involuntary medical living." Second, forgoing or withdrawing this technology is argued as a moral option, not as a mandatory practice. Therefore the conclusion we share with most authors is either that forgoing or withdrawal is not prohibited or it is within the permitted range of moral activities. We also agree with Document E that individuals who conclude that such a practice is morally appropriate should not be prohibited from acting on that conclusion.

We expect that the debate will continue and that different aspects of it will be further examined. Our hope is that this report and presentation of an argument will help structure that process and assist in its resolution.[30]

Notes

1. The longest case of coma is that of Elaine Esposito, who died 37 years and 111 days after falling into coma. See The President's Commission for the Study of Ethical Problems in Medicine and Biomedical and Behavioral Research, *Deciding to Forego Life-Sustaining Treatment: A Report on the Ethical, Medical, and Legal Issues in Treatment Decisions* (Washington, D.C.: U.S. Government Printing Office, 1983) 177 n. 16.

2. Some dioceses may not have received a survey either because the see was vacant or because of error on TAS's part. Additionally, not every respondent answered every question. Thus, in terms of data

analysis there is no constant "n"; yet an overall impression can be gained from the data.

3. Throughout the remainder of this essay we have adopted the terminology used by the Hastings Center in describing the technique by which nutrition and hydration are provided to the PVS patient. As defined by the Hastings Center, "medical procedures for supplying nutrition and hydration are medical enteral procedures and parenteral nutritional procedures. . . ." "Medical enteral procedures are procedures in which nutritional formulas and water are introduced into the patient's stomach or intestine by means of a tube, such as a gastrostomy tube or nasogastric tube." "Parenteral nutritional procedures are procedures in which nutritional formulas and water are introduced into the patient's body by means other than the gastrointestinal tract. Such procedures include total parenteral nutritional support (TPN), in which a formula capable of maintaining the patient for prolonged periods is infused into a vein—usually a large, central vein in the patient's chest—and intravenous procedures in which water and/or a formula supplying limited nutritional support is introduced into a peripheral vein" (Hastings Center, *Guidelines on the Termination of Life-Sustaining Treatment and the Care of the Dying* [Briarcliff Manor, N.Y.: Hastings Center, 1987] 140–41).

4. For a more detailed discussion of the condition of a patient in persistent vegetative state, see Ronald E. Cranford, "The Persistent Vegetative State: The Medical Reality (Getting the Facts Straight)," *Hastings Center Report* 18 (February/March, 1988) 27–32. Also, the President's Report, *Deciding to Forego Life-Sustaining Treatment* 174–81.

5. Cranford, "The Persistent Vegetative State" 29.

6. Ibid. 31.

7. Ibid. In addition, see the recent "Position of the American Academy of Neurology on Certain Aspects of the Care and Management of the Persistent Vegetative State Patient," reprinted in *Medical Ethics Advisor* 4 (August 1988) 111–13.

8. E.g., see George J. Annas, "Quality of Life in the Courts: Earle Spring in Fantasyland," *Hastings Center Report* 10 (August 1980) 9–10; Daniel Callahan, *Setting Limits* (New York: Simon & Schuster, 1987) 187–93; John R. Connery, S.J., "Quality of Life," *Linacre Quarterly* 53 (February 1986) 26–33; Brian V. Johnstone, C.SS.R., "The Sanctity of Life, the Quality of Life and the New 'Baby Doe' Law," ibid. 52 (August 1985) 258–70; Edward W. Keyserlingk, *Sanctity of Life or Quality of Life in the Context of Ethics, Medicine and Law* [a study written for the Law Reform Commission of Canada] (Ottawa: Minister of Supply and Services Canada, 1979) 49–72, 75–105, 185–90; Richard A. McCormick, S.J., "A Proposal for 'Quality of Life' Criteria for Sustaining Life," *Hospital Progress* 59 (1975) 76–79; idem, "The Quality of Life, the Sanctity of Life," *Hastings Center Report* 8 (February 1978) 30–36; Warren T. Reich, "Quality of Life," in *Encyclopedia of Bioethics* 2 (New York: Free Press, 1978) 829–40; idem, "Quality of Life and Defective Newborn Children: An Ethical Analysis," in *Decision Making and the Defective Newborn: Proceedings of a Conference on Spina Bifida and Ethics,* ed. Chester A. Swinyard (Springfield, Ill.: Charles C. Thomas, 1978) 489–511.

9. Joseph Fletcher, "Indicators of Humanhood: A Tentative Profile of Man," *Hastings Center Report* 2 (November 1972) 1–4.

10. Robert Jay Lifton, *The Nazi Doctors: Medical Killing and the Psychology of Genocide* (New York: Basic Books, 1986) 21.

11. For an interesting contrast between the Nazi interpretation of "quality of life" and what contemporary authors tend to mean by this criterion, see Cynthia B. Cohen, " 'Quality of Life' and the Analogy with the Nazis," *Journal of Medicine and Philosophy* 8 (1983) 113–35.

12. Albert R. Jonsen, "Purposefulness in Human Life," *Western Journal of Medicine* 125 (July 1976) 5.

13. E.g., Warren Reich's theological position grounds both the value and the equality of "human life" in the belief that "all men are created as persons in the image of God" ("Quality of Life and Defective Newborn Children" 504). His use of the phrase "human life" is ambiguous here and therefore misleading. The context of his argument is a critique of what he believes to be Richard A. McCormick's position on the value of *physical life,* yet Reich completes his argument by referring to *persons* and their nature and value as images of God.

14. In fact, several contemporary Catholics have given the impression that the value of physical life is dependent on some inherent property or attribute which, when present, gives physical life its value. It is possible that this way of phrasing the value of physical life is due to the lack of a terminology in the contemporary discussion that can mediate between the two traditional categories of value, viz. *bonum honestum* and *bonum utile.* E.g., see Kevin D. O'Rourke, O.P., and Dennis Brodeur, *Medical Ethics: Common Ground for Understanding* (St. Louis: Catholic Health Association of the U.S., 1986) 213; Richard A. McCormick, *How Brave a New World? Dilem-*

mas in Bioethics (Washington, D.C.: Georgetown University, 1981) 405–7; David Thomasma et al., "Continuance of Nutritional Care in the Terminally Ill Patient," *Critical Care Clinics* 2 (January 1986) 66.

15. See James J. Walter, "The Meaning and Validity of Quality of Life Judgments in Contemporary Roman Catholic Medical Ethics," *Louvain Studies* 13 (fall 1988) 195–208, esp. 201.

16. E.g., see John R. Connery, S.J., "Prolonging Life: The Duty and Its Limits," *Linacre Quarterly* 47 (May 1980) 151–65; Johnstone, "The Sanctity of Life, the Quality of Life," esp. 265–69; Reich, "Quality of Life and Defective Newborn Children," esp. 505–9.

17. Keyserlingk also argues a similar position in his report for the Law Reform Commission of Canada. See his *Sanctity of Life or Quality of Life,* esp. 49–72.

18. We agree with the report from the Hastings Center that "All invasive procedures for supplying nutrition and hydration— all enteral and parenteral techniques— should be considered procedures that require the patient's or surrogate's consent . . ." (*Guidelines on the Termination of Life-Sustaining Treatment* 61).

19. See Gerald Kelly, S.J., *Medico-Moral Problems* (St. Louis: Catholic Hospital Association, 1958) 128–41.

20. John R. Connery, S.J., "The Clarence Herbert Case: Was Withdrawal of Treatment Justified? *Hospital Progress* 65 (February 1984) 32–35 and 70.

21. Recently several authors have argued for a patient-centered approach in clinical decision-making: e.g., see Robert M. Veatch, *Death, Dying, and the Biological Revolution: Our Last Quest for Responsibility* (New Haven: Yale University, 1976); James J. Walter, "Food & Water: An Ethical Burden," *Commonweal* 113 (Nov. 21, 1986) 616–19.

22. Though we have refrained from making any judgment about the financial burden either on society or on insurance companies in providing funds for PVS patients, the fact that there are approximately 10,000 of these patients in the U.S. strongly inclines us to agree with Daniel Callahan that "It is hard to see how a debate on that reimbursement issue can be forestalled much longer." See Callahan's "Vital Distinction, Mortal Questions: Debating Euthanasia & Health-Care Costs," *Commonweal* 115 (July 15, 1988) 404. It is important to note here that the *Declaration on Euthanasia* and Document E, both following Pius XII, do permit one to assess the burden on the family or on the community in judging whether a treatment is disproportionate. See the *Declaration on Euthanasia* in *Origins* 10 (Aug. 10, 1980) 16.

23. New Jersey State Catholic Conference Brief, "Providing Food and Fluids to Severely Brain Damaged Patients," in *Origins* 16 (Jan. 22, 1987) 583. The Conference was following the Lutheran theologian Gilbert Meilaender in his "On Removing Food and Water: Against the Stream," *Hastings Center Report* 14 (December 1984) 11–13. An opposing position was taken by Bishop Louis Gelineau of Providence, R.I., in the Marcia Gray court case. See his statement in *Origins* 17 (Jan. 21, 1988) 546–57.

24. E.g., see Daniel Callahan, "On Feeding the Dying," *Hastings Center Report* 13 (October 1983) 22.

25. Hastings Center, *Guidelines on the Termination of Life-Sustaining Treatment* 59.

26. See the *Declaration on Euthanasia,* where the terminology has shifted to a discussion of proportionality between the benefits and the burdens.

27. Jonsen, "Purposefulness in Human Life" 6.

28. Walter, "The Meaning and Validity of Quality of Life Judgments" 207.

29. There have been several court cases recently involving patients in a persistent vegetative state. Two of the more notable cases are Paul Brophy and Nancy Ellen Jobes.

30. Support for the survey was provided by the Research Development Council of Worcester Polytechnic Institute, and the authors acknowledge their gratitude for this assistance.

CARE OF THE ELDERLY

19

Ethical Judgments of Quality of Life in the Care of the Aged

David C. Thomasma

But I have come to see that (dying) is not only something inevitable but will happen to me before long. I keep before me the fact that it is utterly useless to rant and rave against the void. Death is not much of a conversationalist. He won't answer. Neither is he an enemy one can vanquish. Besides, so many people close to my heart have died—some very close—that death has become quite familiar to me. He is a part of my life. The thought that I too shall follow in sleep no longer frightens me. I really have no intention of living on until I'm in my nineties to be confronted with advanced age and all its deficiencies.—*Simone de Beauvoir* [71 years old, from an interview in *De Tijd*, February 23, 1979, author's translation]

Every physician and medical ethicist knows that making quality of life decisions about the lives of aged patients is very difficult. Thus

Hilfiker, in his scrupulously honest description about his care of a nursing home patient with pneumonia, argues that a lack of guidelines renders these judgments subjective, capricious, and guilt-ridden.[1] As Pearlman and Speer argue, our views about the quality of life of others are notoriously off the mark.[2] This is especially true with regard to elderly persons who are incapacitated[3] or cannot speak for themselves.[4] In the face of such uncertainty, therapeutic actions are equally uncertain. Some, like Hilfiker, confess that they "do nothing" or "go slowly," thus limiting easily available interventions and allowing nature to take its course.[1] This approach is contested by those who say it lacks the respect for human life that is essential to the very nature of medicine, or that it shows the lack of a personal philosophy. Still others base their decisions on "positive outcomes," admitting that working on the debilitated aged carries no rewards in

---

Reprinted with permission from the American Geriatrics Society and David C. Thomasma, "Ethical Judgments of Quality of Life in the Care of the Aged," by David C. Thomasma (Journal of the American Geriatrics Society, Vol. 32, No. 7, pp. 525–527, July, 1984).

this respect. Such physicians act as if an avoidance of personal inconvenience were the primary motive for making therapeutic decisions in such cases. Still others claim that philosophical guidelines do exist in such cases, but this claim, even if true, still does not help in making concrete decisions about particular patients.[5]

My view differs from these only in its emphasis on complexity. Reluctance about making quality of life decisions stems from at least three sources.

Legalism

First, in our increasingly litigious society, physicians have become wary of instituting or withholding treatments for fear of lawsuit. Gene Stollerman points out how dangerous it is for medicine and for doctors as moral agents to reduce medical decision-making to a legalistic process. Adoption of the principles embodied in the report of the Law Reform Commission of Canada[6] in the United States would significantly reduce physicians' anxiety about liabilities when they act as advocates for their patients. The mandate to maintain the discretionary space of physician-patient decision-making is made exceptionally clear in the commission's report, while the legal rights and autonomy of the patient remain protected. Nonetheless, a freedom from criminal liability removes only one impediment to making quality of life decisions for patients. More positive guidelines are needed.

Validity

Second, a reluctance to make quality of life decisions about aged patients may stem from a healthy disrespect for the ethical basis of such decisions. In fact, to treat others on the basis of our own judgments of the qualities of their lives is risky. The Law Reform Commission emphasizes that all competent patients may refuse treatment even if such refusal would make death inevitable. Patient autonomy is therefore the primary guideline for treatment decisions. Thus, adoption of the Law Reform Commission Report would not only free physicians from criminal liability in making quality of life decisions, but also provide guidelines for such decisions. In this respect, as Curran notes, there would have to be a reversal of most court decisions in the United States, which have reflected a hesitation to adopt a broadly worded "quality of life" test for removal of life-support systems, focusing instead on a much more narrowly defined brain-death standard.[7]

Of course, the real ethical problems begin when one judges that an aged patient is incompetent. Here the decisions made by the physician become subject to the capriciousness Hilfiker spoke of. The Law Reform Commission Report stresses that incompetent patients have the same right to respect of their life as competent patients. Normally one thinks such a principle would lead to aggressive treatment decisions, but the opposite is actually intended. Here is how the recommendation might be more thoroughly reasoned.

The validity guideline is based on a well-established principle of justice in health care: "Treat equally unless there are morally relevant differences."[8] Normally this principle is used to discuss problems of access to health care, but now it appears to support a *proportionality* judgment in at least three ways:

1. *The physician is not obligated to aggressively treat the seriously ill and incompetent*

aged person if patients who are competent would normally judge the therapy superfluous and refuse it. This judgment requires wisdom and experience. My experience on our ethics consultation service regarding cases of elderly patients is that they seem very capable of assessing a treatment in terms of the meaning of their life. Although most are not as eloquent as Simone de Beauvoir, older patients seem much more resigned to their deaths than those who treat them.

Physicians should spend a lot of their time talking to elderly patients to learn this sense of proportionality. Note, then, that making "substituted judgments" for incompetent patients would rest not on what rational, healthy persons think about the patients' quality of life, or what we ourselves or the family members would want if we were in the patients' shoes, but what other patients of the same age and condition who were competent have tended to choose. This represents a significant refinement of the "substituted judgment" and "reasonable persons" criteria. Its presence is implied in the Law Reform Commission Report and breaks new ground in the care of the debilitated.

2. *The physician is not obligated to prolong aggressive treatment if there is an unreasonable proportion between benefit and intervention.* In effect this second axiom is based on a judgment that it would be cruel to continue treatment considering the medical indications alone. It differs, as I see it, from Paul Ramsey's "medical indications policy" in that it is tempered by the "other debilitated aged" axiom just discussed. Ramsey would have all treatments that are medically indicated instituted on the ground that no one has an absolute right to refuse treatment.[9] Adoption of this policy would lead to an overriding of patients'

autonomous decisions to refuse treatment if they would lead to death, and to providing any medically indicated therapy necessary to sustain life.

3. *The physician is not obligated to continue treatment if it represents a "bottomless pit" with respect to cost and the health benefits received are not significant.*[10] This axiom touches on the economic proportionality of means and ends on the basis of equality of opportunity. While it is the case that the elderly are entitled to support and deserve it for past contributions to life, productivity, and culture,[11,12] this claim does not answer the question about *how much* they deserve. Here it seems best to judge that they deserve as much as needed to bring about comfort and restoration to health, if possible, but with an eye on the fact that they have already been given the opportunity to compete for the goods and resources of society. Expensive treatments that lead to only minor benefits are thus ruled out.

"Ageism"[13] violates the principle of justice that all should be treated equally without considerations of age. For example, an applicant for employment should not be excluded on the basis of age when it has no relevance for ability to perform the position. But, as Norman Daniels has argued so well, age may be a guide for medical suitability. As a consequence, not every appeal to an age criterion for treatment is morally objectionable. In this sense, then, the ratio between treatment and benefit shrinks as one reaches old age and chronic illness.[14]

Although these three proportionality axioms are not explicitly contained in the Law Reform Commission Report, I suggest they are implicitly presumed in the notion that incompetent patients ought to be treated the same as competent patients who have similar conditions and outlooks. As we have seen, this does not mean aggressive treatment must continue at all costs. *There is a morally relevant difference about chronic illness and debilitation that permits us to treat patients suffering these conditions with less intensity than we would others.*

Fear of Death

There is yet a third reason why physicians are reluctant to make quality of life judgments for their patients. The two I have already discussed, fear of legal repercussions and hesitancy about the validity of such judgments in the absence of clear standards, are both addressed by the Law Reform Commission. The third reason is more difficult to correct by policy—it is the fear of one's own death as it peers out at one from the faces of debilitated patients. This fear, I believe, is what makes many physicians so uncomfortable about treating chronically ill and very old people. A physical, stomach-wrenching fear can cause some to withdraw and to "do nothing" and others to continue aggressive therapy beyond the point of making sense. Whether this fear of death comes from personal or social sources, it leads to senseless actions on behalf of patients under one's care.

The only cure for this illness of physicians themselves is courage. Courage to make ethical decisions can be occasioned by legislation along the lines of the Law Reform recommendations. It can be aided by consultation with an ethics advisory service,[15] or with a hospital ethics committee. The latter is suggested not only by the Canadian Report, but also by our own President's Commission,[16] and seems likely to become policy with respect to treat-

ing defective newborns. Courage can be reinforced by superb clinical training of young physicians in geriatrics. But in the end it can come only from a combination of self-awareness and profound discussion with aging patients. For this reason, William May has argued that aged patients teach physicians as much as physicians serve them.[17] In this exchange physicians learn the wisdom to balance the use of therapeutic means to save life with the quality of life, and the patient as well as incompetent confreres is assured respect at the bedside.

Conclusion

I join Gene Stollerman and John Ball in urging adoption by the states of legislation along the lines of the Law Reform Commission of Canada. I suggest more sophisticated guidelines for terminating aggressive treatment of debilitated, incompetent patients. Since the basis of these guidelines is physician judgment about the proportion of means to ends, I encourage formal training programs for young physicians, perhaps conducted by the aged themselves, engaging them in discussion about quality of life treatment decisions. Finally, I support every effort made by role-model teachers of medicine to encourage and reinforce ethical thinking about patient-care judgments with respect to the elderly. In this regard the American Geriatrics Society might consider instituting a subcommittee like the American Board of Internal Medicine's Subcommittee on Evaluation of the Humanistic Qualities of the Internist, whose report was published recently.[18] A comparable report might be generated on the humanistic qualities of the geriatrics specialist. Such reports can, in turn, be useful in designing training programs and guiding and assessing young physicians.

References

1. Hilfiker D: Allowing the debilitated to die: facing our ethical choices. N Engl J Med 308:716, 1983
2. Pearlman R, Speer J Jr: Quality-of-life considerations in geriatric care. J Am Geriatr Soc 31:113, 1983
3. Goldman R: Ethical confrontations in the incapacitated aged. J Am Geriatr Soc 29:214, 1981
4. Gadow S: Medicine, ethics, and the elderly. Gerontologist 20:680, 1980
5. Letters to the Editor. N Engl J Med 308:[April] 1983
6. Law Reform Commission of Canada: Report 20. Euthanasia, Aiding Suicide, and Cessation of Treatment. Law Reform Commission of Canada, Ottawa, Canada, Nov. 1983
7. Curran WG: Law-medicine notes: quality of life and treatment decisions: the Canadian Law Reform Report. N Engl J Med 310:297, 1984
8. Veatch R: What is a "just" health care policy? *in:* Veatch R, Branson R (eds): Ethics and Health Policy. Cambridge, Mass., Ballinger, 1976, pp 127–153
9. Ramsey P: Ethics at the Edges of Life. New Haven, Yale University Press, 1976
10. Wikler D: Philosophical perspectives on access to health care: an introduction *in:* Securing Access to Health Care. President's Commission for the Study of Ethical Problems in Medicine and Biomedical and Behavioral Research. Volume II,

appendix F. The Commission, Washington, D.C. 1983, pp 109–151
11. Morgan JN: The ethical basis of the economic claims of the elderly, *in:* Neugarten BL, Havinghurst RJ, (eds): Social Policy, Social Ethics, and the Aging Society. (Committee on Human Development, University of Chicago). National Science Foundation, Washington, D.C., U.S. Government Printing Office, 1976, pp 67–69
12. Thomasma D: Professional and ethical obligations toward the aged. Linacre Q 48:73, 1981
13. Butler RN: Age-ism: another form of bigotry. Gerontologist 9:243, 1969
14. Daniels N: Am I my parent's keeper? *in:* Securing Access to Health Care. President's Commission for the Study of Ethical Problems in Medicine and Biomedical and Behavioral Research. Volume II, Appendix F. The Commission, Washington, D.C., 1983, pp 265–291
15. Thomasma D: The goals of modern medical education and a required humanities curriculum. Urban Health 12:32, Feb 1983
16. President's Commission for the Study of Ethical Problems in Medicine and Biomedical and Behavioral Research: Deciding to Forego Life-sustaining Treatment: A Report on the Ethical, Medical, and Legal Issues in Treatment Decisions. The Commission, Washington, D.C., March 1983
17. May W: Who cares for the elderly? Hastings Center Rep 12:31, Dec 1982
18. Subcommittee on Evaluation of the Humanistic Qualities of the Internist: ABIM evaluation of humanistic qualities in the internist. Ann Intern Med 99:720, 1983

20

Guiding the Hand that Feeds:
Caring for the Demented Elderly

Bernard Lo
Laurie Dornbrand

The phone message from the patient's daughter is ominous. "Mrs. F. has eaten nothing all weekend. What should we do?" A 70-year-old woman with severe dementia, Mrs. F. rarely speaks, is confined to a wheelchair, and requires diapers because of incontinence. She has been kept out of a nursing home by the efforts of a devoted family and daily attendance at a geriatric day-care center. During the past year, her social interactions have decreased, and her food intake has become increasingly erratic. First, she stopped feeding herself; now, even though she is fed by hand, her intake continues to decline. Once, she required admission to the hospital for dehydration. During the past week, she has been clamping her mouth shut, pushing food away with her hand, or spitting out food. Over the weekend, even coaxing with her favorite foods was unsuccessful. The question that those

who care for her have dreaded must now be faced: If hand feedings continue to fail, should a feeding tube be inserted?

The use of feeding tubes in severely demented patients evokes passionate arguments. If a feeding tube is not used, dehydration, malnutrition, and even death may occur. Proponents of tube feedings contend that without them, patients suffer discomfort from hunger and thirst. Moreover, by not providing adequate nourishment we neglect our moral responsibility to care for the helpless. In contrast, those reluctant to use feeding tubes argue that at the end of a long downhill course, not eating is a natural letting go of life. Feeding tubes cannot reverse the underlying diseases and may only prolong the process of dying. Is it appropriate to try to keep such patients alive with tube feedings, so that they may succumb instead to pneumonia or other conditions?

"Guiding the Hand That Feeds: Caring for the Demented Elderly" by Bernard Lo, M.D. and Laurie Dornbrand, M.D. Reprinted with permission of The New England Journal of Medicine *311 (August 9, 1984): 402–404.*

Moreover, demented patients are often tied down and sedated to prevent them from pulling out the tubes. This practice may compromise what little dignity and independence these patients retain, especially since they cannot comprehend how the treatment benefits them.

There are no easy solutions to these dilemmas. Difficult trade-offs among conflicting values and goals must be made, and reasonable, well-intentioned people may disagree. During a clinical crisis, there is often no opportunity to discuss issues fully; unanalyzed assertions, generalizations, and slogans may pervade discussions. In addition, legal uncertainties may complicate deliberations. The New Jersey Supreme Court will soon rule on a case in which a decision to allow the removal of a feeding tube from an elderly demented patient was reversed on appeal.[1]

The Decision Process

When the patient is incompetent, the physician and family should make a joint decision.[2] If the patient expressed preferences when he or she was competent, those wishes should be followed. Unfortunately, this ideal procedure is usually not possible. Many patients have never indicated their wishes about care. Family members may not be close enough to know the patient's preferences. Moreover, prior statements are often ambiguous and do not address the specific issue of feeding tubes. If patients have said that they would not want to be vegetables or would not want to live on machines, does that mean that they would not want feeding tubes? When these preferences are unclear or unknown, care givers may try to infer them from actions. Such inferences, however, may be controversial. When patients

push away food or pull out feeding tubes, do such actions really mean that they do not want to be fed, or could they be uncomfortable, angry, depressed, or seeking attention?

When the wishes of a patient with severe irreversible illness are unclear or unknown, the family should base decisions on the patient's best interests.[2] Conflicts of interest and emotions such as guilt and grief may complicate family discussions. Moreover, it is often difficult to assess the incompetent patient's quality of life. Family members and health professionals sometimes project their own feelings onto the patient. Life situations that would be intolerable to young, healthy people may be acceptable to older, debilitated patients. Judgments about the quality of life are best based on direct observation of the individual patient rather than on generalizations. Evidence of discomfort, such as moaning and crying, should be given more weight than evidence of lack of pleasure, such as failure to smile or interact with others.

Defining the Goals of Care

In making decisions about tube feedings, physicians and family must determine the goal of such care: Is it to prolong life, deliver calories, or provide comfort?

The goal may be to deliver calories while attempting to identify and treat reversible causes of feeding problems. Decreased intake may result from medical problems, such as intercurrent illness, mouth lesions, or drugs. Feeding problems may also be caused by psychosocial problems, such as a change in care givers or a desire for control. In such situations, temporary use of tube or intravenous feedings may resolve the crisis while the underlying problem is treated. Sometimes, hand feedings may be made more effective by slowing the pace of feeding, offering smaller bites, changing the taste or consistency of the food, or reminding the patient to chew or swallow.

In some patients, feeding problems are irreversible, and for some of these patients, prolonging life with long-term tube feedings is an appropriate goal. However, for those who are severely demented, with a poor quality of life, prolonging life may not be appropriate. Physicians, philosophers, and lawyers agree that life-sustaining treatment is not mandatory simply because it is possible.[2-5] Such judgments are made, for example, when "do not resuscitate" orders are written or when a decision is made not to hospitalize a patient for treatment of pneumonia. It is acceptable for the physician and family to decide that the goal of care is to alleviate symptoms and provide comfort rather than to prolong life.

Benefits and Burdens of Tube Feedings

Nutrition, like provision of a clean, warm bed, is often considered "ordinary" care that must be given rather than "extraordinary" care, such as mechanical ventilation. This belief that feeding is basic, humane care is emotionally compelling, but the distinction between ordinary and extraordinary care may be confusing and misleading.[6,7] All medical treatments, including tube feedings and use of respirators, provide both benefits and burdens. The crucial issue is not the nature of the procedure but whether the benefits of a treatment outweigh the burdens for a particular patient. We suggest that in some cases the burdens of feeding may outweigh the benefits. Instead of being humane care, tube feedings may be painful, invasive, and impersonal for some patients.

Several questions are important in determining the benefits and burdens of tube feedings. First of all, do tube feedings relieve hunger and thirst? Food and water are basic human needs, and those who care for the demented elderly may generalize from their own experience that hunger and thirst are terribly uncomfortable. However, if patients are offered food and fluid by hand and consistently refuse them, it seems unlikely that they are experiencing hunger and thirst.

Secondly, do tube feedings prolong life? If nutrition is the patient's only major problem, it seems reasonable to expect that additional feeding may prolong life. However, this extension of life may be marginal for patients with many other life-limiting medical problems.

Thirdly, do tube feedings cause suffering and complications? Flexible, small-bore nasogastric tubes cause less discomfort than large-bore, stiffer models. Nevertheless, aspiration may occur, and patients may pull out their feeding tubes. If patients remove tubes repeatedly, they may be restrained or sedated. These measures entail more than just indignities; they may also increase the risk of complications, such as pressure sores and pneumonia.

Finally, what are the social and psychological effects of feeding techniques? With tube feedings, the care giver may focus more attention on technical aspects, such as positioning the tube and checking the gastric residual, than on the patient. If feeding proceeds smoothly, contact between the patient and care giver can be minimal. Moreover, the patient has no control over tube feedings except to pull out the tube. In contrast, during hand feedings the care giver may be more attentive and affectionate, talking with the patient or holding his or her hand. Patients with few other ways of exercising control can still determine the timing, pace, and content of hand feeding.[8] Acceptance of such preferences may be a concrete, if unglamorous, example of what philosophers mean when they speak of respecting a person's autonomy. Hand feedings that provide inadequate nutrition may meet more of the patient's needs than tube feedings that deliver adequate calories impersonally. The psychosocial effects of feeding techniques are especially important when the goal is supportive care.

These psychosocial benefits of feeding may seem impractical to harried care givers. Even the most devoted families and staff may be exhausted and frustrated by hand feedings. In busy institutions that provide long-term care, hand feedings may be hurried and impersonal, and it may be difficult to honor individual food preferences. Although the efficiency of tube feedings may allow more time for attention to be paid to the patient, financial constraints may not. If the patient's social and psychological needs are not met, tube feedings may do more to ease the difficulties of care givers than to provide humane care to patients.

Some disadvantages of nasogastric tubes may be obviated by performance of a gastrostomy or jejunostomy for feeding. Since gastrostomy tubes are less obtrusive and more difficult to remove, patients do not need to be sedated or restrained. There are several possible reasons why such feeding stoma are not used more frequently: the operation may seem more invasive than a nasogastric tube, the cost may be considered excessive, or the staff may be unfamiliar with such techniques.

Recommendations

When demented patients stop eating and cannot be fed by hand, physicians and family need to discuss the goals of care and the benefits and burdens of tube feedings. If feeding problems are temporary, tube or even intravenous feedings are appropriate. Long-term tube feedings are indicated in a patient who has no irreversible life-threatening problems, whose quality of life is acceptable, and whose family wants such feedings. However, tube feedings are not indicated when life-threatening medical problems are irreversible, the quality of life is poor, and the family agrees that the appropriate goal is to provide comfort rather than deliver calories or try to prolong life.

In difficult cases that fall in the gray zone rather than at the extremes, a trial of tube feedings may be helpful. If they are well tolerated, the benefits of such feedings probably outweigh the burdens.

If a patient repeatedly pulls out a nasogastric tube, the goal of care needs to be reconsidered. If prolongation of life is still deemed the goal, a gastrostomy or jejunostomy should be considered. Tying the patient down to allow tube feedings is difficult to reconcile with the goal of humane care. Although food and water should still be offered by hand, caring may be better expressed by providing attention and affection than by forcing calories.

Notes

1. In re Conroy. 464 A.2nd 3403 (N.J.Super. A.D. 1983).
2. President's Commission for the Study of Ethical Problems in Medicine and Biomedical and Behavioral Research. Deciding to forego life-sustaining treatment. Washington D.C.: U.S. Government Printing Office, 1983.
3. Jonsen AR, Siegler M, Winslade WJ. Clinical ethics. New York: Macmillan, 1982.
4. Lo B, Jonsen AR. Clinical decisions to limit treatment. Ann Intern Med 1980; 93:764–8.

21

Care of the Elderly Dying

Daniel Callahan

Death, we are told, is no longer a hidden subject. That is at best a half-truth. The aged constitute the majority of those who die, some 70 percent, but a specific discussion of their dying is remarkably scant in legal, ethical, and medical writings. That omission is probably not accidental. The modernization of aging induces a sharp separation between aging and death. The latter is often treated as if it had little to do with the former, a kind of accidental conjunction. In medicine, the long-standing tradition of treating patients regardless of their age works against an open discussion, even though many physicians admit it is a consideration in their actual practice. The courts appear to follow a similar tradition. Despite the large number of decisions in recent years bearing on cases of elderly patients, that fact is typically not mentioned, though it is an obvious feature of the cases.

These inhibitions against explicit discussion of the dying elderly doubtless serve a valuable function. They reflect a sensible fear that the aged might be singled out for unfairly discriminatory treatment. They are a way of acknowledging the difficulty of sharply differentiating the medical conditions of the aged from those of other patients. Yet the pervasiveness of backstage debate about the care of the elderly dying among physicians and nurses, jurists and legislators, and the elderly themselves makes it imperative to now deal explicitly with the issue. There are also other reasons for having such a discussion. If the proper goal of medicine for those who have already lived out a natural life span ought to be the relief of suffering rather than the extension of life, what are the practical implications of that position for the care of the critically ill, or dying, elderly? If the goals of the aging ought to be service to the young and coming generations, what follows for their way of thinking about death? How

---

does the ready availability of technology sway the making of decisions about the dying? I want to start with that last question.

Medical Technology: A House Divided

One of the hardy illusions of the past few decades has been the belief that with a few changes in law and attitudes, the dying can be spared excessive medical treatment and be allowed to die a "death with dignity." Yet the termination of treatment seems to remain almost as hard, if not harder, in practice now than in earlier times. That is true with the old as much as with the young. Despite the public debate and soothing words, both the public and physicians remain profoundly ambivalent about stopping the use of life-sustaining medical technologies. It is often and accurately said that the elderly do not want excessive and useless treatment. They greatly fear a death marked by technological oppressiveness, wrapped in a cocoon of tubes and machines. Yet they have also no less come—as we all have—to expect medicine whenever possible to extend their lives as well as alleviate or cure their diseases. These are not logically incompatible impulses, but they can be psychologically at odds.

The few available public-opinion surveys suggest some of that ambivalence. A 1985 Gallup Poll asked the respondents whether they believed that the law should make possible the withholding of life-sustaining medical treatment if that was what a patient wanted. Those 65 and older were significantly *less* in favor of such a law than younger generations: some 68 percent of those 65 and older favored it, 20 percent were opposed, and 12 percent had no opinion. By contrast, the national average for all age groups was 81 percent in favor, 13 percent opposed, and 6 percent with no opinion.[1]

Two fears seem to compete with each other among the elderly: on the one hand, that they will be abandoned or neglected if they become critically ill or begin to die and that few will care about their fate; or, on the other hand, that they will be excessively treated and their lives painfully extended. Death after a long, lingering illness marked by dementia and isolation in the back room of a nursing home similarly competes as a vision of horror with that of death in an intensive-care unit, a dying constantly interrupted by painful and unwanted interventions. There is reason for such fears. Medicine steadily extends to the elderly the use of drugs, surgery, rehabilitation, and other procedures once thought suitable only for younger patients. Ever-more-aggressive technological means are used to extend the life of the elderly. On the whole, the elderly welcome that development—even as they fear some of its consequences. They want, somehow, that most elusive of all goals: a steadily improving medical technology that will relieve their pain and illness while not leading to overtreatment and to a harmful extension of a life.

The difficulty of making accurate prognoses is part of the problem. In all too many cases, technology is used because it is not known that a patient is dying or in irreversible decline. The prognosis of a terminal illness is difficult to achieve. Moreover, the problem of prognosis is even greater, a government study concluded, when immediate decisions must be made about initiating treatment. Only for patients who have been fully diagnosed can estimates of survival probability be made. Even then, the probabilities are very likely to be insufficient for guiding decisionmaking about withholding or withdrawing treatment for an individual patient."[2]

The ordinary, almost instinctive, tendency of physicians faced with that uncertainty is then to use technology, to treat with vigor. For his or her part, the patient—who will ordinarily want to live, but may also be fearful of useless overtreatment—will be faced with a no less highly uncertain situation. How sick am I? What are my chances? Both patients and families are likely to have the same inclination as the physician, to treat. Given a normal desire to preserve life and to use available technologies, those impulses of both patients and physicians are understandable. The hard question, therefore, is not why technology is used so much by physicians, or why patients want it no less than doctors. We have to ask instead why it is so hard to *stop* using it, even when patient welfare and plain common sense appear to demand just that.

Technology has sometimes been likened to an addiction, or a force, that takes on a life of its own quite apart from human desires or intentions. That is too fanciful, and a more likely story can be offered. Physicians use medical technology because it generally works. They have been accustomed by their own education and experience to its routine efficacy. It works in part because there is faith in it, a faith strengthened and made credible by constant testing and experimentation. That process of innovation and persistent refinement means that technology is usually always changing while simultaneously more is being learned about its use. As a consequence, different results are achieved at different times, and, ordinarily, improved results. Open-heart surgery works better now than ten years ago, and will be even better next year. Physicians begin with the presumption that most technology will do some good until it is proved otherwise. The fact that a technology failed in one case in the past, or even in many cases, does not prove it will fail in other, similar cases at present or in the future. Medical technology may spring

from science, but its use is in great part a matter of art and shifting probabilities. A pervasive ingredient throughout is a psychological imperative to use technology if at all possible. However flawed, however uncertain the outcome, it remains medicine's best, if not only, hope.

We should not see the question of terminating treatment as a sharply focused "yes" or "no" decision to treat vigorously or allow to die, a kind of binary "1" or "0" gateway to life or death. It is more realistically viewed as a continuum in which the odds of effective intervention slowly decline. At age 65, a person (call him Mr. Smith) in otherwise good health who suffers a heart attack will be treated, and the available technology makes the odds of saving him good.[3] Then imagine Mr. Smith being diagnosed for an operable cancer of the colon at age 75, with a 50 percent chance of full recovery. If he is still mentally alert and eager to live, both doctor and patient will most likely choose to go forward with the operation. Imagine still another phase: at 80, he again suffers a heart attack of moderate severity, with the odds of complete recovery if vigorously treated at about 20 percent and partial recovery at about 60 percent. He will probably be treated. Then, at 82, he suffers a moderately severe stroke, one from which his life can most likely be saved but which will almost certainly leave him semiparalyzed and probably only semicompetent thereafter (but amenable to rehabilitation efforts). Thereafter, he gradually declines and suffers a series of other strokes in his mid to late 80s, spending his last years debilitated and demented in a nursing home before dying at 88.

When, in that continuum, was he dying? There is no straight answer to that question, for he was—but for the technology—dying at many points. Each crisis point presented the need to make a choice for or against initiating treatment. A familiar story then unfolded: since physicians generally aim to save life, and since patients ordinarily prefer to live rather than to die, and since at each point there was some realistic hope, treatment was undertaken. The good fight was fought.

Mr. Smith lived on because we expect medicine to continue to devise ever-more-ingenious ways to save our lives. That is why the annual budget of the National Institutes of Health (NIH) has always risen, budget crises or not. Few congressmen can resist the plea to appropriate funds to save lives through medical research. Why should anyone be astonished, much less indignant, that the other message many are trying to deliver—the need to stop treatment—has such a hard time getting through? Unrelenting "wars" against disease are being pursued by thousands of dedicated medical researchers and physicians at the same time that "natural death" legislation is being passed. The former campaigns are much more dedicated and powerful than the latter. We have been told endlessly—and truthfully, with the support of hard data—that more effective emergency care and the improvement of intensive-care units will save additional lives, and that better geriatric rehabilitation services (for which Mr. Smith was an ideal candidate at many points) will help restore the functioning of the lives thus saved. In the meantime, of course, physicians are being exhorted to stop trying so hard to perform technological miracles with those destined—assuming we can know that—to die. The double message is just about perfect, designed for maximum confusion. As a group the elderly dying are to be saved and those diseases which cause death eliminated. As individuals, however, the elderly dying should be allowed to die when it is

right to do so and their diseases allowed to run their course.

Age as a Criterion

Could we not, however, turn to age as a criterion in order to know when to stop, when to say that no more should be done? I want to explore that question in some detail. While there are some good reasons to see age as possibly among the criteria for allowing an elderly person to die, it will remain a delicate and difficult task to accomplish well and with moral safety.

I want to look first at one great source of confusion: the common failure to distinguish between age as a medical or technical criterion, pertinent to prognosis, and age as a person- or patient-centered criterion. By age as a medical criterion, I mean treating chronological age as if it were the equivalent of other physical characteristics of a patient—that is, as the equivalent of such typical medical indicators as weight, blood pressure, or white-cell count. Just as those characteristics would be reasonable considerations in treating a patient, so also would age if it could be treated as a reliable technical consideration. Age as a person-centered characteristic, by contrast, would be understood as the relevance of a person's history and biography, his situation not as a collection of organs but as a person, to be taken into account when that personal situation could legitimately be considered. I will argue that age as a medical standard should be rejected, while age as a person-centered (what I will call a "biographical") standard can be used.

1. Age as a Medical Standard. The principal use of age as a medical standard would be in prognosis of treatment outcome: how well will an elderly person respond to and benefit from a treatment? In that respect, the main problem in using age as a standard is twofold. It is difficult to disentangle age from a wide range of other conditions that may coexist with old age. Do kidneys fail because a person is old, or simply because of the ravages of a disease that anyone could have, whatever his age? It is no less difficult to distinguish between the general characteristics of the aged as a group and the unique characteristics of any given aged person. The OTA report on aging and life-extending technology medicine notes the difficulties in making the necessary distinctions (which I have reordered slightly to bring out the underlying logic):

(a) increasing age is associated with greater likelihood of physical decline, increased co-morbidity, reduced physiological reserve, and cognitive impairment. Clinically, the probability of these decrements increases notably after age 85;[4]

but (b) chronological age turns out to be a poor predictor of the efficacy of a number of life-sustaining technologies (dialysis, nutritional support, resuscitation, mechanical ventilation, and antibiotics);

while (c) efficacy may be lessened for older patients in general;

but (d) improved medical assessment and care could improve that efficacy;

while (e) in any case very little is currently known about differences in treatment outcome that are due to age *per se* and those that are due to increased prevalence or severity of diseases in older ages;

but (f) in some classification systems (for the purposes of, say, admission to an ICU), chronological age functions as a proxy measure for age-associated factors that cannot be easily measured.

I do not cite the OTA material with any intent to amuse. It is a careful set of distinctions based on the best empirical evidence available and makes perfectly clear why age alone is not a good predictor of medical outcome. It also nicely helps explain why physicians can also say that in practice, they do make decisions based on the age of patients—but rarely can give a wholly defensible scientific account of themselves if pressed to do so. The puzzle, I think, is partially explained by the difference between (1) perceiving a patient as a whole person, whose combination, or gestalt, of characteristics makes it evident that he is old rather than young, which makes a difference in his future; and (2) perceiving and medically treating the person part by part, organ by organ. If we look at a person only as a collection of organs, any given characteristic may well be identical with that found in younger persons (some of whom have wrinkled skin, or failing kidneys, or are bald, or have osteoarthritis, for example). Moreover, even if in some cases, with some conditions, we know age to be generally relevant, we may not know where, on a continuum of characteristics of the aged as a group, any particular old person falls in terms of likely medical outcome. For all these reasons, age as a medical criterion is unreliable.

2. Age as a Biographical Standard. If we know someone's age, but nothing else about him, what do we know of significance? If the person is old—say, in his 70s (and certainly by his 80s)—we would know that most of his chronological life is in his past rather than his future, would not expect to find him playing football or climbing trees for recreation, might not be surprised to find that most of his friends are older rather than younger people, and might expect him to have two or more physical impairments, minor or major. Certain "age-associated" traits would almost invariably be present. We would already know something of importance about an old person even before we met him: that he stands much nearer the end than the beginning of the continuum that is his life. Yet we still might not know anything of significance about him in other respects: whether he was happy or sad, relatively healthy or unhealthy for his age, lively or dour, optimistic or pessimistic, bright or dull.

Yet what makes him the person he is, and not someone else, is the combination of his age-associated traits and other, more idiosyncratic personal and social traits. That he was very old, with a statistically short life expectancy, would hardly be irrelevant to him as he thought about his life and his future or to the rest of us for many (even if not all) purposes. As Malcolm Cowley has noted, "we start by growing old in other people's eyes. Then slowly we come to share their judgment."[5] We would not make long-range plans with an elderly person the way we might with a younger person, nor would we likely invite him to take charge of strenuous long-term projects, even if he were highly talented. For his part, he would not be likely to undertake a total change in his way of life, such as immigrating to a new country, or undertaking extensive training for a new career. While age alone would not tell us whether he was lively or dour, bright or dull, we would most likely be far more impressed with great physical vitality in someone that age than in a teenager.

His age would, in other words, surely be a

part of our overall understanding of him—not the whole story, but hardly of no consequence either. While many "age-associated" traits will bear on the functioning of an elderly person, age as a biographical trait does not reduce to that. Age encompasses a relationship to time —less time statistically remains for an old person than a young person, and there is more personal history behind him as well. It encompasses a relationship to self-consciousness— life and its prospects will usually be thought about differently. And it encompasses a relationship to the passing of the generations—the old are next in line to pass as individuals. The old know they are old, and so does everyone else. Age is not an incidental trait of a person. Might the combination of age and other characteristics then be allowed to have a bearing on medical treatment, and particularly termination, decisions?

3. The Morality of Age as a Standard. Before attempting to answer that last question, it is necessary to inquire whether it is moral to make the attempt. Some would say no: age as a criterion for the termination of treatment should be ruled out of bounds altogether. A central strand of medical ethics holds that patients should be treated only on the basis of their strict medical needs, and that age should no more influence the way they are treated than should their race, sex, or ethnic background. Dr. Mark Siegler has pointed to one source of the objection, noting that a failure to retain "need-specific criteria with respect to elderly patients . . . [would] undermine the traditions of clinical medicine, which are based upon medical need and patient preferences . . . and [would] undermine the traditions of our society, which are based upon moral virtues of charity and compassion."[6] The immediate force of such objections is evident. While there has been some toleration in the medical-ethics literature for the idea of rationing by imposing external policy constraints on physicians, there has been little if any toleration for the idea of physician rationing at the bedside. Doctors are enjoined by medical morality to be unstinting advocates for the welfare of their individual patients and no less enjoined to use medical criteria only—"medical need"—in making their decisions. Yet it is precisely that tradition which my approach to limitation of health care for the aged calls into doubt. The high cost of health care, unrelenting technological developments, and the good of the elderly themselves require that it be examined afresh.

"Medical need," in the context of constant technological innovation, is inherently elastic and open-ended; as a guide to what is actually good for patients or what physicians are obliged to give them, it is highly unreliable. Experienced and conscientious physicians do in fact take age into account in termination decisions, and always have. Why should we therefore assume that age is not, and should not be, part of a responsible moral judgment? The problem in responding to this question is in distinguishing between a medical and a moral judgment. That an elderly person should be given a different drug dosage than a younger patient is ordinarily considered a purely medical judgment. By that statement is meant that if the aim is proper physical care of the patient in both cases, then different dosages may be indicated to achieve identical outcomes. A judgment of that kind can be based on scientific evidence. But the use of age as a "medical" indication is ambiguous. If it means that because of a person's age, medical treatment will be futile, do no good whatever, then it may properly be called a medical and not a moral judgment. It is a judgment about medical efficacy only. Yet if a judgment is also being passed about the worth of the life—that the treatment is futile not because it will fail technically but because the life saved is not worth saving because of age—then it has passed into the moral realm. According to the tradition of medical ethics, judgments about the social worth of a patient's life are unacceptable as grounds for terminating care. That is a solid and necessary tradition; but it does not touch the question of whether age as a standard might be defensible.

There is also another possibility for ambiguity. What is medical "need"? If understood as the needs of a patient's organs, or other physiological systems, treatment may (by ordinary standards) be required; otherwise they will fail. But if "need" is understood to be the needs of the patient as a person, not merely as an assemblage of deficient organs, no clear answer about the requirement of "medical need" may be forthcoming. Then the physician may have to make a moral judgment: will meeting the needs of the patient's organs meet his needs as a whole person? They are not necessarily the same needs. It is not clear which need the tradition invoked by Dr. Siegler has in mind. More than that, the technological possibilities of medicine for organ sustenance, quite apart from overall patient welfare, mean that "medical need" can rarely if ever be kept free of moral evaluation and judgment. The good of organs is always subordinate to the good of the person. There is no such thing as pure "medical need"; it always presupposes some value judgment about the desirability of treatment.

Will it necessarily be the case, as James Childress has suggested, that the use of an age standard would symbolize "abandonment and exclusion from communal care"?[7] That would be likely only if it were widely believed or perceived that an age standard for exclusion from care came into use as a manifestation of society's rejection, denigration, or devaluation of elderly people. It would be a different matter if, instead, it emerged from a prudent effort to find an appropriate balance between the needs of the aged and those of younger generations, and from a conscientious effort to determine, in the face of potentially unlimited technological innovation in care for the aged, where a reasonable limit on care could be set. The "symbolic significance" of an age standard depends not on the mere fact of using age but on the meaning attributed to that fact; context, perceived motive, and articulated rationale determine that symbolic meaning. Childress would most likely be right if age were used as a standard in the present situation; but that would not necessarily be the case if its use were transformed so as to be seen as part of an affirmation of old age and not its denigration.

4. Age as a Biographical Standard for Terminating Treatment. How can a combination of age and other characteristics be allowed to have a bearing on the termination of treatment? How, I respond, can it not any longer? If "medical need" is too indeterminate and elastic a concept to be used by itself, then some use of age will be *necessary* to make a judgment about terminating care of the elderly. Since age is an important aspect of the patient as a person, someone who is not just a collection of organs, it falsifies the reality that is part of a person in his fullness to set it aside as irrelevant. Moreover, in addition to being a necessary part of a full and proper medical-moral judgment, age is a valuable and illuminating part, telling us where the patient stands in relation to his own history. There are a large and growing number of elderly who are not imminently dying but who are feeble and declining, often chronically ill, for whom curative medicine has little to offer. That kind of

medicine may still be able to do something for failing organs; it can keep them going a bit longer. But it cannot offer the patient as a person any hope of being restored to good health. A different treatment plan should be in order. That person's history has all but come to an end, and medical care needs to encompass that reality, not try to deny it.

More broadly, even if age is not a good prognosticator for treatment efficacy (that is, physiological efficacy), it is a perfectly reasonable standard for treatment reasonableness or desirability. The mere fact that major surgery, or admission to an ICU, or cardiopulmonary resuscitation might save the life of an elderly person does not mean that it ought to be undertaken. A moral judgment must be made about what ultimately serves the patient's welfare. The "age-associated" fact of multiorgan failure with a poor physical prognosis, for instance, might at the least reasonably incline one to spare an elderly patient such vigorous lifesaving efforts. For many people, beginning with the aged themselves, old age is a reason in itself to think about medical care in a different way, whether in forgoing its lifesaving powers when death is clearly imminent, or in forgoing its use even when death may be distant but life has become a blight rather than a blessing. The alternative is not, as some would have it, respect for life but an idolatrous enslavement to technology.

We should want to know not just what chronological age may tell us about the state of a person's body (as a technical criterion), but also what it morally and psychologically signifies for a person to have an old rather than a young body; or what it means for a person to be old rather than young when considering the prospect of painful treatment; or what it signifies to live life as an old person—or as a sick old person—who cannot expect to recapture the vitality of youth, or even of an earlier old age. When considered in those ways, age becomes a category of evaluation in its own right, something reasonable and proper to wonder and worry about. It bears not only on physical characteristics, but on a person's self-understanding, as something intrinsic (with varying degrees of intensity, to be sure) to a person's individuality and life story. The whole person —and it is that whole person who presents himself or herself for treatment—is a person of a certain chronological age: that determines many characteristics, and much of the coloring, of a person's life. That is the importance of the biographical point of view.

Principles for the Use of Age

How, from a biographical vantage point, should we formulate age as a criterion for the termination of treatment and make use of it in termination decisions? I will begin by proposing some general background principles for the termination of treatment of the aged, each meant to articulate themes developed earlier:

1. *After a person has lived out a natural life span, medical care should no longer be oriented to resisting death.* No precise chronological age can readily be set for determining when a natural life span has been achieved—biographies vary—but it would normally be expected by the late 70s or early 80s. While a person's history may not be complete—time is always open-ended—most of it will have been achieved by that stage of life. It will be a full biography, even if more details are still to be added. Death beyond that period is not now, nor should it be, typically considered premature or untimely. Any greater precision than my "late 70s or early 80s" does not at present seem possible, and extended public discussion

would be needed to achieve even a rough consensus on the appropriate age range. That discussion would also have to consider whether, for policy purposes, it would be necessary to set an exact age or a range only, and that would pose a classic policy dilemma. Too vague a standard of a "natural life span" would open the way for too great a flexibility of application to be fair or workable, while too specific a standard—one indifferent to the unique features of individual biographies—would preclude prudence and appropriate room for discretion.

Problems of that kind, however difficult, should not be used as an excuse to evade the necessity of setting some kind of age standard, or to conclude that any age standard must necessarily mean denying the value of the elderly. The presumption against resisting death after a natural life span would not in any sense demean those who have lived that long or to suggest that their lives are less valuable than those of younger people. To come to the end of life in old age does not diminish the value of the life; that remains until the very end. This is not a principle, in short, for the comparison of lives. It reflects instead an acceptance of the inevitability of death in general and its acceptability for the individual after a natural life span in particular. Death will then take its proper place as a necessary link in the transition of generations.

2. *Provision of medical care for those who have lived out a natural life span will be limited to the relief of suffering.* Medicine is not in a position to bring meaning and significance to the lives of the old. That only they can do for themselves, with the help of the larger culture. Yet medicine can help promote the physical functioning, the mental alertness, and the emotional stability conducive to this pursuit.

These remain valuable goals, even when a natural life span has been attained. The difference at that point is that death should no longer be treated by medicine as an enemy. It may well be, of course, that medical efforts to relieve suffering will frequently have the unintended but foreseeable consequence of extending life expectancy. That is to be expected. A sharp line between relieving suffering and extending life will be on occasion difficult to draw, and under no circumstance would it be acceptable to fail to relieve suffering because of the possibility of life extension. The bias of the principle should be to stop resisting death after a certain age, but not when the price of doing so is unrelievable suffering. At the same time—as the success of the hospice movement proves—it is perfectly possible to relieve suffering while not seeking to extend life.

3. *The existence of medical technologies capable of extending the lives of the elderly who have lived out a natural life span creates no presumption whatever that the technologies must be used for that purpose.* The uses of technology are always to be subordinated to the appropriate ends of medicine: that is, to the avoidance of premature death and to the relief of suffering. The alternative is slavery to the powers of technology—they, not we, will determine our end. Medicine should in particular resist the tendency to provide to the aged the life-extending capabilities of technologies developed primarily to help younger people avoid premature and untimely death. The use of those technologies should be subordinate to what is good for the elderly as individuals, good for them as members of society, good for them as a link in the passing of the generations, and good for the needs of other age groups.

The three principles detailed above are not so radical as they may first appear. They come close to actually articulating what many elderly express as their fears about aging and death. They indicate a wish that their life not be aggressively extended beyond a point at which they still possess a good degree of physical functioning and mental alertness, a life that has value and meaning for them; they are asking not for more years as such (though some would want just that), but for as many *good* years as possible, and that medical technology be limited in its use to those situations in which it will maintain or restore an adequate quality of life, not sustain and extend a deteriorating life.

The old can, of course, be inconsistent and ambivalent; we all can. Neither they nor the rest of us seem fully to understand how to strain out the essence of a desire only to live a full life from an ordinary fear of death, which leads us to grasp at greater longevity even as we recoil from its undesirable consequences. Neither do we seem to understand how to resist the seductions of a medical technology that promises to give us more life as long as we are not prepared to count the costs. Nor do we grasp how to free ourselves from the mistaken worry that a failure to work hard in favor of longer lives for the elderly will be thought tantamount to ageism or to the systematic neglect and abuse of the elderly.

Criteria for Terminating Treatment

How might we put the three principles I have suggested into operation? The appropriate moral and legal standards for terminating treatment of competent adult patients provide a natural point of departure, embodying as they do a commonly expressed ideal, a principle of law, and a base point for understanding the rights of persons and patients. What are our rights as we face death or resist further treatment? To put the matter in its most fundamental terms, both the law and common principles of medical ethics accord competent patients the right to determine when they no longer wish to be treated.[8] The patient is to be the ultimate judge of the benefits and the burdens of life-sustaining treatment, and whether the burdens outweigh the benefits. The right to make such judgments rests upon the principle of patient self-determination. This value reflects our society's long-standing ethical tradition of recognizing the unique moral worth of the individual, and of respecting human dignity by granting individuals the right to make choices about their lives and their bodies in ways consonant with their moral and religious beliefs.[9] The principle of self-determination is the moral basis for the legal doctrine of informed consent, which the courts have determined to include the right to informed refusal of treatment. The right of self-determination is, of course, meant to apply to the elderly as much as to any other patients. Neither the courts nor codes of medical ethics make any age distinctions among competent adults in the application of the principles.

I will not elaborate further on this basic right of self-determination. It has been written about well and at length elsewhere.[10] One should note, however, that the full recognition of that right has met many obstacles in practice and still represents an ideal rather than an achieved reality. An underlying obstacle (in addition to simple paternalism) has been the enormous ambivalence toward lifesaving medicine,

experienced at times by both physicians and patients. Another obstacle is the still-common assumption that a desire for the termination of treatment is symptomatic of depression rather than a free, rational choice. Depression is, of course, a real possibility with the critically ill or debilitated elderly as with any other patient. But it is the automatic assumption of depression in the elderly who express a wish to die that is the greatest source of unfairness. Patients' wishes are simply ignored out of a belief that they do not know what they want. The kind of bias that treats the elderly as children is a closely related obstacle. There the assumption is that the elderly person has already left the world of adult competence and has regressed to a childish state. More properly and fairly, only a clear showing that this has happened should be allowed to overcome the patient's judgment.

For at least two decades now, the right of patients to make known their wishes through advance directives has been understood to be a clear implication of the right of self-determination. These advance directives have been formalized in the legal instrument of "living wills" or use of the durable-power-of-attorney method as recognized by the laws of a growing number of states. Under "living will" statutes, patients may state in advance those conditions under which they want treatment terminated, while the durable-power-of-attorney procedure permits the designation of a specific surrogate to make decisions for a person should he or she become incompetent. A continuing problem with "living wills" has been the unwillingness of many physicians to honor them (out of an often misplaced fear of malpractice suits). Stronger efforts to make those documents more binding on health-care workers would be exceedingly helpful. Such problems with the "living will" approach have made a durable-power-of-attorney strategy seem a more effective one, far more likely to achieve fulfillment of the wishes of the patient.

Strikingly absent in most of the discussion and writings on the competent patient, old or young, are considerations of the appropriate and responsible use of the personal freedom and right to terminate treatment. All too often, moral discussion of competent patients begins and ends with a declaration that they have a right to do with their lives as they please and to terminate their treatment when they choose to do so. That is legally true and long a part of our moral tradition. But why should that be thought, as is often the case, to be the end of moral analysis? What should the individual with that right think about? What moral obligations, for instance, might a person have toward his or her own life and future, toward those friends and family members who could be affected by a voluntary decision to forgo treatment, toward the larger community? These can be difficult, even agonizing questions for the elderly, an aspect of trying to sum up and understand one's life as a whole, and of trying in particular to determine when it should appropriately end, when death should no longer be resisted. I do no more than flag the issue here. It is the great missing link in recent discussions of the rights of competent patients: what should be done with the rights once one has them?

The suggestion is occasionally heard that the elderly may have a duty to die, to relieve their family or society of the costs of their care. This is a dangerous notion, a small step away from declaring the old to be useless; it is a natural child of a utilitarian stance toward the elderly and their social value. The very notion of a duty to die embraces the use of the old as means to the ends of others. That cannot be demanded of anyone. To be sure, I have tried to show that the elderly do not have an unlimited claim on health resources. That is a very different matter from asserting a positive duty not to use resources, and a recourse to death as a means to that end.

There is a related question. Is there a right on the part of a competent, but dying, patient to vigorous life-extending treatment when there is little medical reason to think it will be efficacious? That would be a strange claim. A patient has a right only to ask medicine to do that which is compatible with its proper goals. Those goals cannot encompass an effort to extend a life in the face of a wholly bleak medical prognosis; health cannot thereby be promoted. Discretion and sensitivity in the doctor-patient relationship will be required in a refusal to provide wanted though useless treatment. The physician should make clear that he or she cannot provide useless or inappropriate care which will neither do the patient any good nor bring honor to the practice of medicine.

I now turn to terminal decisions for those incompetent elderly who have lived out a full and natural life span and have left no advance directives, when those caring for the patient do not know what the patient wants or values. A surrogate must then decide what serves the good or welfare of the patient. There are a variety of justifiable moral considerations for a surrogate to have treatment terminated and allow death to occur in the case of the incompetent elderly: when their pain and suffering cannot effectively be relieved; when the physical and psychological burdens of their treatment outweigh its benefits; and when a minimally adequate level of functioning of a person in decline can be neither restored nor maintained by further medical treatment. Note that all three of these criteria imply an important presumption: that an otherwise healthy old person, at least until the late 70s or early 80s, ought to be eligible for government-supported lifesaving medical treatment. I am here concerned not with that policy issue but with treatment standards within those boundaries. An immediate question might next arise about these criteria. Could they not apply to persons of any age? Yes, in one sense they could, but in another sense age will add a particular feature to each, and I will try to bring that out as I move along.

1. Inability to Relieve Pain and Suffering. It is customarily said that with sufficient skill and willingness to use whatever dosage is necessary, most pain can now pharmaceutically be relieved. While that may be true, it still makes little sense to maintain for long a life in such a state that only massive and continuous (and ultimately disorienting and consciousness-reducing) dosages can suffice to make it tolerable. The relief of pain, in any case, is not identical to the relief of suffering. The latter will ordinarily be a manifestation of a realistic hopelessness at the prospect of unending pain, a sense that one's effective life has come to an end, or that the burden to oneself of one's illness or frailty is too great to make life worth continuing. A medicine that can only hold out the prospect of prolonging life in order to extend, but not relieve, suffering has come to the end of its resources and purpose. Where age may make a difference in these cases is that the younger person will still typically not have lived out a full life span and may have significant goals to accomplish (such as support of a family) which might justify, even require, the enduring of pain and suffering. That will not

ordinarily be as true of the aged, and even less so the older they become.

2. Disproportionate Burden of Treatment. Treatment burdens—such as pain, loss of function, and disfigurement—can sometimes out-weigh benefits. There is good evidence that in the case of about 1 in every 6 elderly patients on renal dialysis, treatment is deliberately stopped and death ensues.[11] The thrice-weekly frequency of the dialysis combined with its side effects—mental disorientation, fatigue, physical discomfort, depression—make it a treatment whose personal costs simply seem to some too high. Similarly, surgery is sometimes refused by the elderly because of the pain it would bring, the lasting complications or debilities in its aftermath, and the fact that long survival after the operation is not likely in any case.[12] What difference does age make, particularly since young people sometimes remove themselves from dialysis and also refuse surgery? In this as in other burden-benefit cases, age will bring in two additional considerations: whether a long life can be attained by the burdensome medical procedure; and whether a person still has major life tasks remaining, such that the burdens seem justified or demanded. In both cases, age will ordinarily make a difference.

3. Inability to Restore or Maintain Quality of Life. I have said comparatively little about the burden-benefit problem, and about the relief of suffering, because both shade rapidly into the more encompassing topic of "quality of life."[13] The term itself is not felicitous, lacking clear cultural roots and a precise, well-understood meaning. It invites being stuffed with anything that suits anyone's fancy. Its only, but redeeming, advantage is that we possess no other term or phrase that adequately does its work. That work is ordinarily twofold: to distinguish the condition of human life from the value of that life (often referred to as the sanctity of life), and between the physical state of a person's body and the larger good of the person as a whole. In that latter sense, it has often been used to distinguish between "vitalism"—the view that life in itself, regardless of its condition, ought to be valued and preserved—and the view that the preservation of life should be determined by the condition of that life. A distinction is often also made between the concept of "quality" as referring to individual worth based on some comparative social standard, and quality based on the inherent health and well-being of a person in comparison with his own potential.[14] A great and justifiable fear is that "quality" as a comparative social standard will be used as a way of denying equality to all human beings and of dismissing some lives as not worthy to be lived.[15] That is a view rightly rejected, in the context of the aged no less than with others.

The idea of the sanctity and value of individual life can have no meaning, however, without encompassing some consideration of quality of life. We value human life, and the personhood that is the crowning glory of that life, because it possesses certain capacities that are the distinguishing marks of human beings, those which separate humans from animals and lend them their power to reflect upon their own condition. To be sure, the possession of those capacities forms a continuum, and there has been a justifiable reluctance to exclude borderline cases from the human community. The evils that result from that tendency were displayed all too murderously under the Nazi regime, which coined the term "*Untermensch*" to designate those determined to be subhuman and dispensable and spoke all too readily of "a life not worth living."[16]

However varied its manifestations, and however faint its expression, the essence of a person's "quality of life" will be the possession of certain potentialities for personhood. The "sanctity of life" has to be the sanctity of personhood, not merely the possession of a body. What are the crucial potentialities for personhood? That is a complex and controversial question, but must at least encompass the capacity to reason, to have emotions, and to enter into relationships with others. Of these three potentialities, the most minimal is the capacity to experience emotions (including the sensation of pain); but it has a special importance in the case of the elderly because it may be, locked behind severe dementia, the only capacity some will have remaining. A person who has lost all of these capacities cannot, in any meaningful way, be called a "person" any longer or be said to have a "biographical life" remaining.[17] But a person who has one of these capacities, even the most minimal one of self-enclosed emotions, can still be said to be a person. At the least, lacking access to such a person's inner life, we should give the benefit of the doubt to those who display evidence of emotions (not possible in the case of a permanent vegetative state).

It is also helpful to distinguish between the loss of a potentiality altogether and the presence of severe physical or emotional impediments that may block its expression. Severe and intractable pain and suffering, or the effects of heavy dosages of medication necessary to relieve the pain, can effectively block a person's capacity to reason and to enter into a relationship with others (and severe pain, while producing emotions, could make it impossible for a person to be at one with himself). A consideration in thinking about the burdens and benefits of a proposed medical procedure would be the likelihood of its effects on those potentialities. We need a way also of understanding the possible impact on the capacities of personhood of the loss of such physical functions as movement, speech, sight or hearing. They can make the realization of the inherent capacities difficult.

My definitions and discussion here have been of necessity general and abstract. Let me now turn to the various modes of terminating treatment to give them more specificity.

Determining Appropriate Treatment

In determining morally appropriate care for the elderly, three major types of considerations should come into play: (1) the physical and mental status of the patient; (2) the levels of possible medical and nursing care; (3) the quality of life of the patient. I want to conduct my analysis on the basis of those considerations, but I want also to divide the analysis into two steps. I suggest a number of relatively straightforward ways to make decisions based on quality of life standards.

(I) CLASSIFICATIONS.
  (a) PHYSICAL AND MENTAL STATUS[18]
    (1) Patients with brain death
    (2) Patients in persistent vegetative state
    (3) Patients who are severely demented
    (4) Patients with mild to moderate impairment of competence (or fluctuating competence)
    (5) Severely ill, mentally alert patients

    (6) Physically frail, but not severely ill, mentally alert patients
    (7) Physically vigorous, mentally alert patients

  (b) LEVELS OF CARE
    (1) Emergency lifesaving interventions (example, CPR)
    (2) Intensive care and advanced life support (examples, intensive-care units, respirators)
    (3) General medical care (examples, antibiotics, surgery, cancer chemotherapy, artificial hydration and nutrition)
    (4) General nursing care for comfort and palliation

  (c) QUALITY OF LIFE
    (1) Criteria of quality of life: capacity to think, feel, interact with others
    (2) Impediments to quality: severe pain and suffering (or effects of medication to relieve them), and any other condition that thwarts capacity to think, feel, and interact with others

I want to use this classification system for illustrative purposes. It is not meant to explore all possibilities or to exclude other possibilities that might be consistent with the principles I have proposed. A certain suspicion is in order about tidy charts and clean formulas. As one physician observed in a moving article on the care of the debilitated elderly, "it is simply too difficult to define all the varieties of illness, suffering, prognosis, and treatment with sufficient precision for the definitions to be of much help in the actual situations."[19] Implicit in my analysis will be the assumption that Medicare support would be provided only for the level of care indicated.

In the case of a patient who is *brain dead,* no further care of any kind, medical or nursing, is called for. All potential for being a person is irrevocably lost, and only a pronouncement of death is in order. What are we to make, however, of someone in a *persistent vegetative state (pvs)*—that is, a person whose brain stem is still functioning, but whose higher, neocortical brain functions are clinically judged to have ceased? That being has also lost all capacities for personhood, though clinical death has not occurred. Assuming a careful diagnosis (and occasional errors have been reported), all treatment other than minimal nursing care (level 4) should be terminated.[20] There is no reason to believe that even a minimal capacity for emotion exists. Artificial hydration and nutrition may be terminated also; they serve no purpose, and do no honor to the body or the memory of the person who once inhabited that body. Out of the respect due human bodies prior to clinical death, nursing care should be provided. But death should in no way be resisted.

A more complex situation presents itself with a patient who is *severely demented.* On the one hand, he has lost his capacity for reason and usually—but not always—human interaction. On the other hand, there will be no clear ground for believing that the capacity to experience emotions has been lost. Hence, it would be inappropriate to terminate nursing care (level 4) or nutrition and hydration, either artificial or natural. In general, only nursing care at level 4 should be provided, but I would not eliminate artificial hydration and artificial nutrition, because there is sufficient public

and medical doubt whether their provision should be classified as a form of nursing and ordinary comfort or as a form of medical care. The prognosis for relief from severe dementia is poor at best in the old, and in irreversible cases nonexistent. Death need not be aggressively resisted, although general medical care (level 3) would be justified to reduce suffering. Thus, the death of the person, if not the body, is under way and need not be resisted.

Patients with *mild impairment of competence,* or fluctuating competence, meet the criteria of an acceptable quality of life, even if a low one. They can reason (even if poorly), interact with others (even if erratically), and surely experience emotions. Yet if they have lived out a natural life span and death is therefore not to be rejected, advanced life support (level 2) would not morally be required. While life-extending efforts would not be mandatory, general medical care (level 3) to reduce suffering would be. (A grandfather clause would also be needed in some circumstances: life-extending treatment such as insulin for diabetics or dialysis, if begun in early old age, should not be withdrawn in later old age.)

Severely ill, mentally alert patients who have lived out a full life span should receive care that is limited, as a rule, to general nursing care (level 4), unless there is strong reason to believe that general medical care (level 3) would significantly relieve any suffering. Assuming competence, the patient should make his or her own decisions in these cases. Severe illness—particularly if likely to be terminal without aggressive intervention—should preclude emergency lifesaving interventions (level 1) and intensive care and advanced life support (level 2).

Physically frail, mentally alert patients (apart from being able to make their own decisions in any case) would seem appropriate candidates for general medical care (level 3) and, in some cases, emergency care (level 1). If they have lived a full life, however, extended intensive care and advanced life support would be unwarranted at public expense, an unjustifiable effort (unless necessary to reduce suffering) to extend life. Yet with an elderly and frail person whose death might be counted premature, even general medical care (level 3) should take into account the potential impediments to a decent quality that it may entail. In the case of a younger person, it will be more worth risking in order to allow the living out of a natural life span. However, once medical treatment begins to offer rapidly diminishing returns, and serious deterioration is progressing, then strenuous efforts to prolong life seem out of order.

The care of the *physically vigorous elderly person* poses the fewest problems. All levels of care appear appropriate, at least through the first round of illness and disease, and even for those who have lived a natural life span if there is a solid prospect of a few (say, four or five) more years of good life. It is the one category in which an exception to the cessation of Medicare-supported life-extending treatment to those who have lived a full life span would be justified. Only when such a person deteriorates and falls into one of the other categories would it be appropriate (depending upon the circumstances already discussed) to terminate life-extending treatment. But is it not a contradiction to my age criteria—if a person has lived out a natural life span—to say that all forms of treatment are appropriate? I make an exception in this case because I do not think anyone would find it tolerable to allow the healthy person to be denied lifesaving care. One incident, moreover, does not prove that death or precipitous decline is on its way. A second and further incident will be a different matter.

A concluding comment is required on an issue that frequently arises in the use of age as a criterion for terminating treatment. Is it not unfair to have standards of care, and particularly termination standards, that are different for the old than for the young? If it would be reasonable to terminate medical treatment for an elderly person because of a bleak future, should that not be done with the young as well—for instance, in the case of a severely handicapped newborn? We are not forced to draw such conclusions. The elderly have already lived out a full life. They have not been denied (at least because of their age) the opportunities of living a life; and their death deprives them of less than it does a child or young person who has had no such opportunity. Not only does it seem justifiable to work harder, and to take more chances, to save and rehabilitate the life of a sick child, but also to allocate more resources to those conditions which cause premature death than to those which cause death after a long life. This is not, however, to say that the young should be oppressed by medical treatment in order that they might be saved, or that all technological means for extending the life of handicapped or critically ill children should be used. There are many occasions when that would be cruel and termination of treatment would be morally justified. I am only saying that it is proper to have different standards for young and old.

Notes

1. The Gallup Poll (March 14, 1985).
2. U.S. Congress Office of Technology Assessment, Biological Applications Program, *Life-Sustaining Technologies and the Elderly* (Washington, D.C.: OTA, July 1987), pp. 1–22 *ff.*

3. I have adapted this description from a similar one developed by Jerome L. Avorn, "Medicine, Health, and the Geriatric Transformation," *Daedalus* 115 (Winter 1986), pp. 215–17.

4. This quotation as well as the summaries and further quotations are from OTA, pp. I-39–45.

5. Malcolm Cowley, *The View from Eighty* (New York: Penguin Books, 1982), p. 5. That line was quoted in G. C. Prado's remarkably interesting book *Rethinking How We Age* (Westport, CT: Greenwood Press, 1986) which analyzes psychological and social age, as distinguished from biological age.

6. Mark Siegler, "Should Age Be a Criterion in Health Care?" *Hastings Center Report* 14 (October 1984), p. 27.

7. James F. Childress, "Ensuring Care, Respect, and Fairness for the Elderly," *Hastings Center Report* 14 (October 1984), p. 29.

8. For a full discussion of the rights of competent patients, see President's Commission for the Study of Ethical Problems in Medicine and Biomedical and Behavioral Research, *Deciding to Forgo Life-Sustaining Treatment: Ethical, Medical, and Legal Issues in Treatment Decisions.* (Washington, D.C.: Government Printing Office, 1983). See also Steven A. Levenson, "Ethical Considerations in Critical and Terminal Illness in the Elderly," *Journal of the American Geriatrics Society* 29:12 (December 1981), pp. 563–67.

9. This theme is developed more fully in Susan Wolf, Daniel Callahan, Bruce Jennings, Cynthia Cohen, eds., *Guidelines on the Termination of Life-Sustaining Treatment and the Care of the Dying.* (Briarcliff Manor, N.Y.: The Hastings Center, 1987).

10. A thorough discussion can be found in Jay Katz, *The Silent World of Doctor and Patient* (New York: Free Press, 1984).

11. Steven Neu and Carl M. Kjellstrand, "Stopping Long-Term Dialysis: An Empirical Study of Withdrawal of Life-Supporting Treatment," *New England Journal of Medicine* 314 (January 1986), pp. 14–20.

12. R. Reiss, "Moral and Ethical Issues in Geriatric Surgery," *Journal of Medical Ethics* 6 (1980), pp. 71–77.

13. The most thorough and balanced analysis of the concept of "quality of life" is that of Edward W. Keyserlingk, *Sanctity of Life or Quality of Life* (Montreal: Law Reform Commission of Canada, 1979); see also Richard McCormick, "The Quality of Life, the Sanctity of Life," *Hastings Center Report* (February 1978), pp. 30–36.

14. John D. Arras nicely develops these distinctions in "Quality of Life in Neonatal Ethics" (unpublished paper presented at Hastings Center, May 7, 1986). The difference between patient and physician judgment of "quality of life" is interestingly discussed in T. Jolene Starr et al., "Quality of Life and Resuscitation Decisions in Elderly Patients," *Journal of General Internal Medicine* 1 (November/December 1986), pp. 373–79. See also David C. Thomasma, "Ethical Judgments of Quality of Life in the Care of the Aged," *Journal of the American Geriatrics Society* 32:7 (July 1984), pp. 525–27.

15. See Cynthia B. Cohen, " 'Quality of Life' and the Analogy with the Nazis," *Journal of Medicine and Philosophy* 8 (1983), pp. 113–35.

16. See Robert J. Lifton's chapter (Chapter 2) " 'Euthanasia': Direct Medical Killing," in *The Nazi Doctors* (New York: Basic Books, 1986), pp. 45–56, for a good historical analysis of the origin and nature of Nazi attitudes toward killing the sick and handicapped.

17. James Rachels, in *The End of Life: Eu-*

thanasia and Morality (Oxford: Oxford University Press, 1986), p. 5, makes use of this phrase in a helpful way (though I do not support his analysis of euthanasia).

18. I have adapted this classification system from Sidney H. Wanzer *et al.,* "The Physician's Responsibility Toward Hopelessly Ill Patients," *New England Journal of Medicine* 310 (April 1984), pp. 955–59.

19. David Hilfiker, "Allowing the Debilitated to Die: Facing Our Ethical Choices," *New England Journal of Medicine* 308 (March 1983), p. 718.

20. B. Jennett and F. Plum, "Persistent Vegetative State After Brain Damage: A Syndrome in Search of a Name," *Lancet* 1 (1972), pp. 734–37. *Cf.* Ronald E. Cranford, "Termination of Treatment in the Persistent Vegetative State," *Seminars in Neurology* 4:1 (March 1984), pp. 36–44.

EUTHANASIA AND ASSISTED SUICIDE

22

Declaration on Euthanasia

Sacred Congregation for the Doctrine of the Faith

The rights and values pertaining to the human person occupy an important place among the questions discussed today. In this regard, the Second Vatican Ecumenical Council solemnly reaffirmed the lofty dignity of the human person, and in a special way his or her right to life. The council therefore condemned crimes against life "such as any type of murder, genocide, abortion, euthanasia, or willful suicide" (*Gaudium et Spes*, n. 27).

More recently, the Sacred Congregation for the Doctrine of the Faith has reminded all the faithful of Catholic teaching on procured abortion.[1] The congregation now considers it opportune to set forth the church's teaching on euthanasia.

It is indeed true that in this sphere of teaching the recent popes have explained the principles and these retain their full force,[2] but the progress of medical science in recent years has brought to the fore new aspects of the question of euthanasia, and these aspects call for further elucidation on the ethical level.

In modern society, in which even the fundamental values of human life are often called into question, cultural change exercises an influence upon the way of looking at suffering and death; moreover, medicine has increased its capacity to cure and to prolong life in particular circumstances, which sometimes give rise to moral problems.

Thus people living in this situation experience no little anxiety about the meaning of advanced old age and death. They also begin to wonder whether they have the right to obtain for themselves or their fellowmen an "easy death," which would shorten suffering and which seems to them more in harmony with human dignity.

A number of episcopal conferences have raised questions on this subject with the Sacred Congregation for the Doctrine of the

---

"Declaration on Euthanasia" by the Sacred Congregation for the Doctrine of the Faith. Reprinted from Origins 10 (August, 1980): 154–157.

Faith. The congregation, having sought the opinion of experts on the various aspects of euthanasia, now wishes to respond to the bishops' questions with the present declaration, in order to help them to give correct teaching to the faithful entrusted to their care and to offer them elements for reflection that they can present to the civil authorities with regard to this very serious matter.

The considerations set forth in the present document concern in the first place all those who place their faith and hope in Christ, who through his life, death and resurrection has given a new meaning to existence and, especially to the death of the Christian, as St. Paul says: "If we live, we live to the Lord, and if we die, we die to the Lord" (Rom. 14:8; cf. Phil. 1:20).

As for those who profess other religions, many will agree with us that faith in God the creator, provider and lord of life—if they share this belief—confers a lofty dignity upon every human person and guarantees respect for him or her.

It is hoped that this declaration will meet with the approval of many people of good will who, philosophical or ideological differences notwithstanding, have nevertheless a lively awareness of the rights of the human person. These rights have often in fact been proclaimed in recent years through declarations issued by international congresses,[3] and since it is a question here of fundamental rights inherent in every human person, it is obviously wrong to have recourse to arguments from political pluralism or religious freedom in order to deny the universal value of those rights.

I. The Value of Human Life

Human life is the basis of all goods and is the necessary source and condition of every human activity and of all society. Most people regard life as something sacred and hold that no one may dispose of it at will, but believers see in life something greater, namely a gift of God's love, which they are called upon to preserve and make fruitful. And it is this latter consideration that gives rise to the following consequences:

1. No one can make an attempt on the life of an innocent person without opposing God's love for that person, without violating a fundamental right, and therefore without committing a crime of the utmost gravity.[4]

2. Everyone has the duty to lead his or her life in accordance with God's plan. That life is entrusted to the individual as a good that must bear fruit already here on earth, but that finds its full perfection only in eternal life.

3. Intentionally causing one's own death, or suicide, is therefore equally as wrong as murder; such an action on the part of a person is to be considered as a rejection of God's sovereignty and loving plan. Furthermore, suicide is also often a refusal of love for self, the denial of the natural instinct to live, a flight from the duties of justice and charity owed to one's neighbor, to various communities or to the whole of society—although, as is generally recognized, at times there are psychological factors present that can diminish responsibility or even completely remove it.

However, one must clearly distinguish suicide from that sacrifice of one's life whereby for a higher cause, such as God's glory, the salvation of souls or the service of one's brethren, a person offers his or her own life or puts it in danger (cf. Jn. 15:14).

II. Euthanasia

In order that the question of euthanasia can be properly dealt with, it is first necessary to define the words used.

Etymologically speaking, in ancient times euthanasia meant an easy death without severe suffering. Today one no longer thinks of this original meaning of the word, but rather of some intervention of medicine whereby the sufferings of sickness or of the final agony are reduced, sometimes also with the danger of suppressing life prematurely. Ultimately, the word euthanasia is used in a more particular sense to mean "mercy killing," for the purpose of putting an end to extreme suffering, or saving abnormal babies, the mentally ill or the incurably sick from the prolongation, perhaps for many years, of a miserable life, which could impose too heavy a burden on their families or on society.

It is therefore necessary to state clearly in what sense the word is used in the present document.

By euthanasia is understood an action or an omission which of itself or by intention causes death, in order that all suffering may in this way be eliminated. Euthanasia's terms of reference, therefore, are to be found in the intention of the will and in the methods used.

It is necessary to state firmly once more that nothing and no one can in any way permit the killing of an innocent human being, whether a fetus or an embryo, an infant or an adult, an old person, or one suffering from an incurable disease, or a person who is dying. Furthermore, no one is permitted to ask for this act of killing, either for himself or herself or for another person entrusted to his or her care, nor can he or she consent to it, either explicitly or implicitly. Nor can any authority legitimately recommend or permit such an action. For it is a question of the violation of the divine law, an offense against the dignity of the human person, a crime against life and an attack on humanity.

It may happen that by reason of prolonged and barely tolerable pain, for deeply personal or other reasons, people may be led to believe that they can legitimately ask for death or obtain it for others. Although in these cases the guilt of the individual may be reduced or completely absent, nevertheless the error of judgment into which the conscience falls, perhaps in good faith, does not change the nature of this act of killing, which will always be in itself something to be rejected.

The pleas of gravely ill people who sometimes ask for death are not to be understood as implying a true desire for euthanasia; in fact it is almost always a case of an anguished plea for help and love. What a sick person needs, besides medical care, is love, the human and supernatural warmth with which the sick person can and ought to be surrounded by all those close to him or her, parents and children, doctors and nurses.

III. The Meaning of Suffering for Christians and the Use of Painkillers

Death does not always come in dramatic circumstances after barely tolerable sufferings. Nor do we have to think only of extreme cases. Numerous testimonies which confirm one another lead one to the conclusion that nature itself has made provision to render more bearable at the moment of death separations that would be terribly painful to a person in full health. Hence it is that a prolonged illness, advanced old age, or a state of loneliness or neglect can bring about psychological conditions that facilitate the acceptance of death.

Nevertheless, the fact remains that death, often preceded or accompanied by severe and prolonged suffering, is something which naturally causes people anguish.

Physical suffering is certainly an unavoidable element of the human condition; on the biological level, it constitutes a warning of which no one denies the usefulness; but, since it affects the human psychological makeup, it often exceeds its own biological usefulness and so can become so severe as to cause the desire to remove it at any cost.

According to Christian teaching, however, suffering, especially suffering during the last moments of life, has a special place in God's saving plan; it is in fact a sharing in Christ's passion and a union with the redeeming sacrifice which he offered in obedience to the Father's will. Therefore one must not be surprised if some Christians prefer to moderate their use of painkillers, in order to accept voluntarily at least a part of their sufferings and thus associate themselves in a conscious way with the sufferings of Christ crucified (cf. Mt. 27:34).

Nevertheless it would be imprudent to impose a heroic way of acting as a general rule. On the contrary, human and Christian prudence suggest for the majority of sick people the use of medicines capable of alleviating or suppressing pain, even though these may cause as a secondary effect semiconsciousness and reduced lucidity. As for those who are not in a state to express themselves, one can reasonably presume that they wish to take these painkillers, and have them administered according to the doctor's advice.

But the intensive use of painkillers is not without difficulties, because the phenomenon of habituation generally makes it necessary to increase their dosage in order to maintain their efficacy. At this point it is fitting to recall a declaration by Pius XII, which retains its full force. In answer to a group of doctors who had put the question: "Is the suppression of pain and consciousness by the use of narcotics . . .

permitted by religion and morality to the doctor and the patient (even at the approach of death and if one foresees that the use of narcotics will shorten life)?"

The pope said: "If no other means exist, and if, in the given circumstances, this does not prevent the carrying out of other religious and moral duties: Yes."[5] In this case, of course, death is in no way intended or sought even if the risk of it is reasonably taken; the intention is simply to relieve pain effectively, using for this purpose painkillers available to medicine.

However, painkillers that cause unconsciousness need special consideration. For a person not only has to be able to satisfy his or her moral duties and family obligations; he or she also has to prepare himself or herself with full consciousness for meeting Christ. Thus Pius XII warns: "It is not right to deprive the dying person of consciousness without a serious reason."[6]

IV. Due Proportion in the Use of Remedies

Today it is very important to protect, at the moment of death, both the dignity of the human person and the Christian concept of life against a technological attitude that threatens to become an abuse. Thus some people speak of a "right to die," which is an expression that does not mean the right to procure death either by one's own hand or by means of someone else, as one pleases, but rather the right to die peacefully with human and Christian dignity. From this point of view, the use of therapeutic means can sometimes pose problems.

In numerous cases, the complexity of the situation can be such as to cause doubts about the way ethical principles should be applied. In the final analysis, it pertains to the conscience either of the sick person, or of those qualified to speak in the sick person's name, or of the doctors to decide in the light of moral obligations and of the various aspects of the case.

Everyone has the duty to care for his or her own health or to seek such care from others. Those whose task it is to care for the sick must do so conscientiously and administer the remedies that seem necessary or useful.

However, is it necessary in all circumstances to have recourse to all possible remedies?

In the past moralists replied that one is never obliged to use "extraordinary" means. This reply, which as a principle still holds good, is perhaps less clear today by reason of the imprecision of the term and the rapid progress made in the treatment of sickness. Thus some people prefer to speak of "proportionate" and "disproportionate" means.

In any case, it will be possible to make a correct judgment as to the means by studying the type of treatment to be used, its degree of complexity or risk, its cost and the possibilities of using it, and comparing these elements with the result that can be expected, taking into account the state of the sick person and his or her physical and moral resources.

In order to facilitate the application of these general principles, the following clarifications can be added:

—If there are no other sufficient remedies, it is permitted, with the patient's consent, to have recourse to the means provided by the most advanced medical techniques, even if these means are still at the experimental stage and are not without a certain risk. By accepting them, the patient can even show generosity in the service of humanity.

—It is also permitted, with the patient's consent, to interrupt these means where the results fall short of expectations. But for such a decision to be made, account will have to be taken of the reasonable wishes of the patient's family, as also of the advice of the doctors who are specially competent in the matter. The latter may in particular judge that the investment in instruments and personnel is disproportionate to the results foreseen; they may also judge that the techniques applied impose on the patient strain or suffering out of proportion with the benefits which he or she may gain from such techniques.

—It is also permissible to make do with the normal means that medicine can offer. Therefore one cannot impose on anyone the obligation to have recourse to a technique which is already in use but which carries a risk or is burdensome. Such a refusal is not the equivalent of suicide; on the contrary, it should be considered as an acceptance of the human condition, or a wish to avoid the application of a medical procedure disproportionate to the results that can be expected, or a desire not to impose excessive expense on the family or the community.

—When inevitable death is imminent in spite of the means used, it is permitted in conscience to take the decision to refuse forms of treatment that would only secure a precarious and burdensome prolongation of life, so long as the normal care due the sick person in similar cases is not interrupted. In such circumstances the doctor has no reason to reproach himself with failing to help the person in danger.

Conclusion

The norms contained in the present declaration are inspired by a profound desire to serve people in accordance with the plan of the Creator. Life is a gift of God, and on the other hand, death is unavoidable, it is necessary therefore that we, without in any way hastening the hour of death, should be able to accept it with full responsibility and dignity. It is true that death marks the end of our earthly existence, but at the same time it opens the door to immortal life. Therefore all must prepare themselves for this event in the light of human values, and Christians even more so in the light of faith.

As for those who work in the medical profession, they ought to neglect no means of making all their skill available to the sick and the dying; but they should also remember how much more necessary it is to provide them with the comfort of boundless kindness and heartfelt charity. Such service to people is also service to Christ the Lord, who said: "As you did it to one of the least of these my brethren, you did it to me" (Mt. 25:40).

At the audience granted to the undersigned prefect, His Holiness Pope John Paul II approved this declaration, adopted at the ordinary meeting of the Sacred Congregation for the Doctrine of the Faith, and ordered its publication.

Rome, the Sacred Congregation for the Doctrine of the Faith, May 5, 1980.

Cardinal Franjo Seper
Prefect
Archbishop Jerome Hamer, O.P.
Secretary

Notes

1. "Declaration on Procured Abortion," Nov. 18, 1974: AAS 66 (1974), pp. 730–747.
2. Pius XII, "Address to those attending the Congress of the International Union of Catholic Women's Leagues," Sept. 11, 1947: AAS 39 (1947), p. 483; "Address to Midwives," Oct. 29, 1951: AAS 43 (1951), pp. 835–854; "Speech to the Members of the International Office of Military Medicine Documentation," Oct. 19, 1953: AAS 45 (1953), pp. 744–754; "Address to those taking part in the ninth Congress of the Italian Anaesthesiological Society," Feb. 24, 1957: AAS 49 (1957), p. 146; cf. also "Address on Re-animation," Nov. 24, 1957: AAS 49 (1957), pp. 1027–1033; Paul VI, "Address to the Members of the U.N. Special Committee on Apartheid," May 22, 1974: AAS 66 (1974), p. 346; John Paul II: "Address to the Bishops of the United States of America," Oct. 5, 1979: AAS 71 (1979), p. 1225.
3. One thinks especially of Recommendation 779 (1976) on the rights of the sick and dying, of the Parliamentary Assembly of the Council of Europe at its 27th ordinary session; cf. Sipeca, no. 1, March 1977, pp. 14–15.
4. We leave aside completely the problems of the death penalty and of war, which involve specific considerations that do not concern the present subject.
5. Pius XII, "Address" Feb. 24, 1957: AAS 49 (1957), p. 147.
6. Pius XII, *ibid.*, p. 145, cf. "Address," Sept. 9, 1958: AAS 50 (1958), p. 694.

23

Euthanasia and the Quality of Life

Michael D. Bayles

The judgments and attitudes of many contemporary secular moral philosophers towards euthanasia diverge sharply from those of many enlightened leaders of society. Most people disapprove of euthanasia although they may not be willing to punish those who commit it—witness the tendency of juries to acquit in the rare instances in which trials are held. Leaders in the field of medical ethics usually approve allowing a patient to die, at least by withholding extraordinary treatment, but oppose intentional, direct killing of a dying patient even upon his request.[1] Yet, many philosophers are favorably disposed towards euthanasia in certain contexts.

There are three central issues with respect to the morality of euthanasia, defined as the intentional killing of another person from motives that include concern for his quality of life. (1) Is there a morally significant intrinsic difference between killing and allowing to die?

(2) Is the consent of the patient necessary for euthanasia to be morally permissible? (3) What standards and criteria should be used to determine the value of continued life and thereby the rightness of euthanasia? When is life no longer worth living?

This paper focuses on the first and third of these issues. The issue of consent is too complicated to be adequately discussed here. However, there are certain types of cases, e.g., infants, in which consent of the patient is not possible. The first section of this paper argues that there is no intrinsic moral difference between killing and allowing to die. The second section examines the practical import of this conclusion with respect to euthanasia of consenting adults and infants. The final section discusses standards for evaluating the quality of life and criteria for judging the value of its continuation. Throughout, the discussion concerns the morality, not the legality, of eu-

"Euthanasia and the Quality of Life" by Michael D. Bayles in Medical Treatment of the Dying: Moral Issues, eds. Michael D. Bayles and Dallas M. High, 1978, pp. 128–152. Reprinted with permission of Schenkman Books.

thanasia. The legal issue undoubtedly involves other considerations.

Killing versus Allowing to Die

John Ladd argues that ethics operates under the *Onus Probandi* Principle, that anyone who claims that one has a moral obligation to do or forbear from an action has the burden of proof to show why.[2] He thus places the burden of proof upon opponents of euthanasia. While one who claims that people have moral duties generally has the burden of proof, this interpretation of the *Onus Probandi* Principle does not work for all situations. The burden of proof is context dependent. In the context of moral dispute, someone who claims an exception to a mutually accepted moral rule or principle has the burden of proof. A more adequate interpretation of the *Onus Probandi* Principle is that one who claims a moral distinction has the burden of proof. The burden of proof thus falls upon those who claim there is a moral difference between allowing a patient to die and killing one. And if one assumes, as Ladd does, that most actions are morally permissible (or neutral), the burden of proof falls upon one who claims some actions are not permissible.[3]

Several points need to be clarified before particular arguments for a moral difference between killing and allowing to die may be examined. First, Ladd suggests that the distinction between killing and allowing to die is between withdrawing and withholding treatment, the former being a form of killing.[4] However, all major supporters of a moral difference classify withdrawal of treatment as allowing to die. The distinction is not between mere performance and non-performance. Moreover, whether a non-performance counts as an action is usually undisputed, because the non-performances in issue are intentional ones which almost everyone counts as responsible actions. Thus, developing a precise classification of those non-performances which count as actions attributable to a person does not significantly advance the argument.

Second, one must distinguish between various forms or kinds of treatment which may, however, be combined in one treatment regimen. One kind is treatment which cures a disease, e.g., antibiotics which usually cure pneumonia. Another kind of treatment does not cure a disease but sustains a patient's health by compensating for the disease and preventing debilitating effects, e.g., insulin for diabetes. Another kind of treatment neither cures nor compensates for a disease; instead, it retards the course of a disease, e.g., therapies which delay the progress of cancer or produce remissions. Yet another type of treatment merely sustains life, e.g., artificial respirators. The final kind of treatment simply alleviates symptoms, e.g., pain-killers and cough medicine.

The expression "allowing to die" is sometimes used for this kind of symptomatic treatment—only caring for the dying. Herein "allowing to die" does not mean this type of treatment although it does not exclude it; "care" is used in the very restricted sense of such symptomatic treatment which does not prolong life (or does so only incidentally by reducing stress caused by symptoms). "Allowing to die" is used to mean withholding or withdrawing treatment when it is probable that its institution or continuation would prolong a patient's life however briefly. It thus includes failure to provide cures, compensating treatments, disease-retarding therapies, and artificial life sustaining treatment.

Third, one must distinguish two forms of

the claim that there is a moral difference between killing and allowing to die. One form holds that there is an intrinsic moral difference. Usually, it is held that there is an absolute duty not to kill but only a prima facie duty not to allow to die. However, it may be held that while both are only prima facie duties, the duty not to kill is stronger than that not to allow to die. Or, it may be held that there is a prima facie duty not to kill but no duty not to allow to die. Hence, even if there is an intrinsic moral difference, it need not always be dispositive of the overall moral evaluation of instances of killing and allowing to die. All of these versions agree that there is an intrinsic moral difference between killing and allowing to die which is always morally relevant. It always takes stronger reasons to justify killing (if it can be done at all) than it does to justify allowing to die. The second form of the claim that there is a moral difference between killing and allowing to die merely holds that usually there is a moral difference between the two. Hence, while usually there is a stronger duty not to kill than to allow to die, in some cases there is not. This form of the claim is a generalization from particular cases evaluated by considerations extrinsic to a difference between killing and allowing to die. The following discussion concerns only the first, not this second, form of the claim.[5]

To establish an intrinsic moral difference between killing and allowing to die, two conditions must be shown. (1) A logical or intrinsic difference must be shown between the two. (2) This difference must be shown to be morally significant. Ladd's argument against the distinction appears to be aimed at the first point, for he suggests that "letting him die" might generate "killing him."[6] His example of this generation, letting the patient die by starving him, is not persuasive. Supporters of the dis-

tinction may argue that "starving" is ambiguous between "failing to provide food" and "actively preventing from obtaining food." If the latter is meant, then one has not "let the person die" but "killed him"; while if the former is meant, one has "let the patient die" but not "killed him." Moreover, as certain facts in addition to having "let the patient die" are necessary to generate "killed him," the two are logically distinct. Finally, even if both descriptions may apply to "one act," it does not follow that no moral difference may be found. One may simply claim that when both apply, the duty not to kill is the more significant although one may violate two duties—not to kill and not to let die (if there is such a duty). In short, duties may be attached to descriptions of actions; and if two or more descriptions apply, one may have duties (or a duty and no duty) *qua* each description.

Five different grounds may be suggested for an intrinsic moral difference between killing and allowing to die. Each of them is frequently used in moral discussions. They are (1) the doctrine of double effect, and the distinctions between (2) actions and their consequences, (3) commissions and omissions, (4) sufficient and necessary conditions, and (5) positive and negative duties. Grounds (1) and (2) fail both to correlate with the difference between killing and allowing to die and to establish its moral significance. Grounds (3) and (4) fail to be morally significant, while ground (5) fails to correlate with the difference although it may be morally significant.

The doctrine of double effect permits performing actions which have a bad or evil effect that normally ought not be produced. The doctrine can be stated as follows: An action having both a good and a bad effect is permissible if (1) the bad effect is not intended as an end or means, and (2) the good effect outweighs the bad.[7] This definition needs to be clarified in several respects. First, it is assumed that the person knows the bad effect will occur. No moral consideration can be made if the bad effect is an unknown consequence, e.g., an unexpected effect of an experimental drug. Second, while the bad effect is known to occur, it is not intended as a conscious object of the action. Instead, the good effect is the conscious object. Third, since the bad effect cannot be intended as a means, it must be a known but unintended side effect.

The doctrine of double effect does not always distinguish between killing and allowing to die, nor is it morally acceptable. For example, suppose a physician withholds a life-prolonging treatment in order to bring about the early death of a patient and thus relieve his suffering. Since the physician intends the early death of the patient to end his suffering, he intends the patient's death as a means and the doctrine of double effect does not permit it. Essentially, the doctrine of double effect distinguishes between direct and indirect killing, not between killing and allowing to die. Moreover, the doctrine is not morally acceptable. Suppose both a woman and her unborn child will die unless she has an abortion, but the only possible procedure for the abortion involves intentionally killing the fetus. The doctrine of double effect does not permit the abortion even though the fetus will die whatever is done. In short, when a person will die whatever is done, the doctrine of double effect forbids deliberately hastening that person's death by killing as a means to saving the lives of others, no matter how many. A correct morality cannot be so impervious to consequences.

The intentions of an actor may be relevant to distinguishing an action from its consequences. When one intentionally produces the death of a person, then the person's death is part of the action. When one does not intend the death of a person but merely foresees it, the person's death may not be part of the action but a (mere) consequence of it. This distinction between an action and its consequences is not identical to either the distinctions between killing and allowing to die or between direct and indirect killing. As construed, the consequences of an action may include either indirect killing or allowing to die. However, it is worth considering whether the distinction is morally significant, because if it is, there is a moral difference between direct killing and allowing to die.

Jonathan Bennett has penetratingly considered whether the difference between an action and its consequences is always morally significant.[8] While not disputing the distinction, he contends that there is no moral significance always (intrinsically) attached to it. Bennett shows that several features which might be thought relevant to the difference will not suffice. He frames his discussion in terms of the following example: A woman in labor will die unless an abortion involving a craniotomy is performed. If the abortion is not performed, then the fetus can be safely delivered. Performing the operation involves directly killing the fetus, but not performing it involves allowing the mother to die. If there is a moral difference between killing and allowing to die, then assuming the fetus and mother have equal rights, it is wrong to perform the abortion.

Consideration of this example shows that the action/consequence distinction will not support a moral difference between killing and allowing to die. Several features which may be morally relevant do not necessarily attend the distinction between an action and its consequences. For example, there is no difference in the expectation or inevitability of death whether the abortion is performed or not. Nor is there a difference in the ultimate aim; for in either case, the ultimate aim is not to kill the mother or the fetus.[9] Thus, the difference must, Bennett claims, lie either in the immediacy of death upon the physician's movements or the difference between doing and refraining from doing. Under the concept of immediacy, Bennett includes a number of factors such as temporal or spatial proximity and complexity of causal connection. None of these factors is morally relevant. Philosophers generally agree that no preference is to be given for the temporal proximity of events. Nor is there any obvious reason why spatial proximity between movements and effects should count any more than temporal proximity. The same applies to the complexity of the causal connections. These factors may make a difference in the certainty of the outcome, but when the effects are known to occur in either case, these differences do not have any moral significance. With these other factors shown to be irrelevant, the only difference left is that between doing and refraining from doing. But that is precisely the point at issue here, so the distinction between actions and consequences could not support that point even if it did correlate with it.

Before considering other grounds for an intrinsic moral difference between killing and allowing to die, it is useful to follow Philippa Foot and distinguish two senses of "allow."[10] In one sense, to allow something is to enable it to happen. For example, one pulls the plug in the tub and allows the water to drain. In another sense, one allows something to happen by not interfering. These two senses are closely related, for the first is ceasing to prevent while the second is not preventing. Moreover, they correspond to the two types of situations

usually referred to as allowing a patient to die. The first sense, ceasing to prevent, corresponds to withdrawing treatment, while the second sense corresponds to withholding treatment.

Several writers consider the distinction between killing and allowing to die to be a distinction between commissions and omissions. Foot suggests that the second sense of "allow" requires an omission. Moreover, George Fletcher has claimed that for legal purposes the first sense should also be considered an omission. It is sufficient for classifying conduct as an omission, he claims, if people would describe it as permitting harm rather than causing it.[11] Since withdrawing treatment permits harm, it is an omission. If both senses of "allow" involve omissions rather than commissions, then the distinction between commissions and omissions does correspond to that between killing and allowing to die.[12]

However, the distinction between commissions and omissions does not provide a basis for an intrinsic moral difference between killing and allowing to die. First, as von Wright has satisfactorily shown, there is no logical difference between the consequences of acts (commissions) and forbearances (omissions).[13] Second, in order to classify withdrawal of treatment as an omission, Fletcher argues that it merely permits (allows) the event (death) to occur. If the basis of a distinction between commissions and omissions is between causing death (killing) and permitting (allowing) it, then it cannot in turn be used to support a moral difference between killing and allowing to die. Third, one is morally responsible for omissions if one has a duty to act. Since a moral difference between commissions and omissions depends upon one's duties, one cannot use the distinction to support there being no duty or a lesser one to provide treatment in the case of omissions.

The distinction between the two senses of "allow" may suggest another ground for morally differentiating killing and allowing to die. The notion of nonintervention involved in allowing to die presupposes an ongoing process which will result in death. Allowing a person to die of cancer implies a process which will result in the patient's death unless something is done. Forbearance from intervention is a necessary but not sufficient condition for death. Killing a person, however, does not presuppose an ongoing process which will bring about death. Instead, the action in killing a person is, in any situation, a sufficient, not a necessary, condition for the person's death. ("Killing," being a success word, logically entails death. "Attempting to kill" does not logically entail death, but it merely brings in the element of certainty which has already been shown to be insufficient to establish an intrinsic moral difference between killing and allowing to die. Hence, "the action in killing" is used to suggest that the logical connection is not intended and yet ignores the issue of certainty.) Thus, there is a "causal" difference between killing a person and allowing one to die. The action in killing is a sufficient condition for a person's death, but nonintervention (allowing to die) is only a necessary, not a sufficient, condition for a person's death.[14]

Nonetheless, this difference between necessary and sufficient conditions does not support an intrinsic moral difference between killing and allowing to die. People are generally held responsible for providing necessary as well as sufficient conditions for events. For legal responsibility, one does not usually require conduct to be a sufficient condition although it will suffice. The usual requirement is that the conduct be sine qua non for the result. Not everything which is a necessary condition for a result establishes causal responsibility in legal contexts, but in almost every instance in the particular situation the conduct is necessary for the event.[15] Since in the relevant sorts of situations a physician's not providing life-prolonging treatment is necessary for the death of the patient (at least sooner than would otherwise be the case), there is no reason on that ground for removing responsibility or claiming a moral difference between allowing to die and killing.

David Meyers has suggested a variation of the distinction between necessary and sufficient conditions for death. In the context of terminating extraordinary treatment, he distinguishes between causing the patient's death and not prolonging his death. The difference lies in the likely effects of the treatment, whether it preserves the patient's life and improves his living conditions or merely maintains certain bodily functions that have no independent viability without hope of improving his living conditions. If a physician terminates treatment in the latter situation, he does not cause the patient's death, "for it would already have come and claimed his patient but for the treatment being ceased."[16]

However, this distinction fares worse than the previous one. First, even with ordinary treatment, e.g., antibiotics for pneumonia, frequently the patient would already be dead *but for* the treatment. This factor holds for any life-prolonging or saving treatment. Second, Meyers rests much of the difference upon whether the patient can be restored to health. While such a consideration is obviously relevant, it has nothing to do with the distinction between killing and allowing to die. Instead, it concerns the prognosis and the physician's duties. Hence, if there is an intrinsic moral difference between killing and allowing to die, it must be found in a difference between the duties to treat and not to kill.

Foot believes that there is a significant difference in these duties which supports a moral difference between killing and allowing to die. She distinguishes between positive and negative duties. Roughly, negative duties are not to injure a person while positive duties are to benefit a person.[17] Negative duties are more basic or stronger than positive ones. Killing involves injuring or harming a person, whereas allowing to die is not benefiting a person. Since there is a stronger obligation not to injure a person than there is to benefit one, there is a stronger obligation not to kill a person than there is not to allow one to die.

This distinction between negative and positive duties obviously has some general appeal. It is wrong to steal $5000 from a person, but not to fail to give him $5000. Nonetheless, the distinction is incapable of bearing the significance Foot attaches to it. First, it is sometimes quite difficult to distinguish between nonbenefit and injury. Moreover, it raises the issue of who ultimately judges that something is a nonbenefit or injury—the patient, his family, or the physician. However, that issue may be ignored for now.

The second and more crucial point is that the judgments to support an intrinsic moral difference between killing and allowing to die must be such that killing always involves injury and allowing to die always involves nonbenefit. That is, killing must always violate a negative duty and allowing to die at most violate a positive duty. Foot does not retain the necessary correlations. She imagines not giving food to a beggar and allowing him to die so his body can be used for medical research. But, she comments, "presumably we are inclined to see this as a violation of negative rather than positive duty."[18] Consequently, as there are no strict correlations of negative duties with killing and positive duties with allowing to die, the distinction between negative and positive duties does not support an intrinsic moral difference between killing and allowing to die.

The upshot is that no intrinsic moral difference between killing and allowing to die has been established. Various proposed grounds for it have been examined—the doctrine of double effect and the distinctions between actions and consequences, commissions and omissions, necessary and sufficient conditions, and negative and positive duties. Consequently, various types of situations must be examined on their merits. Simplistic moral thinking based upon an intrinsic difference is no more satisfactory here than elsewhere. In the following section, the practical import of this conclusion will be considered.

Unjustified Practices

The practical import of the conclusion that there is no intrinsic moral difference between killing and allowing to die will be considered with respect to two common practices. The first is denying voluntary euthanasia to dying adult patients while respecting their requests not to receive extraordinary life-prolonging treatment. The second practice is allowing infants with birth defects to die by withholding ordinary treatment.

Not everyone believes it is permissible to comply with the wishes of an adult patient that he be allowed to die. Those who deny that it is ever right to withhold or withdraw life-prolonging or saving treatment agree that there is no intrinsic moral difference between killing and allowing to die. Consequently, only those people who believe that in some situations it may be right to allow a patient to die but not to kill him disagree with the above conclusion. All of them agree that in some situations it is permissible for a physician to comply with a patient's request to be allowed to die by withholding extraordinary as opposed to ordinary life-prolonging treatment. The distinction between extraordinary and ordinary life-prolonging treatment is subject to much debate by physicians and moralists. For present purposes, the precise nature of this distinction is irrelevant. The arguments below hold whenever treatment is classified as extraordinary. In general, extraordinary treatment may be taken as involving any medicine, operation, or equipment which is unusual and expensive, painful, or otherwise very inconvenient.[19]

If it is right to comply with an adult patient's voluntary, sincere request to be allowed to die by withholding or withdrawing extraordinary life-prolonging treatment, then the patient is the ultimate judge of the value of the extra life which the treatment might provide. That it may only be right to comply with such a request under certain circumstances, e.g., one believes the patient can not live much longer anyway, does not negate this point. Under whatever circumstances one wishes to define, the patient's judgment is authoritative. Consequently, under similar circumstances the patient's judgment that he should die now must be accepted. That is, if under similar circumstances the patient voluntarily and sincerely requests that he be killed, then one must accept his judgment that whatever future life he might have left would be a burden to him rather than a benefit. Sometimes attempts are made to avoid this conclusion by the question-begging assertion that any patient who makes such a request *must be* incapable of rational choice.

If it is right to allow the patient to die in the one case, it is also right to kill him in the other because there is no intrinsic moral difference between killing and allowing to die. Indeed, since by hypothesis the patient's judgment is authoritative in the situation, to deny either request is wrong. It is morally equivalent to inflicting upon the patient the hardship which he undergoes during the time he lives but would not have undergone had one complied with his request. In short, in these circumstances not to comply with a patient's request for euthanasia (killing) is morally equivalent to inflicting on him as torture whatever he suffers the rest of his life.

A patient may rationally decide to forgo extraordinary life-prolonging treatment but not request to be killed. He may determine that while if given care his life is not such that he would prefer to die, neither is it of sufficient value to be prolonged. Or, he may judge that the extra life he would gain from an extraordinary life-prolonging procedure would come at the end when his condition would have so deteriorated that life would no longer be worth living even if given care. However, it is also possible that extraordinary life-prolonging treatment extends the time when, given care, life is of a quality worth living and the patient therefore requests it.

Perhaps in recognition of this symmetry between killing and allowing to die, arguments against voluntary euthanasia have emphasized untoward effects of a policy permitting voluntary euthanasia.[20] But these arguments also apply to allowing a patient to die by withholding or withdrawing extraordinary life-prolonging treatment. The three major ones will be briefly examined.

The first argument is the "wedge" argument. Essentially, it contends that permitting voluntary euthanasia would be to admit the thin edge of the wedge. Once voluntary euthanasia is permitted, there is no stopping short of killing all those whom society thinks are unfit or unhappy.[21] Logically, the argument is balderdash. F. M. Cornford described it as the principle "that you should not act justly now for fear of raising expectations that you may act still more justly in the future. . . ."[22] It might be made valid by adding an empirical premise that the undesired extensions will probably occur. However, a similar claim may be made concerning allowing to die by not using extraordinary means of life-prolongation. Without scientific studies supporting either claim, neither provides any basis for a conclusion against either practice. It would be worth investigating the point at which distinctions become too fine to be useful in moral rules. Nevertheless, it is implausible that ordinary people cannot distinguish between killing dying patients upon their request and killing relatively healthy persons without their consent.

A second argument, or set of arguments, rests upon uncertainty. A physician may misdiagnose as terminal an illness which is not. A cure may be found before the patient would otherwise have died. And it is difficult to establish that the patient does make a fully voluntary and sincere request that his life be ended. Indeed, this last point is sometimes turned into a certainty that the patient cannot voluntarily consent to having his life terminated because of pain, effects of drugs, etc. Surely this last ploy is taking the argument too far. However, no one is ever certain (in the sense sought) about empirical matters relevant to moral judgments. If a cancer patient has metastases throughout his body, one can be quite sure he will not live much longer. In any case, the very same points apply to allowing to die by not using extraordinary means of life-prolongation. The diagnosis might be mistaken, a cure might be found in the extra time provided, or the patient may object to its not being used.

Mistake-proof medicine and morals are not human medicine and morals.

The final objection to be considered is that euthanasia would undermine the doctor-patient relationship. The patient would no longer trust his doctor not to "do him in."[23] This objection is plausible for compulsory euthanasia, but it applies equally to allowing patients to die without their consent. When both procedures are based on the wishes of the patient, there is little reason to believe that the relation of confidence will be undermined. Indeed, noncompliance with patients' wishes for euthanasia might well undermine the relationship more than compliance.

Consequently, the practice of complying with adult patients' requests to die by not having life-prolonging treatment but not complying with similarly circumstanced patients' requests for euthanasia is morally unjustified. The patients' judgments as to the value of their continued life must be respected equally in both situations. The arguments from untoward consequences of the practice of voluntary euthanasia apply equally well or poorly to the practice of not using extraordinary life-prolonging treatment. Finally, it is sometimes suggested that only a very few patients request to be killed. Even if true, that is certainly not a reason against its moral rightness. The moral rightness of an action does not depend upon the frequency of the occasion for it.

The second unjustified practice is allowing defective newborn infants to die by withholding or withdrawing what in at least some cases is ordinary treatment. There has recently come to public attention a number of cases where treatments which are usual for the disease or problem and likely to prolong life have been withheld or withdrawn from newborn infants.[24] Generally, in these cases the infant has two or more genetic or congenital defects, such as Down's syndrome (mongolism) and an obstruction or defect of the gastrointestinal tract. If the latter defect is not repaired by surgery, then the infant will soon die; if it is repaired, then the infant may live for an indefinite period of time—perhaps a number of years.

In several cases, the parents have refused to consent to the operation. Intravenous feeding, etc., have been discontinued and after a time the infant has died. In the famous Johns Hopkins case, the infant lingered fifteen days before dying. Some commentators believe that sometimes it is permissible not to provide the life-prolonging treatment but wrong to kill the infant. On what grounds one may decide not to "save" or prolong the life of such an infant is not in dispute at this point. What is in dispute is leaving the infant to a lingering death rather than killing it.

As there is no intrinsic moral difference between killing and allowing to die, once a decision is made in such cases not to prolong life, the infant should be killed. The decision not to prolong life implies *ceteris paribus,* a judgment that the future life the infant might have were the treatment given is not of sufficient quality to be worth living. Consequently, the extra time lived in allowing to die rather than killing is not worth living. While it may be rational for an adult to forgo life-prolonging treatment but not be killed because the period of life gained by the treatment might only come at the end when, despite care, life is not worth living, with infants such a judgment does not seem generally reasonable. The longer an infant lives, the more it will develop whatever limited capacities it may have. Hence, the latter part of its life is apt to be of higher, not lower, quality and so more worth living. The only plausible ground for a contrary judgment is that the infant, as it developed, would be more aware of its defects or pain and so suffer more. However, there is no reason to believe that an older infant is more conscious of physical pain than a newborn one. If it becomes more aware of its defects, then it might be killed at a later time. If the infant suffers sufficiently at the time to render further life not worth living, then in not killing it one merely inflicts further days of suffering upon it.

Moreover, there is an added burden on adults involved in not killing an infant. Those who decide not to treat may view the remaining life as one of suffering and thus suffer more themselves. Those who disagree with the decision will be upset by the sight or knowledge of the dying baby. This burden upon others is greater with infants than it is with adults upon whose request treatment is forgone. An adult has consented to die in such a fashion, so others may be comforted with the view that he is at least dying as he desires.

The case of such infants is empirically similar to that of injured animals. Newborn infants, unlike adults, have conscious capacities similar to animals. They are primarily restricted to consciousness of their physical state. If anything, newborn infants have less consciousness of their environment than do many adult mammals. Yet it would be deemed wantonly cruel, even criminal, to allow a fatally injured animal to die rather than kill it. This parallel with animals is frequently drawn in discussions of euthanasia, but it is most relevant in the case of infants. The stock (false) objection is that people are not animals. As Antony Flew has replied, "This is precisely not a ground for treating people worse than brute animals."[25]

The general point being made cuts both ways. As there is no intrinsic moral difference between killing and allowing to die, if it is wrong to kill a defective infant, it is as wrong to allow it to die by withholding life-prolonging treatment except for the small amount of extra life in the latter case. People cannot assuage their consciences by asserting that they did not kill an infant but only allowed it to die. Whatever the criteria as to when one should or should not prolong the life of infants, if there are sufficient reasons not to prolong an infant's life, then it ought to be killed; and if it is wrong to kill it, it is also wrong to allow it to die. In either case, allowing an infant to die is unjustified.

This section has not considered the substantive criteria as to when life may not be worth living or prolonging. Instead, it has been restricted to issues about how people die once a judgment is made or recognized that life is not worth prolonging. The final section considers grounds for judgments that a life is not worth living or prolonging.

Value of Life Judgments

As Hudson correctly points out, semantic and conceptual precision cannot be achieved as to quality of life.[26] However, the reason is not, as he suggests, the uniqueness of each biological situation. On the one hand, everything in the universe is unique in that it is different from everything else. On the other hand, biological situations are sufficiently similar for physicians to develop general practices and therapies of choice which apply to many people and situations. Rather, the difficulty is that the judgments require the application of standards which admit of degrees. But just as the legal standards of due care, fair rate, and good faith may be indisputably applied over a wide

range of cases despite uncertainty in others, so likewise, allowing for their greater abstractness, may standards as to the quality and value of life.

While "quality of life" is much in vogue, the expression is ambiguous. Different ethical theories provide different standards and criteria for evaluating the quality of life and whether it is worth living. In particular, utilitarian and perfectionist standards of quality of life are quite distinct. The rest of this section briefly sketches these standards and considers criteria using them in making judgments about the value of continued life.

The utilitarian standard of the quality of life is simply the net happiness (degree of happiness minus the degree of unhappiness) experienced at a moment.[27] The quality of life is good or has positive value as long as happiness exceeds unhappiness; it is bad when unhappiness exceeds happiness. Nonexistence is ascribed the same value as zero net happiness. In short, the quality of life at a moment is simply the overall happiness or unhappiness one then experiences.

There are two utilitarian criteria for evaluating the value of life. One criterion is to maximize the "total amount of happiness" in a life, which is simply the sum of the net happiness experienced during the time lived. (One must allow for variation in the quality of life over time.) This criterion has a common sense basis in the ideas that the more net happiness in a life, the better it is; and that as long as one is happy, the longer one lives the better. By this criterion, a life is not worth continuing when its total happiness will not be increased.

The other utilitarian criterion is to maximize the "average level of happiness" in a life which is simply the average of the quality of life at the various moments. For example, if one had a net happiness of two units at a moment for one week and four units for the next, the average level for the two weeks would be three units. The common sense basis of this criterion is that it is not the length of life which counts but how good it is while it lasts. It is better to live a shorter, more eventful, and intensely happy life than a long, relatively dull one of moderate happiness even if there is more total happiness in the latter. By this criterion, as long as the expectable level of happiness is as high as the average for one's previous life, it is worth living. When the rest of one's life is likely to involve a significantly lower average level of happiness, it is not worth living. This criterion thus allows for some decline from a peak level of happiness, but if in advancing years one's level of happiness declines permanently below the average of one's previous life, it is not worth continuing to live.

Perfectionist standards of quality of life provide the main alternatives to the utilitarian standard. Perfectionist standards specify certain qualities (activities and actualizations of capacities) which determine the quality of life. Generally, certain qualities or a minimum number are thought necessary for a quality of life worth living, and the more such qualities in addition to the minimum or necessary ones the higher the quality of life. Perfectionist standards vary depending upon the qualities specified. They are often closely tied to the concept of personhood, specifying qualities such as self-awareness, memory, love, communication, conceptual thinking, and physical mobility.[28] If a person has prospects for the development or continued use of the necessary or minimum number of qualities, his life is worth living. If he cannot have such qualities, then his life is not worth living even if it will involve

positive net happiness. A variation or addition to perfectionist standards involves considerations of the overall coherence of a life. Samuel Gorovitz's conception of a life as a biography, with appropriate and inappropriate possible endings, is an example of such a perfectionist criterion for evaluating a whole life.[29]

Dallas High correctly claims that attention should be paid to a dying patient's quality of life and the possibilities of providing care. But he misleadingly suggests that the choice between life prolongation, euthanasia, and allowing to die is a false issue.[30] If life-prolongation is possible, these alternatives are exhaustive; one either provides life-prolonging treatment or not, in which case one either allows the patient to die or kills him. High's valid point is that in choosing between these alternatives each must be evaluated on the assumption that care will be provided to maintain as high a quality of life as possible. However, one must not assume, as High appears to do, the context of advanced Western medicine. For most people of the earth, medical personnel, supplies, and facilities are simply not available to provide even the type of care High recommends. Of course, these conditions also obviate worries about drastic attempts to prolong life. The rest of this section considers when, given the best possible care, termination of life is appropriate on the different criteria for the value of continued life.

The specific factors for determining the quality of life are likely to be similar on the utilitarian and perfectionist standards, because the qualities included in the latter also usually increase happiness. In judging the quality and value of continued life, three types of specific factors are predominant: mental capacity, physical capacity, and pain. Proponents of euthanasia have usually emphasized pain as the primary factor indicating termination of life. Such an emphasis implies a utilitarian standard of quality of life. On a perfectionist standard, pain need not imply a quality of life not worth continuing unless it interferes unduly with other factors, e.g., impairs mental functioning. And as High suggests, it may now be possible to control pain in most cases.[31]

However, even in the absence of pain, mental or physical incapacity may indicate that life is no longer worth living. By the total happiness criterion, the incapacity must be such that there is negative net happiness. By perfectionist criteria, the incapacity need only be such that one no longer has the necessary or minimum number of qualities. For example, if one classifies physical mobility as necessary, then paralysis from the neck down may deprive one of a quality of life sufficient to make it worth living. Finally, by the average level of happiness criterion, one's life may no longer be worth living even though one has considerable mental and physical capacity. One's incapacity need only be such that the expectable average level of happiness for any subsequent period of life is below the average level to that time. Consequently, by any one of these criteria a patient free from pain may correctly judge that future life is not worth living.

In making a judgment to end one's life, one may also consider duties to others. Tristram Engelhardt argues that, because one is excused from most duties by incapacitation, duties to others do not usually present grounds for judging that a dying person ought to live longer.[32] But incapacity excuses only when it renders one incapable of fulfilling a duty; if one can obtain substitute performance, one is not excused. For example, an ill teacher may

be able to get someone else to take over his classes. Moreover, one may have a duty not to impose a great burden on others. If so, and one's continued life would be a great burden on others, then one may have a duty to end it. Thus, one may properly judge that one's life should be ended, even though were it not for the burden it would place upon others it would be of sufficient quality to be worth living. As such a judgment needs to be made upon a realistic appraisal of the burden imposed on others, a patient should be frankly told about the financial and emotional burden being shouldered by his family or friends.

The differences between the criteria of the value of continued life are most marked when one must judge whether the lives of others are worth prolonging. When the other person is an adult, one should probably use the criterion that person would use. If one uses a different criterion, then one may terminate life which the patient would find worth living or extend life the patient finds not worth living. When, however, the other person is a newborn infant, one must decide which criterion is appropriate, and it need not be the same criterion one would use for one's own life.

The total happiness per life criterion rarely supports killing a defective infant or allowing it to die. The question is whether the infant experiences more happiness than unhappiness. If it does, then its life is worthwhile. The difficulty is in determining whether it experiences more happiness than unhappiness. However, if it suffers no or little pain (does not cry frequently, etc.), then as it has few other sources of unhappiness, its happiness is probably greater than its unhappiness.

The average level of happiness criterion is somewhat more difficult to use. Infants have little or no previous life to establish an average level of happiness. Moreover, as their life has been at such a primitive level, any significant development is likely to increase their level of happiness. For example, a week old infant with Down's syndrome is likely to develop enough mentally and physically to greatly increase its average level of happiness. Being retarded, it is not likely to experience anguish from a realization of its incapacity as compared to normal children.

At this point, it is tempting to use an interpersonal criterion of average level of happiness —is this infant likely to have an average level of happiness comparable to that of normal children? But this interpersonal criterion of average level of happiness is fatally defective. Applied to the normal population, it implies that the lives of all those below the average level of happiness in the society are not worth living. If all those lives which are not worth living are eliminated, then one has a new average level of happiness in society and another set of lives which are not worthwhile. By successive applications of the criterion and elimination of worthless lives, one may reduce a population to its happiest member (assuming the loss of the other lives would not decrease his happiness).

Perfectionist criteria are most likely to support a judgment that a defective infant's life is not worth prolonging. How many infants would be so judged and how defective they must be depends upon the qualities used in the standard of quality of life. But suppose, with minimal plausibility, that the necessary qualities for positive value are those required for living on one's own in society. Then any infant which does not have the potentiality of developing into a self-sufficient member of society does not have a sufficiently high expectable quality of life to make it worth living. Of course, this standard is pretty high, probably the highest a non-Nietzschean would set, but even lower standards may imply that the lives of many defective infants are not worth living.

This analysis has only considered whether an infant's life is worth living. A decision upon termination might take into account benefits or burdens of others. It is ethically questionable whether possible benefits or burdens of others should be considered. Considering benefits would make a difference only if one judged that the life in question was not in itself worth living but would benefit others. For example, on a high perfectionist standard of quality of life, the life of an infant with Down's syndrome might not be worth living, but it might bring considerable happiness to its parents. However, one would then be prolonging a worthless life for the benefit of others—using the infant as a mere means (because it does not benefit at all) to the ends of others. The same objection would arise if an infant's life would be worth living but terminated because it would be a burden to others.

This objection to considering the burdens and benefits of others arises only on a nonutilitarian ethical view, which is unlikely to use a utilitarian standard of quality of life. Utilitarians would consider the benefits and burdens of others. A crucial problem in considering burdens and benefits of others is the extent to which public monies are used to pay for medical care. If public monies are used, then the burdens of continuing an infant's life may be acceptable to its parents; but if they are not available, the combined financial and emotional strain might overwhelm a family. This issue cannot be pursued further here.[33]

It has thus been shown that there is no basis for an intrinsic moral difference between killing and allowing to die. Thus, the practices of honoring requests by adults not to receive extraordinary life-prolonging treatment while denying requests of similarly circumstanced adults for euthanasia and of allowing defective infants to die instead of killing them are morally unjustifiable. These practices take as given judgments about the value of prolonged life. There are at least two kinds of standards for evaluating the quality of life and various criteria for judging the value of its continuation. While the different criteria result in varying judgments as to when life is of sufficient quality to be worth living, they all support the claim that in some contexts life is no longer of value. Since benefits and burdens of others are not always significant, each criterion implies that sometimes a life is not worth prolonging. Consequently, euthanasia of dying adults and defective infants is morally justified in some contexts.

Notes

1. House of Delegates of the American Medical Association, *Journal of the American Medical Association* 227 (1974):728; Pope Pius XII, *New York Times,* 25 November 1957, p. 1; Edwin F. Healey, S.J., *Medical Ethics* (Chicago: Loyola University Press, 1956), pp. 67, 266; and Arthur J. Dyck, "An Alternative to the Ethic of Euthanasia," in *To Live and To Die: When, Why, and How,* ed. Robert H. Williams (New York: Springer-Verlag, 1973), p. 104. While it is not completely settled, this distinction also appears in the law: David W. Meyers, "The Legal Aspects of Medical Euthanasia," *BioScience* 23 (1973): 467–68; Survey, "Euthanasia: Criminal, Tort, Constitutional and Legislative Considerations," *Notre Dame Lawyer* 48 (1973): 1207–10, 1242–44; and George P.

Fletcher, "Prolonging Life: Some Legal Considerations," in *Euthanasia and the Right to Death,* ed. A. B. Downing (New York: Humanities Press, 1970), pp. 75–76, 84 [hereinafter this book is cited as *Euthanasia*]. Moreover, it reflects physicians' attitudes: Diana Crane, "Physicians' Attitudes Toward the Treatment of Critically Ill Patients," *BioScience* 23 (1973):472; Robert H. Williams, "Propagation, Modification, and Termination of Life: Contraception, Abortion, Suicide, Euthanasia," in *To Live and To Die,* pp. 90–91.

2. "Positive and Negative Euthanasia."

3. A complete analysis of the allocation of the burden of proof in arguments generally, and those about euthanasia in particular, would be much more complex than that given in the text.

4. Ladd, "Positive and Negative Euthanasia," pp. 107, 122.

5. A confusion between these two forms of the claim may be seen in the writing of Paul Ramsey. In a justly famous discussion of care of the dying, he at first asserts that the distinction between allowing to die and killing, which he treats as that between omissions and commissions, "must be taken into account" and "is of first importance." *The Patient as Person: Explorations in Medical Ethics* (New Haven: Yale University Press, 1970), pp. 118, 151. However, as the discussion proceeds, he considers it less important. Instead, he emphasizes providing care and suggests that as the treatment would be useless, withholding or withdrawing it is only incidentally not doing something (pp. 151, 159); it is primarily substituting care when life cannot be prolonged. Finally, he clearly makes the difference a generalization and not an intrinsic one, because if care for the dying should no longer be possible, as with a comatose patient, "the basic reason for

a significant moral distinction between omission and commission is abrogated" (p. 162; see also p. 163). Thus, the difference between killing and allowing to die is not itself morally significant but rather which option may benefit the patient.

6. "Positive and Negative Euthanasia," p. 120.

7. Healey, *Medical Ethics*, p. 98; Norman St. John-Stevas, *Life, Death and the Law* (Cleveland: World Publishing Company, Meridian Books, 1961), p. 190; John C. Ford, S.J., "The Morality of Obliteration Bombing," in *War and Morality*, ed. Richard A. Wasserstrom (Belmont, Cal.: Wadsworth Publishing Company, 1970), p. 26. How one determines whether an effect is intended is a difficult issue but not relevant here.

8. "Whatever the Consequences," in *Moral Problems*, ed. James Rachels (New York: Harper & Row, 1971), pp. 42–66.

9. *Ibid.*, p. 48.

10. "The Problem of Abortion and the Doctrine of the Double Effect," in *Moral Problems, op. cit.*, pp. 35–36.

11. "Prolonging Life," pp. 77, 79.

12. Some physicians may believe there is a moral difference between withholding and withdrawing treatment, being less inclined to do the latter (Ramsey, *Patient as Person*, p. 121). The distinction between commissions and omissions does not support that difference since both withholding and withdrawing treatment are classified as omissions.

13. Georg Henrik von Wright, *Norm and Action: A Logical Enquiry* (London: Routledge & Kegan Paul, 1963), p. 48.

14. This analysis differs from that of Bennett. He claims that the only difference is that in killing, of all the movements a physician might perform, few result in death; while in allowing to die, of all the movements a physician might perform, almost all result in death. "Whatever the

Consequences," pp. 57–58. The distinction in the text essentially agrees with that by Daniel Dinello, "On Killing and Letting Die," in *Ethics and Public Policy*, ed. Tom L. Beauchamp (Englewood Cliffs, N.J.: Prentice-Hall, 1975), p. 357. Dinello claims there is an intuitive moral difference, but his claim is open to Ladd's criticisms of relying on intuitions ("Positive and Negative Euthanasia.")

15. See generally, H. L. A. Hart and A. M. Honoré, *Causation in the Law* (Oxford: Clarendon Press, 1959), chap. 5. In The Queen v. Instan, [1893] 1 Q.B. 450, a woman was convicted of felonious homicide for failing to provide her aunt food and care which "substantially accelerated" death from exhaustion caused by gangrene.

16. "Legal Aspects," p. 469. There is a tendency for those who discuss such cases to assume the patient is already dead by brain death criteria. Meyers' example of not prolonging death is "cessation of mechanical respiration wherein cerebral hemorrhage has caused irreversible cessation of the patient's spontaneous brain function, assuming the latter to be a medically acceptable, conclusive criterion of death." See also Crane, "Physicians' Attitudes," p. 473. Such an assumption may be very misleading, for the dead can neither be killed nor allowed to die.

17. "Problem of Abortion," p. 37. See also W. D. Ross, *The Right and the Good* (Oxford: Clarendon Press, 1930), pp. 21–22.

18. "Problem of Abortion," p. 38. Michael Tooley suggests that the reason one is tempted to correlate negative and positive duties with killing and allowing to die concerns plausible motivational inferences and the effort involved in action as opposed to inaction; "Abortion and Infanticide," *Philosophy & Public Affairs* 2 (1972):59–60.

19. See Ramsey, *Patient as Person*, pp. 121–22; St. John-Stevas, *Life, Death and the Law*, p. 275; Healey, *Medical Ethics*, p. 67.

20. See Yale Kamisar, "Euthanasia Legislation: Some Non-Religious Objections," in *Euthanasia*, pp. 85–133; St. John-Stevas, *Life, Death and the Law*, pp. 271–75; and Sissela Bok, "Euthanasia and the Case of the Dying," *BioScience* 23 (1973):462–63.

21. See, for Example, James F. Toole, "The Concept of Brain Death as Viewed by a Neurologist," in this volume, p. 58; and Robert P. Hudson, "Death, Dying, and the Zealous Phase."

22. Quoted in Paul A. Freund, *On Law and Justice* (Cambridge: Harvard University Press, Belknap Press, 1968), p. 55.

23. Hudson, "Death, Dying, and the Zealous Phase," p. 76. His claim that medical skills and judgment are needed for passive euthanasia (allowing to die) is surely false; it takes no medical skill not to administer treatment. What may require medical skill is providing care to a patient not receiving life-prolonging treatment.

24. See, for example, the cases discussed in David H. Smith, "On Letting Some Babies Die," *Hastings Center Studies* 2 (May 1974):37–46; Richard A. McCormick, S.J., "To Save or Let Die: The Dilemma of Modern Medicine," *Journal of the American Medical Association* 229 (1974):172–76; Anthony Shaw, "Dilemmas of 'Informed Consent' in Children," *New England Journal of Medicine* 289 (1973):885–90; and Raymond S. Duff and A. G. M. Campbell, "Moral and Ethical Dilemmas in the Special-care Nursery," *New England Journal of Medicine* 289 (1973):890–94.

25. "The Principle of Euthanasia," in *Euthanasia*, p. 34.

26. "Death, Dying, and the Zealous Phase," pp. 68–71.

27. This discussion of the utilitarian standard and criteria has benefited from an unpublished paper by Lawrence N. Davis. He has shown how the standard and criteria for the value of a life may be given mathematical expression clearly indicating their differences.

28. See Hudson, "Death, Dying, and the Zealous Phase," p. 69.

29. "Dealing with Dying."

30. "Quality of Life and Care of the Dying Person."

31. *Ibid.*, p. 101.

32. H. Tristram Engelhardt, Jr., "Rights and Responsibilities of Patients and Physicians."

33. I develop a principle for the appropriateness of using public monies for certain types of health care in "National Health Insurance and Noncovered Services," *Journal of Health Politics, Policy and Law* 2 (Fall 1977).

24

The Physician's Responsibility Toward Hopelessly Ill Patients: A Second Look

Sidney H. Wanzer, Daniel D. Federman, S. James Adelstein, Christine K. Cassel, Edwin H. Cassem, Ronald E. Cranford, Edward W. Hook, Bernard Lo, Charles G. Moertel, Peter Safar, Alan Stone, and Jan van Eys

Some of the practices that were controversial five years ago[1] in the care of the dying patient have become accepted and routine. Do-not-resuscitate (DNR) orders, nonexistent only a few years ago, are now commonplace. Many physicians and ethicists now agree that there is little difference between nasogastric or intravenous hydration and other life-sustaining measures. They have concluded, therefore, that it is ethical to withdraw nutrition and hydration from certain dying, hopelessly ill, or perma-nently unconscious patients. The public and the courts have tended to accept this principle. Most important, there has been an increase in sensitivity to the desires of dying patients on the part of doctors, other health professionals, and the public. The entire subject is now dis-cussed openly. Various studies and reports from governmental bodies, private founda-tions, the American Medical Association, and state medical societies reflect these advances in thinking.[2-9]

"The Physician's Responsibility Toward Hopelessly Ill Patients: A Second Look" by Sidney H. Wanzer, M.D. et al. Reprinted with permission of The New England Journal of Medicine 320 (March 30, 1989): 844–849.

The increased awareness of the rights of dying patients has also been translated into new laws. Thirty-eight states now have legislation covering advance directives ("living wills"), and 15 states specifically provide that a patient's health care spokesperson, or proxy, can authorize the withholding or withdrawal of life support.[10,11]

The courts have continued to support patients' rights and have expanded the legal concept of the right to refuse medical treatment, upholding this right in more than 80 court decisions.[12] As a general rule, the cases in the early 1980s involved terminally ill patients whose death was expected whether or not treatment was continued, and the treatment at issue—for instance, prolonged endotracheal intubation, mechanical ventilation, dialysis, or chemotherapy—was often intrusive or burdensome. The courts recognized the patient's common-law right to autonomy (to be left alone to make one's own choices) as well as the constitutional right to privacy (to be protected from unwanted invasive medical treatment).

Currently, the courts are moving closer to the view that patients are entitled to be allowed to die, whether or not they are terminally ill or suffering. Many recent cases have permitted treatment to be terminated in patients who are permanently unconscious, indicating that the right to refuse treatment can be used to put an end to unacceptable conditions even if the patients are not perceptibly suffering or close to death. In such court opinions, many of which have dealt with artificial feeding, the cause of the patient's death continues to be attributed to the underlying disease, rather than to the withholding or withdrawal of treatment.[13]

Popular attitudes about the rights of dying patients have also changed, often in advance of the attitudes of health care providers, legislators, and the courts. The results of one public-opinion poll indicated that 68 percent of the respondents believed that "people dying of an incurable painful disease should be allowed to end their lives before the disease runs its course."[14]

Health professionals have also become much more aware of patients' rights. In states with laws legitimizing living wills, hospitals have become responsive to patients' wishes as expressed in their advance directives, and hospital accreditation by the Joint Commission on Accreditation of Health Care Organizations now requires the establishment of formal DNR policies. The frequency with which DNR orders are used in nursing homes has also increased. In 1987 the California Department of Health Services became the first state agency to develop clear guidelines for the removal of life support, including tube feeding, in the state's 1500 nursing homes and convalescent hospitals.[15]

Gaps between Accepted Policies and Their Implementation

Many patients are aware of their right to make decisions about their health care, including the refusal of life-sustaining measures, yet few actually execute living wills or appoint surrogates through a health care proxy. Although such documents can be very helpful in clarifying the patient's wishes, they are all too infrequently discussed in standard medical practice. Furthermore, at present, advance directives do not exert enough influence on either the patient's ability to control medical decision making at the end of life or the physician's behavior with respect to such issues in hospitals, emergency rooms, and nursing homes. There remains a considerable gap between the acceptance of the directive and its implementation. There is also a large gap between what the courts now allow with respect to withdrawal of treatment and what physicians actually do. All too frequently, physicians are reluctant to withdraw aggressive treatment from hopelessly ill patients, despite clear legal precedent.

Physicians have a responsibility to consider timely discussions with patients about life-sustaining treatment and terminal care. Only a minority of physicians now do so consistently.[16] The best time to begin such discussions is during the course of routine, nonemergency care, remembering that not all patients are emotionally prepared, by virtue of their stage in life, their psychological makeup, or the stage of their illness. Nevertheless, as a matter of routine, physicians should become acquainted with their patients' personal values and wishes and should document them just as they document information about medical history, family history, and sociocultural background. Such discussions and the resultant documentation should be considered a part of the minimal standard of acceptable care. The physician should take the initiative in obtaining the documentation and should enter it in the medical record.

These issues are not sufficiently addressed in medical schools and residency programs. Medical educators need to recognize that practitioners may not sufficiently understand or value the patient's role in medical decision making or may be unwilling to relinquish control of the decision-making process. The interests of patients and physicians alike are best served when decisions are made jointly, and

medical students and residents should learn to pursue this goal. These topics ought to be specifically included as curriculums are revised.

In general, health care institutions must recognize their obligation to inform patients of their right to participate in decisions about their medical care, including the right to refuse treatment, and should formulate institutional policies about the use of advance directives and the appointment of surrogate decision makers. Hospitals, health maintenance organizations, and nursing homes should ask patients on admission to indicate whether they have prepared a living will or designated a surrogate. It seems especially important that nursing homes require a regular review of patient preferences, with each patient's physician taking responsibility for ensuring that such information is obtained and documented. In the case of patients who lack decision-making capacity, surrogate decision makers should be identified and consulted appropriately. (We prefer the term "decision-making capacity" to "competency" because in the medical context, the patient either has or does not have the capacity to make decisions, whereas competency is a legal determination that can be made only by the courts.)

Although we advocate these approaches, we recognize that the mechanisms of appointing a surrogate and executing a living will do present certain problems. Obviously, it may happen that a surrogate appointed previously is unavailable for consultation when problems arise in the treatment of a patient who lacks decision-making capacity. In addition, there is the problem of determining what constitutes an outdated living will or surrogate appointment and how often they need to be reaffirmed. Laws in most states provide that a living will is valid until it is revoked, but patients need to be encouraged to update and reconfirm such directives from time to time.

Settings for Dying

Home

Dying at home can provide the opportunity for quiet and privacy, dignity, and family closeness that may make death easier for the patient and provide consolation for the bereaved. Assuming that a stable and caring home environment exists, emotional and physical comfort is most often greatest at home, with family and friends nearby.

Patients and their families need reassurance that dying at home will not entail medical deprivation. They should be carefully instructed in the means of coping with possible problems, and appropriate community resources should be mobilized to assist them. The provision of care should be guided by the physician and implemented with the help of well-trained, highly motivated personnel from the hospice units that now serve many communities in this country, since home care often becomes too difficult for the family to handle alone. Hospice, a form of care in which an interdisciplinary team provides palliative and support services to both patient and family, is a concept whose time has come.

Recent cost-containment measures for expensive hospital care have given the home hospice movement considerable impetus, resulting in an emphasis on alternatives such as home care.[17] On the other hand, hospice care at home, which should be adequately financed by insurance as a cost-effective way to care for the patient, is often poorly reimbursed, and many hospice programs struggle to stay solvent. There is too much emphasis on reimbursement for high-technology care in the home, as opposed to hands-on nursing care. More adequate financing is clearly indicated for hospice and other home care providers, since it is clear that, overall, care at home usually costs much less than in other settings.

Nursing Home

When an admission to a nursing home is planned for a terminally ill patient, it is important to specify the treatment plans and goals at the outset. The nursing home should inquire about the patient's wishes with regard to life-sustaining procedures, including DNR orders and artificial nutrition and hydration. The patient should be encouraged to execute an advance directive, appoint a surrogate, or both. The possibility that it may be necessary to transfer the patient to a general hospital should be discussed in advance (transfer may become indicated, but usually it is not). All parties should anticipate that the final phases of the dying process will occur in the nursing home without a transfer to the hospital, unless the patient cannot be kept reasonably comfortable in the nursing home.

Even though care can clearly be given more cost-effectively in the nursing home setting than in the general hospital, a major drawback to using the nursing home as a place for dying is that often insurance does not cover the cost of the nursing home care (just as it often does not cover the cost of care at home). Currently, there is almost no private insurance for nursing home care, and Medicare now covers only about 3 percent of nursing home days. The rest must be covered by a combination of Medicaid, to be eligible for which a patient must be pauperized, and private pay. It is essential that federal and private health care plans be modified to make nursing home care more accessible to patients of limited means.

Hospital

As much as one third of the patients cared for at home and expected to die there actually die in the hospital, even when hospice techniques of home care are used. The symptoms or anxiety generated by an impending death may overwhelm the family, and recourse to the hospital is appropriate whenever any treatment program, including a psychosocial one, cannot palliate the distress felt by the patient, the family, or both.

To accommodate such families and patients, hospitals should consider the development of specialized units, with rooms appointed so as to provide pleasant surroundings that will facilitate comfortable interchange among patient, family, and friends. The presence of life-sustaining equipment would be inappropriate in such an environment.

The intensive care unit should generally be discouraged as a treatment setting for the hospitalized patient who is dying, unless intensive palliative measures are required that cannot be done elsewhere. Too often, life-sustaining measures are instituted in the intensive care unit without sufficient thought to the proper goals of treatment. Although the courts have held that in the treatment of the hopelessly ill there is no legal distinction between stopping treatment and not starting it in the first place, there is a bias in the intensive care unit toward continuing aggressive measures that may be inappropriate. Though difficult, it is possible for a patient to die in the intensive care unit with dignity and comfort, since medical hardware itself has no capacity to dehumanize anyone. The important point is that the physician set a tone of caring and support, no matter what the setting.

Although the physicians and nurses in intensive care units may be less prepared than other professionals to switch from aggressive curative care to palliation and the provision of comfort only, they have all seen many situations in which clear decisions to limit treatment have brought welcome relief. Since these care givers often have considerable emotional energy invested in patients who have previously been receiving aggressive curative treatment, they may need consultation with colleagues from outside the intensive care unit to decide when to change the treatment goals.

Treating the Dying Patient —The Importance of Flexible Care

The care of the dying is an art that should have its fullest expression in helping patients cope with the technologically complicated medical environment that often surrounds them at the end of life. The concept of a good death does not mean simply the withholding of technological treatments that serve only to prolong the act of dying. It also requires the art of deliberately creating a medical environment that allows a peaceful death. Somewhere between the unacceptable extremes of failure to treat the dying patient and intolerable use of aggressive life-sustaining measures, the physician must seek a level of care that optimizes comfort and dignity.

In evaluating the burdens and benefits of treatment for the dying patient—whether in the hospital, in a nursing home, or at home—the physician needs to formulate a flexible and adjustable care plan, tailoring treatment to the patient's changing needs as the disease progresses. Such plans contrast sharply with the practice, frequent in medicine, in which the physician makes rounds and prescribes, leaving orders for nurses and technicians, but not giving continual feedback and adjustment. The physician's actions on behalf of the patient should be appropriate, with respect to both the types of treatments and the location in which they are given. Such actions need to be adjusted continually to the individual patient's needs, with the physician keeping primarily in mind that the benefits of treatment must outweigh the burdens imposed.

When the patient lacks decision-making capacity, discussing the limitation of treatment with the family becomes a major part of the treatment plan. The principle of continually adjusted care should guide all these decisions.

Pain and Suffering

The principle of continually adjusted care is nowhere more important than in the control of pain, fear, and suffering. The hopelessly ill patient must have whatever is necessary to control pain. One of the most pervasive causes of anxiety among patients, their families, and the public is the perception that physicians' efforts toward the relief of pain are sadly deficient. Because of this perceived professional deficiency, people fear that needless suffering will be allowed to occur as patients are dying.[18] To a large extent, we believe such fears are justified.

In the patient whose dying process is irreversible, the balance between minimizing pain and suffering and potentially hastening death should be struck clearly in favor of pain relief. Narcotics or other pain medications should be given in whatever dose and by whatever route is necessary for relief. It is morally correct to increase the dose of narcotics to whatever dose is needed, even though the medication may contribute to the depression of respiration or blood pressure, the dulling of consciousness, or even death, provided the primary goal of the physician is to relieve suffering. The proper dose of pain medication is the dose that is sufficient to relieve pain and suffering, even to the point of unconsciousness.

Dying patients often feel isolated and doubt seriously that their physician will be there to relieve their pain when the terminal phase is near. Early in the course of fatal disease, patients should be offered strong reassurance that pain will be controlled and that their physician will be available when the need is greatest. Both the patient and the family should be told that addiction need not be a source of concern and that the relief of pain will have nothing but a salutary effect from both the physical and the emotional standpoint. When possible, pain medication should be given orally to maximize patient autonomy, but usually a continuous parenteral route is needed for the adequate medication of patients in the near-terminal or terminal state. Under no circumstances should medication be "rationed." For episodic pain, patients should be encouraged to take medication as soon as they are conscious of pain, instead of waiting until it becomes intense and far more difficult to control. For continuous or frequently recurring pain, the patient should be placed on a regular schedule of administration. Some patients will choose to endure a degree of pain rather than experience any loss of alertness or control from taking narcotics—a choice that is consistent with patient autonomy and the concept of continually adjusted care.

If pain cannot be controlled with the commonly used analgesic regimens of mild or moderate strength, the patient should be switched quickly to more potent narcotics. It is important that doses be adequate: the textbook doses recommended for short-term pain are often grossly inadequate for long-term pain in the patient dying of cancer. The physician should be familiar with two or three narcotics and their side effects and appropriate starting dosages. Doses should be brought promptly to levels that provide a reliable pain-free state. Since adequate narcotic management seems to be an unfamiliar area to many physicians, we urge that educational material be distributed to them from a noncommercial source.[19] To allow a patient to experience unbearable pain or suffering is unethical medical practice.

Legal Concerns

The principles of medical ethics are formulated independently of legal decisions, but physicians may fear that decisions about the care of the hopelessly ill will bring special risks of criminal charges and prosecution. Although no medical decision can be immune from legal scrutiny, courts in the United States have generally supported the approaches advocated here.[20-23] The physician should follow these principles without exaggerated concern for legal consequences, doing whatever is necessary to relieve pain and bring comfort, and adhering to the patient's wishes as much as possible. To withhold any necessary measure of pain relief in a hopelessly ill person out of fear of depressing respiration or of possible legal repercussions is unjustifiable. Good medical practice is the best protection against legal liability.

Preparing for Death

As sickness progresses toward death, measures to minimize suffering should be intensified. Dying patients may require palliative care of an intensity that rivals even that of curative efforts. Keeping the patient clean, caring for the skin, preventing the formation of bed sores, treating neuropsychiatric symptoms, controlling peripheral and pulmonary edema, aggressively reducing nausea and vomiting, using intravenous medications, fighting the psychosocial forces that can lead to family fragmentation—all can tax the ingenuity and equanimity of the most skilled health professionals. Even though aggressive curative techniques are no longer indicated, professionals and families are still called on to use intensive measures—extreme responsibility, extraordinary sensitivity, and heroic compassion.

In training programs for physicians, more attention needs to be paid to these aspects of care. Progress has been made in persuading house staff and attending physicians to discuss DNR orders and to include clear orders and notes in the chart about limits on life-sustaining therapies, but patients are too rarely cared for directly by the physician at or near the time of death. Usually it is nurses who care for patients at this time. In a few innovative training programs, most notably at the University of Oregon, the hands-on aspects of care of the dying are addressed,[24] and such techniques should be presented at all training institutions.

Assisted Suicide

If care is administered properly at the end of life, only the rare patient should be so distressed that he or she desires to commit suicide. Occasionally, however, all fails. The doctor, the nurse, the family, and the patient may have done everything possible to relieve the distress occasioned by a terminal illness, and yet the patient perceives his or her situation as intolerable and seeks assistance in bringing about death. Is it ever justifiable for the physician to assist suicide in such a case?

Some physicians, believing it to be the last act in a continuum of care provided for the hopelessly ill patient, do assist patients who request it, either by prescribing sleeping pills with knowledge of their intended use or by discussing the required doses and methods of administration with the patient. The frequency with which such actions are undertaken is unknown, but they are certainly not rare. Suicide differs from euthanasia in that the act of bringing on death is performed by the patient, not the physician.

The physician who considers helping a patient who requests assistance with suicide must determine first that the patient is indeed beyond all help and not merely suffering from a treatable depression of the sort common in people with terminal illnesses. Such a depression requires therapeutic intervention. If there is no treatable component to the depression and the patient's pain or suffering is refractory to treatment, then the wish for suicide may be rational. If such a patient acts on the wish for death and actually commits suicide, it is ethical for a physician who knows the patient well to refrain from an attempt at resuscitation.

Even though suicide itself is not illegal, helping a person commit suicide is a crime in many states, either by statute or under common law. Even so, we know of no physician who has ever been prosecuted in the United States for prescribing pills in order to help a patient commit suicide.[25] However, the potential illegality of this act is a deterrent, and apart from that, some physicians simply cannot bring themselves to assist in suicide or to condone such action.

Whether it is bad medical practice or immoral to help a hopelessly ill patient commit a rational suicide is a complex issue, provoking a number of considerations. First, as their disease advances, patients may lose their decision-making capacity because of the effects of the disease or the drug treatment. Assisting such patients with suicide comes close to performing an act of euthanasia. Second, patients who want a doctor's assistance with suicide may be unwilling to endure their terminal illness because they lack information about what is ahead. Even when the physician explains in careful detail the availability of the kind of flexible, continually adjusted care described here, the patient may still opt out of that treatment plan and reject the physician's efforts to ease the dying process. Also, what are the physician's obligations if a patient who retains decision-making capacity insists that family members not be told of a suicide plan? Should the physician insist on obtaining the family's consent? Finally, should physicians acknowledge their role in a suicide in some way—by obtaining consultation, or in writing? Physicians who act in secret become isolated and cannot consult colleagues or ethics committees for confirmation that the patient has made a rational decision. If contacted, such colleagues may well object and even consider themselves obligated to report the physician to the Board of Medical Licensure or to the prosecutor. The impulse to maintain secrecy gives the lie to the moral intuition that assistance with suicide is ethical.

It is difficult to answer such questions, but all but two of us (J.v.E. and E.H.C.) believe that it is not immoral for a physician to assist in the rational suicide of a terminally ill person. However, we recognize that such an act represents a departure from the principle of continually adjusted care that we have presented. As such, it should be considered a separate alternative and not an extension of the flexible approach to care that we have recommended.

Clearly, the subject of assisted suicide deserves wide and open discussion.

Euthanasia

Some patients who cannot carry out suicide plans themselves, with or without assistance, may ask their physicians to take a more active part in ending their lives. In the case of suicide, the final act is performed by the patient, even when the physician provides indirect assistance in the form of information and means. By contrast, euthanasia requires the physician to perform a medical procedure that causes death directly. It is therefore even more controversial than assisted rational suicide, and various arguments have been mustered through the years for and against its use.[26,27]

In the Netherlands, the practice of euthanasia has gained a degree of social acceptance. As a result of a 1984 decision by the Dutch Supreme Court, euthanasia is no longer prosecuted in certain approved circumstances. The Dutch government authorized the State Commission on Euthanasia to study the issue, and the commission's report favored permitting doctors to perform euthanasia with certain safeguards, but the Dutch parliament, the States-General, has not yet acted to change the law.

Many Dutch physicians believe, however, that the medical treatments and actions needed to keep dying patients comfortable may at times be extended to include the act of euthanasia. Some of them hold that a continuum of measures can be brought into play to help the patient, and occasionally the injection of a lethal dose of a drug (usually a short-acting barbiturate, followed by a paralyzing agent) becomes necessary, representing the extreme end of that continuum. This occurs between 5000 and 10,000 times a year in the Netherlands, according to van der Werf[28] (and Admiraal P: personal communication).

The medical community in the Netherlands has developed criteria that must be met for an act of euthanasia to be considered medically and ethically acceptable.[29] The patient's medical situation must be intolerable, with no prospect of improvement. The patient must be rational and must voluntarily and repeatedly request euthanasia of the physician. The patient must be fully informed. There must be no other means of relieving the suffering, and two physicians must concur with the request.

In recent years, euthanasia has been discussed more openly in the United States, and the public response has been increasingly favorable. When a Roper poll asked in 1988 whether a physician should be lawfully able to end the life of a terminally ill patient at the patient's request, 58 percent said yes, 27 percent said no, and 10 percent were undecided. (This poll, taken for the National Hemlock Society by the Roper Organization of New York City, surveyed 1,982 adult Americans in March 1988.)

Presumably, the majority of physicians in the United States do not favor the Dutch position. Many physicians oppose euthanasia on moral or religious grounds, and indeed it raises profound theological questions. All religions address the matter of whether it is proper to decide the time of one's death. Whatever attitudes society may develop toward assisted suicide or euthanasia, individual physicians should not feel morally coerced to participate in such approaches. Many physicians oppose euthanasia because they believe it to be outside the physician's role, and some fear that it may be subject to abuse. (Some physicians and laypersons fear that active voluntary euthanasia, as practiced in the Netherlands, could lead to involuntary euthanasia and to murder, as practiced by the Nazis. Ethically, however, the difference is obvious.) In addition, the social climate in this country is very litigious, and the likelihood of prosecution if a case of euthanasia were discovered is fairly high—much higher than the likelihood of prosecution after a suicide in which the physician has assisted. Thus, the prospect of criminal prosecution deters even the hardiest advocates of euthanasia among physicians.

Nevertheless, the medical profession and the public will continue to debate the role that euthanasia may have in the treatment of the terminally or hopelessly ill patient.

Notes

1. Wanzer SH, Adelstein SJ, Cranford RE, et al. The physician's responsibility toward hopelessly ill patients. N Engl J Med 1984; 310:955–9.
2. President's Commission for the Study of Ethical Problems in Medicine and Biomedical and Behavioral Research. Deciding to forego life-sustaining treatment: a report on the ethical, medical and legal issues in treatment decisions. Washington, D.C.: Government Printing Office, 1983.
3. Office of Technology Assessment. Life-sustaining technologies and the elderly. Washington, D.C.: Government Printing Office, 1987.
4. Senate Special Committee on Aging. A matter of choice: planning ahead for health care decisions. Washington, D.C.: Government Printing Office, 1987.
5. Guidelines on the termination of life-sustaining treatment and the care of the dying: a report by the Hastings Center. Briarcliff Manor, N.Y.: Hastings Center, 1987.
6. Current Opinions of the Council on Ethical and Judicial Affairs of the American Medical Association — 1986. Withholding or withdrawing life-prolonging treatment. Chicago: American Medical Association, 1986.
7. Executive Board of the American Academy of Neurology. Position of the American Academy of Neurology on certain aspects of the care and management of the persistent vegetative state patient. Minneapolis: American Academy of Neurology, 1988.
8. Ruark JE, Raffin TA. Stanford University Medical Center Committee on Ethics. Initiating and withdrawing life support. N Engl J Med 1988; 318:25–30.
9. Safar P, Bircher N. Cardiopulmonary cerebral resuscitation: an introduction to resuscitation medicine. 3rd ed. Philadelphia: W.B. Saunders, 1988.
10. Society for the Right to Die. Handbook of living will laws. New York: Society for the Right to Die, 1987.
11. Appointing a proxy for health care decisions. New York: Society for the Right to Die, 1988.
12. Adult right to die case citations. New York: Society for the Right to Die, 1988.
13. Right to die court decisions: artificial feeding. New York: Society for the Right to Die, 1988.
14. Associated Press/Media General. Poll no. 4. Richmond, Va.: Media General, February 1985.
15. California Department of Health Services. Guidelines regarding withdrawal or withholding of life-sustaining procedure(s) in longterm care facilities, August 7, 1987.
16. Bedell SE, Pelle D, Maher PL, Cleary PD. Do-not-resuscitate orders for critically ill patients in the hospital: how are they used and what is their impact? JAMA 1986; 256:233–7.

17. Bulkin W, Lukashok H. Rx for dying: the case for hospice. N Engl J Med 1988; 318:376–8.

18. Angell M. The quality of mercy. N Engl J Med 1982; 306:98–9.

19. Payne R, Foley KM, eds. Cancer pain. Med Clin North Am 1987; 71:153–352.

20. Bartling v. Superior Court (Glendale Adventist Medical Center), 163 Cal. App. 3d 186, 209 Cal. Rptr. 220 (Ct. App. 1984).

21. Bouvia v. Superior Court (Glenchur), 179 Cal. App. 3d 1127, 225 Cal. Rptr. 297 (Ct. App. 1986), review denied (Cal. June 5, 1986).

22. Brophy v. New England Sinai Hosp., Inc., 398 Mass. 417, 497, N.E. 2d 626 (1986).

23. In re Culham, No. 87-340537-AC (Mich. Cir. Ct., Oakland County, Dec 15, 1987) (Breck J).

24. Tolle SW, Hickham DH, Larson EB, Benson JA. Patient death and housestaff stress: Clin Res 1987; 35:762A. abstract.

25. Glantz LH. Withholding and withdrawing treatment: the role of the criminal law. Law Med Health Care 1987–88; 15:231–41.

26. Van Bommel H. Choices for people who have a terminal illness, their families and their caregivers. Toronto: NC Press, 1986.

27. Angell M. Euthanasia. N Engl J Med 1988; 319:1348–50.

28. van der Werf GT. Huisarts en euthanasie. Medisch Contact 1986; 43:1389.

29. The Central Committee of the Royal Dutch Medical Association. Vision on euthanasia. Utrecht, the Netherlands, 1986.

Part 3

PUBLIC POLICY

part 3

Introduction

The use of quality of life considerations in treatment decisions does not only affect the individuals involved in the medical setting. Their use also has implications and ramifications at the level of public policy in our society. It is not all that infrequent that medical personnel are sued in a court of law because of their decisions and actions in a particular case. It is almost commonplace today to pick up a newspaper or to watch a news broadcast and discover yet another instance in which a "Baby Doe" or a patient in a persistent vegetative state has died because a decision was made not to treat them due to their low "quality of life."

Some believe that decisions to forgo or to withdraw medical treatment based on quality of life considerations are strictly between the physician and the patient or the surrogate decisionmaker. On the other hand, others in society argue that the government should involve itself heavily in the health-delivery system especially where incompetent or vulnerable patients are involved, e.g., newborns and the senile elderly in nursing homes. Neither extreme may be helpful in the public debate about the use of quality of life judgments, but what is clear is that society needs to formulate some kind of public policy on the issue. What is also clear is that individual court decisions have produced a body of contrary law, and many lawyers and physicians find it increasingly difficult to apply these decisions to concrete cases which they face.

Several governmental agencies and presidential commissions have begun to study this issue in some depth over the past few years, but again it appears that these studies have produced almost contrary conclusions in some instances, e.g., critically-ill newborns. Various professional groups have also entered the debate by writing guidelines for the medical care of certain patients, e.g., patients in a persistent vegetative state. The debate has become so widespread at the public policy level that it is not unusual to find representatives from various church groups presenting *amicus curiae* briefs before legal tribunals and testimony before Congressional subcommittees. All these activities by different groups are necessary to establish a broad-based social, legal and political consensus on such a delicate issue as the use of quality of life judgments in medical decision making.

Several important issues begin to be raised at the public policy level of this debate. Questions of justice and the protection of human rights of the vulnerable in society will inevitably be raised. Have we come to the point where medical technologies now have more legal rights than the patients who are forced to accept their application? Who should decide whether quality of life judgments are appropriate in a given medical situation? Finally, what is the relation between morality and public policy? Once again, answers to these questions are at least partially dependent upon theological, ethical, medical and social considerations that are frequently overlooked or neglected.

Further Readings

Annas, George J. "Do Feeding Tubes Have More Rights Than Patients?," *Hastings Center Report* 16(February, 1986):26–28.

————. "Termination of Life Support Systems in the Elderly: Legal Issues: The Cases of Brother Fox and Earle Spring," *Journal of Geriatric Psychiatry* 14(1981):31–43.

Armstrong, Paul W. and Colen, B.D. "From Quinlan to Jobes: The Courts and the PVS Patient," *Hastings Center Report* 18(February/March, 1988):37–40.

Braithwaite, Susan and Thomasma, David C. "New Guidelines on Foregoing Life-Sustaining Treatment in Incompetent Patients: An Anti-Cruelty Policy," *Annals of Internal Medicine* 104(1986):711–715.

Connery, John R., S.J. "The Clarence Herbert Case: Was Withdrawal of Treatment Justified?," *Hospital Progress* 65(February, 1984):32–35 and 70.

Dresser, Rebecca S. and Boisaubin, Eugene V., Jr. "Ethics, Law, and Nutritional Support," *Archives of Internal Medicine* 145(January, 1985):122–124.

Gelineau, Bishop Louis. "On Removing Nutrition and Water From Comatose Woman," *Origins* 17(January 21, 1988): 545 and 547.

McCormick, Richard A. "Caring or Starving?: The Case of Claire Conroy," *America* 152(April 6, 1985):269–273.

National Conference of Catholic Bishops Committee for Pro-Life Activities. "The Rights of the Terminally Ill," *Origins* 16(September 4, 1986):222–224.

National Conference of Commissioners on Uniform State Laws. *Uniform Rights of the Terminally Ill Act* (Chicago: National Conference of Commissioners on Uniform State Laws, June 10, 1987).

Pontifical Academy of Sciences. "The Artificial Prolongation of Life," *Origins* 15(December 5, 1985):415–417.

PRECEDENTS

25

Quality of Life and the Withholding or Withdrawing Life-Prolonging Medical Treatment

AMA Council on Ethical and Judicial Affairs

2.17: QUALITY OF LIFE. In the making of decisions for the treatment of seriously deformed newborns or persons who are severely deteriorated victims of injury, illness or advanced age, the primary consideration should be what is best for the individual patient and not the avoidance of a burden to the family or to society. Quality of life is a factor to be considered in determining what is best for the individual. Life should be cherished despite disabilities and handicaps, except when the prolongation would be inhumane and unconscionable. Under these circumstances, withholding or removing life supporting means is ethical provided that the normal care given an individual who is ill is not discontinued. (I,III,IV)

2.20: WITHHOLDING OR WITHDRAWING LIFE-PROLONGING MEDICAL TREATMENT. The social commitment of the physician is to sustain life and relieve suffering. Where the performance of one duty conflicts with the other, the preferences of the patient should prevail. If the patient is incompetent to act in his own behalf and did not previously indicate his preferences, the family or other surrogate decisionmaker, in concert with the physician, must act in the best interest of the patient.

For humane reasons, with informed consent, a physician may do what is medically necessary to alleviate severe pain, or cease or omit treatment to permit a terminally ill patient to die when death is imminent. However, the

"Quality of Life and the Withholding or Withdrawing Life-Prolonging Medical Treatment" by the American Medical Association Council on Ethical and Judicial Affairs in 1989 Current Opinions of the Council on Ethical and Judicial Affairs of the American Medical Association, *Nos. 2.17, 2.20 and 2.21. Reprinted with permission of the American Medical Association.*

physician should not intentionally cause death. In deciding whether the administration of potentially life-prolonging medical treatment is in the best interest of the patient who is incompetent to act in his own behalf, the surrogate decisionmaker and physician should consider several factors, including: the possibility for extending life under humane and comfortable conditions; the patient's values about life and the way it should be lived; and the patient's attitudes toward sickness, suffering, medical procedures, and death.

Even if death is not imminent but a patient is beyond doubt permanently unconscious, and there are adequate safeguards to confirm the accuracy of the diagnosis, it is not unethical to discontinue all means of life-prolonging medical treatment.

Life-prolonging medical treatment includes medication and artificially or technologically supplied respiration, nutrition or hydration. In treating a terminally ill or permanently unconscious patient, the dignity of the patient should be maintained at all times. (I,III,IV,V)

2.21: WITHHOLDING OR WITHDRAWING LIFE-PROLONGING MEDICAL TREATMENT—PATIENTS' PREFERENCES.

A competent, adult patient may, in advance, formulate and provide a valid consent to the withholding or withdrawal of life-support systems in the event that injury or illness renders that individual incompetent to make such a decision. The preference of the individual should prevail when determining whether extraordinary life-prolonging measures should be undertaken in the event of terminal illness. Unless it is clearly established that the patient is terminally ill or permanently unconscious, a physician should not be deterred from appropriately aggressive treatment of a patient. (I,III,IV,V)

26

Patients with Permanent Loss of Consciousness

President's Commission for the Study of Ethical Problems in Medicine and Biomedical and Behavioral Research

The general public probably first became aware of the issues addressed in this chapter following the tragedy that began for a New Jersey family on April 15, 1975. On that day, Karen Ann, the 21-year-old daughter of Joseph and Julia Quinlan, lapsed into a coma from which she has never recovered.[1] [Editor's Note: Karen Ann Quinlan died, June, 1985.] In the years since, as her situation ceased being solely a private, family concern and—because of legal proceedings[2]—became front-page news, people across the country have confronted such difficult questions as:

- what is the relationship of permanent unconsciousness to life and death?
- how reliable is the medical prognosis of permanence of unconsciousness?

- what life-extending care should be considered unnecessary in the context of patients with little or no chance of regaining cognitive functions?

Uncertainties regarding the care of long-term unconscious patients have been raised with increasing frequency,[3] though the number of such patients whose care has become the subject of judicial scrutiny still represents only a fraction of the total number of permanently unconscious patients.

The Commission's involvement with the issues raised by this group of patients began with its Congressionally mandated study of the "definition" of death.[4] In an empirical investigation conducted as part of that study, the

---

"Patients with Permanent Loss of Consciousness," by the President's Commission for the Study of Ethical Problems in Medicine and Biomedical and Behavioral Research. Reprinted from Deciding to Forgo Life-Sustaining Treatment: A Report on the Ethical, Medical, and Legal Issues in Treatment Decisions, *1983, pp. 171–186 and 192–196.*

Commission found that although two-thirds of the patients who are supported by an artificial respirator during a coma of at least six hours duration are dead within a month, about 6% remained indefinitely in a "persistent vegetative state."[5] The Commission was especially interested in this group for two reasons. First, for many years the leading set of clinical criteria for the determination of "brain death" were those published in 1968 under the title "A Definition of Irreversible Coma."[6] Using this term as synonymous with death unfortunately served to perpetuate a confusion in the medical field between the state of being permanently unconscious, as are patients in a persistent vegetative state, and that of being dead.[7] Second, and more importantly, once it is acknowledged that permanently unconscious patients are not dead, difficult questions are raised about the type and extent of care that should be provided for them.

Since permanently unconscious patients raise issues at least as difficult as those considered in *Defining Death,* the Commission resolved to give this group special attention in the present study. Two major issues are presented: Who are these patients exactly? And what issues arise during their care that are different from those of other incompetent patients? The first section of this chapter addresses the theoretical concerns in making a diagnosis of permanent loss of consciousness and identifies the major groups of patients in this state, though the Commission leaves to the appropriate biomedical experts the task of providing working guidelines for making the medical diagnosis. After establishing that some patients' unconsciousness can be reliably predicted to be permanent, the chapter attempts to clarify what should be considered permissible care of these patients. The second section

evaluates the considerations that would justify continued treatment of these patients. . . . The final section presents the Commission's recommendations for decisionmaking processes that encourage both justifiable assignment of authority to decide and ethically defensible decisions.

Identifying Patients

Unconsciousness. No one can ever have more than inferential evidence of consciousness in another person. A detailed analysis of the nature of consciousness is not needed, however, when considering the class of patients in whom *all* possible components of mental life are absent—all thought, feeling, sensation, desire, emotion, and awareness of self or environment.[8] Retaining even a slight ability to experience the environment (such as from an ordinary dose of sedative drugs, severe retardation, or the destruction of most of the cerebral cortex) is different from having no such ability, and the discussion in this chapter is limited to the latter group of patients.

Most of what makes someone a distinctive individual is lost when the person is unconscious,[9] especially if he or she will always remain so. Personality, memory, purposive action, social interaction, sentience, thought, and even emotional states are gone.[10] Only vegetative functions and reflexes persist. If food is supplied, the digestive system functions and uncontrolled evacuation occurs; the kidneys produce urine; the heart, lungs, and blood vessels continue to move air and blood; and nutrients are distributed in the body.

Exceedingly careful neurologic examination is essential in order for a diagnosis of complete unconsciousness to be made. Application of noxious stimuli to the nerve endings of an unconscious patient leads to simple, unregulated reflex responses at both the spinal and the brain stem levels. Reflexes may allow some eye movement, grimacing, swallowing, and pupillary adjustment to light. If the reticular activating system in the brain stem is intact, the eyes can open and close in regular daily cycles. The reflex activity can be unsettling to family and other observers, but the components of behavior that produce this appearance are "accompanied by an apparent total lack of cognitive function."[11] In order to have awareness, a person must have an integrated functioning of the brain stem's activating system with the higher "thinking" functions from the thalamus and cerebral hemispheres.[12] Many patients whose brain dysfunctions cause unconsciousness nevertheless have a fairly intact brain stem and, if provided extensive nursing care, are able to remain alive without respirator support for many years.

Permanence. The other essential property of this category of patients is that their unconsciousness is permanent,[13] which means "lasting . . . indefinitely without change; opposed to temporary."[14] Three sources of uncertainty should be acknowledged about any judgment that a particular patient's unconscious state is permanent.

The first uncertainty affects any scientific proposition about as-yet-unobserved cases. No matter how extensive the past evidence is for an empirical generalization, it may yet be falsified by future experience. Certainty in prognosis is always a matter of degree, typically based upon the quantity and quality of the evidence from which a prediction is made.

Second, this empirical qualification is especially serious in predictions about unconsciousness because the evidence relevant to a prognosis of permanence is still quite limited. The overall number of such patients is small,[15] and most cases have not been carefully studied or adequately reported. Furthermore, the number of variables affecting prognosis (for example, the cause of unconsciousness, the patient's age and other diseases, the length of time the patient has been unconscious, and the kinds of therapy applied) is large and imperfectly understood.

Finally, any prediction that a patient will not regain consciousness before dying, regardless of the treatment undertaken, contains an implicit assumption about future medical breakthroughs. Since some such patients can be maintained alive for extended periods of time (often years rather than days, weeks, or months),[16] this assumption about treatment innovations can be a long-range one. At the moment, however, it introduces only a very small uncertainty, since the possibility of repairing the neurologic injuries that destroy consciousness is exceedingly remote.

Given these three qualifications on the meaning and basis of any judgment regarding permanence, such a judgment is always a matter of probability about whether a particular patient will remain unconscious until he or she dies despite any treatment that might be undertaken. Nevertheless, the Commission was assured that physicians with experience in this area can reliably determine that some patients' loss of consciousness is permanent.[17]

Disease Categories. Only a few fairly uncommon diseases cause permanent loss of consciousness. The pathophysiology of an unconscious state that becomes permanent entails severe disruption of the coordinated functioning of the cerebral hemispheres and the midbrain but with retention of sufficient brainstem activity to sustain vegetative functions.

Most commonly, this occurs when the cerebral hemispheres are profoundly injured but the brain stem is nearly entirely spared. Diagnosis in these cases typically involves extensive physical examination, special radiographic and other imaging procedures, and circulation studies of the brain.

Although many individuals with such an injury survive only briefly, some stay alive for an indefinite period and die of some other illness, often contracted while they are unconscious. Nearly all such long-term survivors are in the diagnostic category of "persistent vegetative state" (PVS).[18] This syndrome usually arises from head injury (as from fights, gunshots, or automobile accidents), intracranial hypoxia (as from cardiac arrest, asphyxiation, or hypotensive shock), or intracranial hypoglycemia (as from insulin overdose). If a patient who is initially comatose from a head injury fails to become responsive and aware within a few weeks, the prognosis for any recovery becomes extremely remote. The absence of all responsiveness, vocalization, or purposive action one month after the trauma makes a lack of recovery virtually certain, despite vigorous therapy.[19] The incidence of head injuries leading to permanent coma or vegetative state is unclear, as there is no central registry, but preliminary evidence seems to point to at least a few cases each year at each large referral hospital.[20]

As with head injury, hypoxic and hypoglycemic damage to the brain often initially causes loss of function in areas of the brain that might recover with time and treatment. However, probably 12% of patients with nontraumatic coma develop reliably diagnosed PVS.[21] Two patients recovered consciousness after a year of PVS from hypoxia.[22] Recovery of consciousness is very unlikely, however, for patients with hypoxia who remain comatose or in PVS for more than one month.[23] Certainly, extended observation is appropriate before making a diagnosis of permanent unconsciousness, at least for hypoxic injuries in otherwise healthy young people.[24]

In addition to those with PVS, four other groups of patients might be diagnosed to be permanently unconscious. First are those who are unresponsive after brain injury or hypoxia and who do not recover sufficient brain-stem function to stabilize in a vegetative state before dying. Most of these die within a few weeks after the brain damage. Although the number of patients in this category is uncertain, it is probably large; more than half the individuals for whom cardiac resuscitation is initially successful die without recovering consciousness, mostly in the first few days.[25]

Second, the end-stage victims of such degenerative neurologic conditions as Jakob-Creutzfeldt disease and severe Alzheimer's disease are permanently unconscious. Only in their final stages do these illnesses become so severe as to bring on complete unconsciousness, and the life span thereafter is only a few weeks or months, depending in part on the extensiveness of support given. Again, the incidence of this source of irreversible unconsciousness is unknown.

A third group of permanently unconscious patients who are in a coma rather than in persistent vegetative state are those who have intracranial mass lesions from neoplasms or vascular masses. If the lesion is correctable, some of these unconscious patients might have restoration of some consciousness. However those for whom there is no effective therapy will be unconscious until they die. Such states usually last only for a few days or weeks, and their frequency is unknown.

The fourth source of permanent unconsciousness is congenital hypoplasia of the central nervous system (anencephaly). Various degrees of hypoplasia and dysplasia are possible and some engender brief vegetative life without development of any mentation or cognition. Usually such conditions are apparent because of abnormalities of the cranium at birth. Sometimes the infant is fairly normal, however, and only the failure to achieve the usual developmental landmarks or the appearance of other medical complications leads to detection. Most babies whose anencephaly precludes development of any consciousness die within a few days of birth, and none survive for more than a few months. This condition afflicts one of every 850 births, for an annual incidence of 4000 in the United States.[26]

Reasons for Continued Treatment

Physicians arrive at prognoses of permanent unconsciousness only after patients have received vigorous medical attention, careful observation, and complete diagnostic studies, usually over a prolonged period. During this time when improvement is thought to be possible, it is appropriate for therapies to be intensive and aggressive, both to reverse unconsciousness and to overcome any other problems. Once it is clear that the loss of consciousness is permanent, however, the goals of continued therapy need to be examined.

The Interests of the Patient. The primary basis for medical treatment of patients is the prospect that each individual's interests (specifically, the interest in well-being) will be promoted. Thus, treatment ordinarily aims to benefit a patient through preserving life, relieving pain and suffering, protecting against disability, and returning maximally effective functioning. If a prognosis of permanent unconsciousness is correct, however, continued treatment cannot confer such benefits. Pain and suffering are absent, as are joy, satisfaction, and pleasure. Disability is total and no return to an even minimal level of social or human functioning is possible.[27]

Any value to the patient from continued care and maintenance under such circumstances would seem to reside in the very small probability that the prognosis of permanence is incorrect.[28] Although therapy might appear to be in the patient's interest because it preserves the remote chance of recovery of consciousness, there are two substantial objections to providing vigorous therapy for permanently unconscious patients.

First, the few patients who have recovered consciousness after a prolonged period of unconsciousness were severely disabled.[29] The degree of permanent damage varied but commonly included inability to speak or see, permanent distortion of the limbs, and paralysis. Being returned to such a state would be regarded as of very limited benefit by most patients; it may even be considered harmful if a particular patient would have refused treatments expected to produce this outcome. Thus, even the extremely small likelihood of "recovery" cannot be equated with returning to a normal or relatively well functioning state. Second, long-term treatment commonly imposes severe financial and emotional burdens on a patient's family, people whose welfare most patients, before they lost consciousness, placed a high value on. For both these reasons, then, continued treatment beyond a minimal level will often not serve the interests of permanently unconscious patients optimally.

The Interests of Others. The other possible

sources of an interest in continued care for a permanently unconscious patient are the patient's family, health care professionals, and the public. A family possessing hope, however slim, for a patient's recovery shares that individual's interest in the continuation of treatment, namely, the possibility that the prognosis of permanent unconsciousness will prove wrong. Also, families may find personal meaning in attending to an unconscious patient, and they have a substantial interest in that patient's being treated respectfully.[30]

Health care professionals undertake specific and often explicit obligations to render care. People trust these professionals to act in patients' best interests. This expectation plays a complex and crucial part in the professionals' ability to provide care. Failure to provide some minimal level of care, even to a permanently unconscious patient, might undermine that trust and with it the health care professions' general capacity to provide effective care. Furthermore, the self-identity of physicians, nurses, and other personnel is bound in significant ways to the life-saving efforts they make; to fail to do so is felt by some to violate their professional creed.[31] Consequently, health care providers may have an interest in continued treatment of these patients.[32]

Finally, society has a significant interest in protecting and promoting the high value of human life.[33] Although continued life may be of little value to the permanently unconscious patient, the provision of care is one way of symbolizing and reinforcing the value of human life so long as any chance of recovery remains.[34] Moreover, the public may want permanently unconscious patients to receive treatment lest reduced levels of care have deleterious effects on the vigor with which other, less seriously compromised patients are treated. Furthermore the public has reason to support appropriate research on the pathophysiology and treatment of this condition so that decisions always rely upon the most complete and recent data possible.

There are, on the other hand, considerations for each of these parties—the family, health care professionals, and society—that argue against continued treatment of permanently unconscious patients. As mentioned, long-term treatment commonly imposes substantial financial burdens on a patient's family and on society[35] and often creates substantial psychological stresses for family members and providers.[36] Health care professionals must devote scarce time and resources to treatment that is nearly certain to be futile. Any alternate useful allocation of the resources and personnel is likely to benefit other patients much more substantially.

In sum, the interests of the permanently unconscious patient in continued treatment are very limited compared with other patients. These attenuated interests in continuing treatment must be weighed against the reasons to choose nontreatment in order to arrive at sound public policy on the care of the permanently unconscious. . . .

The Decisionmaking Process

Recommending a single management scheme would be neither possible nor desirable because of the great variations in the situations of permanently unconscious patients, the nature of the institutions and persons providing care, and the desires of the families involved. First, the values and beliefs of health care professionals and the policies of the institution may place limits on the treatment options made available, even when all providers try to avoid idiosyncratic thinking or unreasonable rigidity; transfer to other care givers may not be a possibility. Second, decisions are often constrained by legal uncertainty about the effects particular courses of treatment might have for the rights and liabilities of the parties involved.[37] Third, the people who love and care about the patient should have a voice in decisions. Certain options that are morally, medically, and legally valid might be quite unacceptable to them.[38] Finally, realistic possibilities may be curtailed by the unavailability of funds and resources.

Although a single scheme is not feasible, procedures for deciding among possible alternatives can still be endorsed. Sometimes, though infrequently, a patient will have indicated his or her preferences before losing consciousness.[39] A reasonably specific advance directive to withhold care should be honored by those responsible for a permanently unconscious patient.[40] A directive requesting continued treatment should guide those responsible but it cannot supersede their obligation to decide on management of the patient's care in light of all the circumstances, some of which may not have been foreseen by the patient when the directive was given.

When there are several treatment options that are acceptable to all interested parties and there is no advance directive from the patient, the option actually followed should generally be the one selected by the family.[41] When no alternative is acceptable to all concerned, an attempt to reach an acceptable compromise is preferable to forcing a confrontation. If substitution of another provider, institution, or funding would achieve accord and is possible, such a course should be followed.[42] Where institutional ethics committees exist, their assis-

tance should be sought since the advice of a group of concerned but disinterested people may foster understanding and agreement.[43]

If disagreement between at least two of these parties—the health care professionals, the family members, and the institution—persists after institutional review, recourse to the courts for the appointment of a guardian may be both appropriate and unavoidable.[44] Any physician involved in such a proceeding is under a strong moral obligation to assist in educating the lawyers and the court about the complexities of the situation. Courts ought to avoid deciding among treatment options, however, because explicit judicial decisions may prematurely rigidify the options available and paralyze the exercise of judgment by the parties directly involved. Rather, the court should appoint a responsible surrogate who is charged with collecting and considering the relevant information and making a decision, which might then be reported to the court.

In general, the courts have followed this course. The New Jersey Supreme Court, for example, held that the constitutional right of privacy of an unconscious patient in a situation like that of Karen Quinlan is broad enough to encompass a right to refuse the application of a mechanical respirator and that her father, as guardian, could make such a choice on her behalf.[45] A number of other cases of permanently unconscious patients have come before the courts in the seven years since the *Quinlan* decision, and guardians have uniformly been allowed to consent to withdrawal of treatment for patients whose status is comparable to hers.[46] Most of these civil cases relied largely upon a constitutional claim of privacy on behalf of the unconscious patient against which the state had no substantial contravening interests.[47] In one criminal case, the court decided that responsibility for the permanently unconscious patient's death rested with the robber whose battery caused the unconsciousness, not the physicians who, without prior court sanction, removed a respirator.[48]

In sum, the Commission finds good decisionmaking regarding patients who have permanently lost consciousness to be possible without changes in law or other public policy. The medical profession should continue to carry its weighty obligation to establish diagnoses well and to help families understand these tragic situations. Health care institutions need to provide good policies to govern decisionmaking, including appropriate sources of consultation and advice. Family and friends of the permanently unconscious patient bear not only the protracted tragedy of their loss but also the substantial responsibility of collaborating in decisionmaking. When families can direct the care of an unconscious family member, practices and policies should encourage them to do so and should restrict the degree to which outsiders may intervene in these matters. Courts and legislatures should not encourage routine resort to the judicial system for the actual decisionmaking. Instead, courts ought to ensure that appropriate surrogates are designated and that surrogates are allowed an appropriate range of discretion.

Notes

1. Sometime after she ceased breathing for unknown reasons, Karen Quinlan was brought, unconscious, to a hospital emergency room. After her condition stabilized, feeding required a nasogastric tube and breathing required a respirator. She never experienced irreversible cessation of all brain functions (that is, death) but rather retained function of the brain stem and was diagnosed as being in a "persistent vegetative state," a condition that has not changed. Joseph Quinlan and Julia Quinlan, with Phyllis Battelle, KAREN ANN: THE QUINLANS TELL THEIR STORY, Doubleday & Co., Garden City, N.Y. (1977).

2. Karen Quinlan's father sought court appointment as guardian of her person for the express purpose of authorizing the removal of her respirator, whether or not she died as a consequence. He was opposed not only by Karen's physicians but by the local prosecutor and the state attorney general. The New Jersey Supreme Court, however, granted his request. Her physicians gradually discontinued the respirator during May of 1976 and she was able to breathe on her own; at this writing she is alive, cared for in a New Jersey nursing home. *In re* Quinlan, 70 N.J. 10, 355 A. 2d 647, *cert. denied* 429 U.S. 922, (1976); IN THE MATTER OF KAREN QUINLAN (2 vol.), Univ. Publications of America, Frederick, Md. (1977).

3. See, e.g., Lawrence K. Altman, *Princess Death: U.S. Physicians Raise Questions,* N.Y. TIMES, Sept. 21, 1982, at C-1; Glenn Collins, *When Life is a Matter for Debate,* N.Y. TIMES, Aug. 16, 1982, at B-12.

   In addition to the well-known *Quinlan* case, there have been several other court reviews of the case of comatose patients. Dockery v. Dockery, 559 S.W. 2d 952 (Tenn. App. 1977) (appeal of chancery court order, which appointed husband as guardian for purposes of authorizing removal of respirator from comatose wife, mooted by wife's death); *In re* Piotrowicz, No. 1948 (Essex Cty., Mass. Probate Ct., Dec. 23, 1977) (husband appointed guardian of 56-year-old comatose wife for purposes of authorizing withdrawal of respirator); *In re* Nichols, No. A99511, Orange Cty. Calif. Super. Ct. (March 21, 1979) discussed in Note, *Comatose Conservatee—Restrictions of Legal Capacity—Substance or Procedure?*, 7 WASH ST. U. L. REV. 205 (1980); Leach v. Akron General Medical Center, 426 N.E.2d 809 (Ohio Com. Pl. 1980) (family sought directive to disconnect life support); *In re* Storar 52 N.Y.2d 363, 420 N.E.2d 64 (1981), *modifying* Eichner v. Dillon, 426 N.Y.S.2d 527 (App. Div. 1980) (in which a comatose Catholic priest, Brother Joseph Fox, was allowed to have treatment stopped because he had given strong advance directives); Severns v. Wilmington Medical Center, Inc., 421 A.2d 1334 (Del. 1980) (comatose woman with substantial advance deliberation allowed to stop all treatment); *In re* Lydia Hall Hospital, No. 23730182 (Special Term, Part II, Sup. Ct., Nassau County, N.Y., Oct. 22, 1982) (Peter Cinque, while competent, asked to cease dialysis and then became comatose after a resuscitation effort and court ordered discontinuation of treatment on family request); *In re* Cruse, No. J914419 and *In re* Guardianship of Cruse No. P645318 (Sup. Ct., Los Angeles, Cal., Feb. 15, 1979) (3-year-old child in coma, life-support discontinuance authorized); *In re* Young, No. A100863 (Sup. Ct., Orange County, Cal., Sept. 11, 1979) (removal of respirator allowed for comatose automobile accident victim).

4. President's Commission for the Study of Ethical Problems in Medicine and Biomedical and Behavioral Research, DEFINING DEATH, U.S. Government Printing Office, Washington (1981).

5. About 12%, typically those whose coma was due to drug intoxication, made a good to moderate recovery, and about an equal number were left with severe disability, though they regained consciousness. *Id.* at 94.

6. Ad Hoc Committee of the Harvard Medical School to Examine the Definition of Brain Death, *A Definition of Irreversible Coma*, 205 J.A.M.A. 377 (1968).

7. *See* Julius Korein, *Terminology, Definitions and Usage*, 315 ANNALS N.Y. ACAD. SCI. 6 (1978); testimonies of Dr. Lawrence Pitts, Dr. Robert Kaiser, and Mr. Leslie Rothenberg, transcript of 12th meeting of the President's Commission (Sept. 12, 1981) at 348-65; testimony of Dr. David Levy, transcript of 15th meeting of the President's Commission (Dec. 12, 1981) at 275-82.

8. A determination of unconsciousness will therefore generally be based upon evidence that the person lacks any responsiveness to the internal or external environment (excepting unmodulated reflex responses), does not engage in purposive action, and manifests no other signs of mental activity.

9. Two other terms could have been used: "coma" and "vegetative state." But "coma" has often been used imprecisely and both terms might connote only a subset of the relevant group. Sometimes coma is graded to reflect all possible degrees of impaired consciousness. *See, e.g.*, Graham Teasdale and Bryan Jennett, *Assessment of Coma and Impaired Consciousness—A Practical Scale*, 1 LANCET 81 (1974); Bruce D. Snyder *et al.*, *Neurologic Prognosis after Cardiopulmonary Arrest: II. Level of Consciousness*, 30 NEUROLOGY 52 (1980). Others have insisted upon a more restrictive definition that includes absence of eye opening. "Coma is complete unresponsiveness with eyes closed." Fred Plum, *Consciousness and Its Disturbances: Introduction,*

in Paul B. Beeson, Walsh McDermott, and James B. Wyngaarden, eds., CECIL TEXTBOOK OF MEDICINE, W.B. Saunders Co., Philadelphia (15th ed. 1979) at 640. The first usage is overly inclusive for the present discussion, as it includes responsive and sentient individuals; the second definition is overly restrictive as it excludes unconscious patients whose eyes open, like those in a "vegetative state," a large subgroup of patients with permanent unconsciousness.

The term "vegetative state" (or, more anatomically, "apallic syndrome") denotes unconsciousness with persistent brain-stem functions that maintain subsistence functions and often wakefulness. It includes patients with the appearance of wakefulness but conversely excludes those who are more deeply comatose with closed eyes. *See* David H. Ingvar *et al., Survival after Severe Cerebral Anoxia with Destruction of the Cerebral Cortex: The Apallic Syndrome,* 35 ANNALS N.Y. ACAD. SCI. 184 (1978). The term needed for the discussion in this Report was selected to include deep coma and vegetative state but to exclude patients with partial impairments of consciousness. "Permanent loss of consciousness" accomplishes this.

10. Some hold that such a patient ought not to be considered a "person." *See* Joseph Fletcher, *Indicators of Humanhood,* 2 HASTINGS CTR. REP. 1, 3 (Nov. 1972); Lawrence C. Becker, *Human Being: The Boundaries of the Concept,* 4 PHIL. & PUB. AFFAIRS 334 (Summer 1975); John Lachs, *Humane Treatment and the Treatment of Humans,* 294 NEW ENG. J. MED. 838 (1976). Rather than attempt to define "person," the Commission has concentrated on delineating the obligations to provide care to patients who have permanently lost consciousness,

since it had earlier concluded that such patients are living human beings. DEFINING DEATH, *supra* note 4, at 7, 38–41.

11. Fred Plum and Jerome B. Posner, THE DIAGNOSIS OF STUPOR AND COMA, F.A. Davis Co., Philadelphia (3rd ed. 1980) at 6.

12. Medical science has been unable to detect or postulate neurologic damage to the brain that would result in a functioning cerebrum capable of consciousness but able to perform absolutely no purposeful actions. At the least, to have consciousness a person must have some functioning cerebrum connected to adequate activating structures in the midbrain. Neurological findings indicate that having that much of a functioning central nervous system entails having at least the ability to blink voluntarily or move the eyes deliberately, and usually much more. Patients with the rare neurologic syndrome termed "locked-in state" retain only the ability to control movements of the eyes or eyelids. *See, e.g.,* Martin H. Feldman, *Physiological Observations in a Chronic Case of "Locked-in Syndrome,"* 21 NEUROLOGY 459 (1971); Plum and Posner, *supra* note 11, at 6, 24.

13. The term "permanent" could have been replaced by "persistent," "irreversible," or "judged to be permanent." "Persistent" was rejected because it can apply to situations that are not permanent. Ordinarily a situation is persistent when it lasts a long time, but not necessarily forever. However, repeated evaluations over a period of persistence is often essential to a reliable prognostication of permanence.

"Irreversible" not only conveys permanence but also focuses upon the prognostication of therapeutic possibilities, which might be a beneficial additional nuance. However, using "irreversible" to refer to this class of patients is virtually precluded by its inappropriate use in the phrase "irreversible coma" to describe neurologically dead bodies maintained on artificial circulatory and respiratory support. *See* notes 6 and 7, *supra.*

The phrase "judged to be permanent" would highlight the irreducible element of probabilistic judgment that is part of the diagnosis of permanent unconsciousness. However, since such judgment is an essential part of every scientific prognostication, it is redundant and unnecessarily awkward. *See, e.g.,* Alvan R. Feinstein, CLINICAL JUDGMENT, Robert Kreiger Pub. Co., Huntington, N.Y. (1967); Mark Siegler, *Pascal's Wager and the Hanging of Crepe,* 292 NEW ENG. J. MED. 853 (1975).

14. COMPACT EDITION OF THE OXFORD ENGLISH DICTIONARY, Oxford University Press, New York (1971) at 710.

15. The only prevalence survey available estimates that Japan has about 2000 permanently unconscious patients in long-term care, which, if the prevalence were the same (and if differing definitions of terms did not cause substantial error), would imply less than 5000 at any one time in the United States. S. Sato *et al., Epidemiological Survey of Vegetative State Patients in Tokuhu District in Japan,* 8 NEUROLOGIA MEDICO-CHIRURGIA (Tokyo) 141 (1978). *See also,* Peter Perl, *Silent Epidemic: Modern Medicine Saves Victims of Crash but Creates Dilemma: Coma,* WASH. POST, March 18, 1982, at A-1; William D. Kalsbeek *et al., National Head Injury and Spinal Cord Injury Survey: Major Findings,* 53 J. NEUROSURG. 19 (Supp. 1980); DEFINING DEATH, *supra* note 4, at 92–95. Dr. Ake Grenvik reports between 500 and 1000 patients at Presbyterian-University Hospital in Pittsburgh have had life-sustaining treatment

withdrawn because of permanent loss of the important cortical layers of the brain. Letter to Joanne Lynn, Dec. 14, 1981.

16. The longest case of coma on record is that of Elaine Esposito, who never recovered consciousness after receiving general anesthesia for surgery on August 6, 1941. She died 37 years and 111 days later. Norris McWhirter, ed., THE GUINNESS BOOK OF WORLD RECORDS, Bantam Books, New York (1981) at 42. *See also* the description of a woman injured at age 27 who neither regained consciousness nor left the hospital during the remaining 18 years of her life. Robert E. Field and Raymond J. Romanus, *A Decerebrate Patient: Eighteen Years of Care,* 151 ILL. MED. J. 121 (1977).

17. Letter from Dr. Fred Plum, Neurologist-in-Chief, New York Hospital-Cornell Medical Center, New York, Dec. 22, 1981, *reprinted in* Appendix G, pp. 459–60 *infra. See also, Predicting Outcome After Severe Brain Damage* (Editorial), 1 LANCET 523 (1973); Eichner v. Dillon, 426 N.Y.S.2d 517, 527–529, *modified in, In re* Storar, 420 N.E.2d 64 (1981).

18. Bryan Jennett and Fred Plum, *The Persistent Vegetative State: A Syndrome in Search of a Name,* 1 LANCET 734 (1972); K. Higashi *et al., Epidemiological Studies on Patients with a Persistent Vegetative State,* 40 J. NEUROL., NEUROSURG. & PSYCHIATRY 876 (1977); Plum and Posner, *supra* note 11, at 338–40.

19. Testimony of Dr. Lawrence Pitts, transcript of 12th meeting of the President's Commission (Sept. 12, 1981) at 348-64; Bryan Jennett *et al., Severe Head Injuries in Three Countries,* 40 J. NEUROL., NEUROSURG., & PSYCHIATRY 291 (1977).

20. Bryan Jennett *et al., Prognosis of Patients with Severe Head Injury,* 4 NEUROSURGERY 283 (1979); Thomas W. Langfitt, *Measuring the Outcome from Head Inju-*

ries, 48 J. NEUROSURG. 673 (1978); DE-FINING DEATH, *supra* note 4, at 89–107.

21. *See* David Bates *et al., A Prospective Study of Nontraumatic Coma: Methods and Results in 310 Patients,* 2 ANNALS NEUROL. 211 (1977); David E. Levy *et al., Prognosis in Nontraumatic Coma,* 94 ANNALS INT. MED. 293 (1981); Higashi, *supra* note 18; DEFINING DEATH, *supra* note 4, at 92–95.

22. In one case, cognitive abilities became normal, although the patient suffered from emotional instability and paralysis of three limbs and remained completely dependent upon others for the rest of his life. Gary A. Rosenberg, Stephen F. Johnson, and Richard P. Brenner, *Recovery of Cognition after Prolonged Vegetative State,* 2 ANN. NEUROL. 167 (August 1977). The other case has recovered only to a locked-in status, with all communication by eyeblink. Lewis Cope, *Doctors Think Mack "in vegetative state,"* MINNEAPOLIS TRIBUNE, March 20, 1980, at A-1; David Peterson, *Shooting Case Turns into Vigil,* MINNEAPOLIS TRIBUNE, March 7, 1980, at A-1; telephone interviews with Ronald Cranford, M.D., consultant neurologist on this case, Hennepin County Hospital, Minneapolis, Minn., March 8, 1982, and Dec. 2, 1982.

23. *Outcome of Non-Traumatic Coma* (Editorial), 2 LANCET 507 (1981); J.A. Bell and H.J.F. Hodgson, *Coma after Cardiac Arrest,* 97 BRAIN 361 (1974); Fred Plum and John J. Caronna, *Can One Predict Outcome of Medical Coma?, Outcome of Severe Damage to the Central Nervous System,* CIBA Foundation Symposium #34, Elsevier-North Holland, Amsterdam, (1975) at 121; Bruce D. Snyder, Manuel Ramirez-Lassepas, and D.M. Lippert, *Neurologic Status and Prognosis after Cardiopulmonary Arrest: I. A Retrospective Study,* 27 NEUROLOGY 807

(1977); Bruce D. Snyder, *et al., Neurologic Prognosis after Cardiopulmonary Arrest: II. Level of Consciousness,* 30 NEUROLOGY 52 (1980). Jorgensen and Malchow-Moller contend that recovery of consciousness before death can be reliably predicted from careful attention to the time course of EEG and brain stem reflex activity in the first 10 to 36 hours. E.O. Jorgensen and A. Malchow-Moller, *Natural History of Global and Critical Brain Ischaemia: Part III: Cerebral Prognostic Signs After Cardiopulmonary Resuscitation. Cerebral Recovery Course and Rate during the First Year after Global and Critical Ischaemia Monitored and Predicted by EEG and Neurological Signs,* 9 RESUSCITATION 175 (1981). Snyder *et al.* state that "Reliable predictions of survival and outcome can often be based up on LOC [level of consciousness] within 2 days after CPA [cardiopulmonary arrest]." Bruce D. Snyder *et al., Neurologic Prognosis after Cardiopulmonary Arrest: II. Level of Consciousness,* 30 NEUROLOGY 52 (1980). Evoked potentials may add to the reliability of these early prognostications. Richard Paul Greenberg and Donald Paul Becker, *Clinical Applications and Results of Evoked Potential Data in Patients with Severe Head Injury,* 26 SURG. FORUM 484 (1975).

24. This caution might be especially appropriate in children. *See, e.g.,* "The brains of infants and young children have increased resistance to damage and may recover substantial functions even after exhibiting unresponsiveness on neurological examination for longer periods compared with adults." Medical Consultants on the Diagnosis of Death to the President's Commission for the Study of Ethical Problems in Medicine and Biomedical and Behavioral Research, *Guidelines*

for the Determination of Death, 246 J.A.M.A. 2184, 2186 (1981).

25. *See, e.g.,* Snyder, Ramirez-Lassepas, and Lippert, *supra* note 22; Bell and Hodgson, *supra* note 22; DEFINING DEATH, *supra* note 4, at 92–95.

26. *See* Gayle C. Windham and Larry D. Edmonds, *Current Trends in the Incidence of Neural Tube Defects,* 70 PEDIATRICS 333 (1982); Lewis B. Holmes, *The Health Problem: Neural Tube Defects,* in National Center for Health Care Technology, MATERNAL SERUM ALPHA-FETOPROTEIN: ISSUES IN PRENATAL SCREENING AND DIAGNOSIS OF NEURAL TUBE DEFECTS, U.S. Government Printing Office, Washington (1980). The annual number of live births used to calculate incidence is from U.S. Department of Health and Human Services, *Health United States 1981,* U.S. Government Printing Office, Washington (1981).

27. One recent court case points out the conceptual and practical conundrums that arise in defining the interests of a person devoid of all mental life or conscious experience. The suit was brought on behalf of such a plaintiff, seeking damages for loss of enjoyment of life as a result of loss of customary activities. One of the questions for the court was whether it must be shown that the plaintiff is conscious of the fact that he has lost any enjoyment of life. The court answered that, under the disability law, conscious awareness of injuries need not be shown. Flannery v. U.S., 51 U.S.L.W 2293, 2293 (W. Va. Sup. Ct., 1982).

However, other legal questions are even more vexing:

Someone who has died cannot be said to have "rights" in the usual sense; although a person may have a right to determine how her body is dealt with after death, even that is a troublesome concept. . . . To be sure, Karen Quinlan was not "dead" in most of the increasingly multiple senses of that term, but the task of giving content to the notion that she had rights, in the face of the recognition that she could make no decisions about how to exercise any such rights, remains a difficult one.

Laurence H. Tribe, AMERICAN CONSTITUTIONAL LAW, Foundation Press, Mineola, N.Y. (1978) at 936, n 11.

28. There is a small, finite chance that she [Karen Quinlan] could recover, so keeping her alive for that reason might be a benefit to her, for it at least leaves open the possibility of recovery. This is not to say that Karen Quinlan has a very great chance of recovery, but even a small possibility suggests that it may be in her interests to continue to be alive.

John A. Robertson, *The Courts and Non-treatment Criteria,* in Cynthia B. Wong and Judith P. Swazey, eds., DILEMMAS OF DYING: POLICIES AND PROCEDURES FOR DECISIONS NOT TO TREAT, G.K. Hall Med. Pub., Boston (1981) at 105.

29. *See* note 22 *supra. See also* Martin Lasden, *Coming Out of Coma,* N.Y. TIMES, June 27, 1982 (Magazine) at 29.

30. Testimony of Earl Appleby, transcript of 25th meeting of the President's Commission (Oct. 9, 1982) at 383–85.

31. When, some six weeks after the New Jersey Supreme Court opinion authorizing the discontinuance of the respirator for Karen Quinlan, the family asked her attending physician, Dr. Robert J. Morse, why the respirator care was still being continued, Dr. Morse explained, "I have tried to explain to you, I am following

medical protocol." When asked how long he would keep her on the respirator if she could not successfully be weaned, Dr. Morse replied, "For as long as it takes. Forever." Quinlan and Quinlan, *supra* note 1, at 287.

Dr. Marshall Brumer, Abe Perlmutter's physician when Perlmutter requested the Florida courts to authorize removal of his life-supporting ventilator, told the Commission: "[The Court-ordered removal of the respirator] was an execution, as the day, location, time, and mode of death were all chosen by the court." When asked how he would have treated a respirator-dependent Karen Quinlan, Dr. Brumer replied, "My opinion of the Karen Ann Quinlan case is that I would support her with whatever technologies are available." Testimony of Dr. Marshall Brumer, transcript of 8th meeting of the President's Commission (April 19, 1981) at 16.

32. The New Jersey Supreme Court recognized this interest, in a case involving a blood transfusion for a 23-year-old Jehovah's Witness who had been rendered incompetent and in need of blood as a result of an accident: "The medical and nursing professions are consecrated to preserving life. That is their professional creed. To them, a failure to use a simple established procedure in the circumstances of this case would be malpractice." John F. Kennedy Memorial Hospital v. Heston, 279 A.2d 670, 673 (1971).

More recently, however the Massachusetts Supreme Judicial Court denied that an independent interest of health professionals exists that would go against what patients want or will find beneficial:

Recognition of the right to refuse necessary treatment in appropriate circumstances is consistent with existing medical mores; such a doctrine does not threaten either the integrity of the medical profession, the proper role of hospitals in caring for such patients or the State's interests in protecting the same. It is not necessary to deny a right of self-determination to a patient in order to recognize the interests of doctors, hospitals, and medical personnel in attendance on the patient. Also, if the doctrines of informed consent and right of privacy have as their foundations the right to bodily integrity and control of one's own fate, then those rights are superior to the institutional considerations.

Superintendent of Belchertown School v. Saikewicz, 370 N.E.2d 417, 426 (1977) (citation and footnote omitted).

33. Two unusual circumstances present additional considerations for the interests of others. First, occasionally a permanently unconscious woman is pregnant. If the pregnancy can be continued to the stage of viability for the infant, the interests of the child and the family would usually provide adequate justification for vigorous life-support and therapy until delivery. *See* WASH. POST, March 2, 1982, at A-2, noting the case of a 23-year-old Oregon woman who gave birth to a 7 lb. 13 oz. child after being comatose and on life-support systems for four months. *But see* Pettit v. Chester County Hospital, No. 322, August Term 1982 (Court of Common Pleas, Chester County, Pa.); Mark Butler, *Judge Rules Comatose Woman Can Have Abortion*, PHIL. INQUIRER, Aug. 26, 1982, at A-1. *See generally* William P. Dillon et al., *Life Support and Maternal Brain Death During Pregnancy*, 248 J.A.M.A. 1089 (1982).

Second, permanently unconscious patients may be desirable subjects for research. When the research offers prospect of even distant benefit to the subject, it might be approved in the usual way. When the research is not intended to benefit the subject, it would probably be very difficult to secure legally effective consent from a surrogate. *See* President's Commission, PROTECTING HUMAN SUBJECTS, U.S. Government Printing Office, Washington (1981) at 74–76; Task Force on Research on Senile Dementia, Vijaya Melnick, ed., *Guidelines for Research on Senile Dementia of the Alzheimer's Type,* submitted to National Institutes on Aging (Nov. 1982). Since it would be so easy to overuse these patients in research, great caution is probably appropriate before considering any weakening of the protection involved in the requirement for valid consent.

34. At least one court has specifically denied a state interest in preserving such a patient's life: "Such a patient has no health and, in the true sense, no life for the state to protect." Eichner v. Dillon, 426 N.Y.S.2d 517, 543 (1980) *modified in, In re* Storar, 420 N.E.2d 64 (1981).

35. In 1968 Henry Beecher estimated it would cost $25,000 to $30,000 per year for hospital care for each permanently unconscious patient. Henry K. Beecher, *Ethical Problems Created by the Hopelessly Unconscious Patient,* 278 NEW ENG. J. MED. 1425 (1968). While these costs are mitigated by providing care in a skilled nursing facility, inflation must also be taken into account. Even skilled nursing facilities can now cost over $25,000 per year. Telephone survey of Washington, D.C., area nursing homes (Dec. 1982).

Reported cases provide striking cost estimates. A comatose Tennessee woman who was maintained on a respirator

because her death without it might lead to a murder prosecution was costing $1000 per day. David Meyers, *The California Natural Death Act: A Critical Appraisal,* 52 CAL. ST. BAR J. 326 (1977). Four months of care for a comatose child cost about $40,000. *In re* Benjamin Cruse. Nos. J9 14419 and P6 45318 (Los Angeles Superior Ct., Feb. 15, 1979). The first two years of care for an adolescent with persistent vegetative state cost $280,000. Ronald E. Cranford and Harmon L. Smith, *Some Critical Distinctions between Brain Death and Persistent Vegetative State,* 6 ETHICS IN SCI. & MED. 199, 203 (1979). *See also* note 115, Chapter Four *supra.*

36. The disruption of family life, together with the emotional drain on families which elect to care for these patients at home, can be very significant. Moreover, sensational but unverified reports from the lay literature regarding miraculous recovery in patients with irreversible brain damage are often unsettling to the families and a source of false hope and further emotional turmoil.

Cranford and Smith, *supra* note 35, at 206.

37. One case went to court for this reason alone:

The attending physicians testified that in their opinion the proper course of action to follow would be to turn off the respirator and let Benjamin die. They also testified that this was the standard of medical conduct in the community and was in conformity with generally accepted medical practice. They further testified that the reason they refused to do this when the parent asked them to was because of the uncertain state of law. That is, the doctors were afraid of any resulting civil and criminal liability that might follow their actions.

In re Benjamin Cruse. Nos. J914419 and P645318, Slip op. at 5 (Los Angeles County Super. Ct. Feb. 15, 1979).

38.　Joseph and Julia Quinlan have written:

We understand that conceivably *all* treatment of Karen Ann is extraordinary. That means the antibiotics and the food and the respirator. However, we personally have moral problems with our conscience, with regard to the food and the antibiotics. We have problems with it now, and we realize we would have more problems with it ten years from now.

Quinlan and Quinlan, *supra* note 1, at 282 (emphasis in original).

Others have, however, recognized that distinguishing feeding as more obligatory to provide for these patients is psychologically rather than ethically based. Donald G. McCarthy, *Care of Persons in the Final Stage of Terminal Illness or Irreversibly Comatose,* in Donald G. McCarthy and Albert S. Moraczewski, eds., in MORAL RESPONSIBILITY IN PROLONGING LIFE DECISIONS, Pope John Center, St. Louis, Mo. (1981) at 196.

39.　Formalization and standardization of action for patients in prolonged noncognitive states would invade the area of personal belief in a way that would harm freedom of choice. While the patient can no longer express a choice, families and physicians can. If well-documented statements from the patient, either verbal or in the form of a so-called living will, are available, the position so stated can be taken into consideration. My belief is that the end result of such reasoning together will, in most instances, provide an acceptable solution to a tragic problem.

Stuart A. Schneck, *Brain Death and Prolonged States of Impaired Responsiveness,* 58 DENVER L.J. 609, 621–22 (1981).

Living wills, whether or not drafted under natural death acts, (*see* pp. 139–45 *supra*) are unlikely to apply to this situation. The permanently unconscious patient is probably not terminally ill within the meaning of the statutes, and the measures at issue are not highly intrusive and artificial, both of which are common requirements of living wills. *But see* N.C. Gen. Stat. §90-322 (Cum. Supp. 1979) Appendix D, pp. 357–62 *infra*. It may be instructive, however, that many people feel that there is a large and growing consensus that life as a permanently unconscious patient is more horrible than death. *See* Eichner v. Dillon, 426 N.Y.S. 2d 517, *modified in, In re* Storar, 420 N.E. 2d 64 (1981).

40.　In *Eichner,* the New York State Superior Court and Court of Appeals relied on Brother Fox's statements in discussions of morals and high school teaching that he would not want to be kept alive in Karen Quinlan's situation. *See In re* Storar, 420 N.E.2d 64, 71 ff. (1981).

41.　In one District of Columbia case, the court specifically declined to require formal guardianship or petition to the court. Parker v. U.S., 406 A2d 1275, 1282 (D.C. Ct. App., 1979).

42.　"You see, if the Quinlans had changed the doctor before they brought this case to court, it might never have come to court." Koichi Bai, *Around the Quinlan*

Case-Interview with Judge R. Muir, 1, INT'L. J. MED. 45, 55 (Summer 1979).

43. *See* pp. 161–65 *supra*.

44. It may be best to require, where any doubt or disagreement of any kind or degree exists on the part of the physician or the family as to the appropriate course of action, recourse to the courts for conservatorship powers. . . . Where no such doubt or disagreement exists between family or physician and where the hopeless diagnosis has been confirmed by an independent consultant after all clinical trials have failed, it would seem unnecessary to involve the courts in any way in decisions to terminate any or all life-support systems.

Meyers, *supra* note 41, at 171–72.

45. Unfortunately, the court went beyond appointment of the guardian and seemed occasionally to step into the role of guardian itself, giving an opinion on what Karen Ann Quinlan would want were she capable of expressing herself. The court clearly recognized that Karen Quinlan's situation differed from other cases where courts have been asked to rule on the propriety of medical treatments. The court's decision in large measure turned on to the nature of the patient's condition, the degree of invasiveness of the medical care, and the minimal hope for recovery.

The nature of Karen's care and the realistic chances of her recovery are quite unlike those of the patients discussed in many of the cases where treatments were ordered. In many of those cases the medical procedure required (usually a transfusion) constituted a minimal bodily invasion and the chances of recov-

ery and return to functioning life were very good. We think that the State's interests *contra* weakens and the individual's right to privacy grows as the degree of bodily invasion increases and the prognosis dims.

In re Quinlan, 70 N.J. 10, A.2d 647, 664, *cert. denied* 429 U.S. 922 (1976).

The court was careful to note that in the future such decisions must continue to be made on the basis of reliable prognoses to ensure that there is no reasonable possibility of return to a cognitive, sapient state. For this reason it assigned the task of confirming the prognosis to an "ethics committee." *Id.* at 67. *See, New Jersey Guidelines for Health Care Facilities to Implement Procedures Concerning the Care of Comatose Non-Cognitive Patients, reprinted in* Appendix G, pp. 463–66 *infra*.

46. *See* note 3, *supra*. In one Ohio case, the court specified certain requirements to assure the diagnosis and to notify the county coroner and prosecutor. Leach v. Akron General Medical Center, 426 N.E.2d 809 (Ohio Com. Pl. 1980).

In the case of Mary Severns, the Delaware Supreme Court, after hearing evidence that Mrs. Severns, now permanently unconscious, would not have wanted to have treatment continued and that her husband and family were in accord, ruled that treatment could be foregone. Yet the court reserved a final decision until after an evidentiary hearing before a chancery court to confirm the medical facts (which had only been presented as stipulations from unnamed physicians). Severns v. Wilmington Medical Center, Inc., 421 A. 2d 1334, 1349–50 (Del. 1980). The resulting chancery court order was quite broad, explicitly extending to authorizing refusal of resuscitation, feeding tubes, and antibiotics. *In re* Severns, No. C.M. 3722 (Ct. of Ch., New Castle County, Del., Dec. 31, 1980).

In the Brother Fox case the intermediate court ruling would have required confirmation of the prognosis of terminal illness and "irreversible, permanent or chronic vegetative coma," with "extremely remote" prospects of recovery by the majority vote of a three-member committee. This would be followed by court review, including appointment of a guardian *ad litem* and notification of the Attorney General and appropriate District Attorney. Eichner v. Dillon, 426 N.Y.S. 2d 527, 550 (1980). The court of appeals overruled the procedural aspects of the case, holding that court review is optional: "[A] mandatory procedure of successive approval by physicians, hospital personnel, relatives and the courts . . . should come from the Legislature." *In re* Storar, 420 N.E.2d 64, 74 (1981).

47. *But see, In re* Storar, 420 N.E.2d 64 (1981).

48. Parker v. U.S., 406 A.2d 1275 (D.C. Ct. App., 1979).

27

Quality of Life in the Courts: Earle Spring in Fantasyland

George J. Annas

The term "quality of life," like "right to life," means many things to many people. It can conjure up notions of genocide or of a "good death"; it can be favorably compared with "quantity" of life, and unfavorably contrasted to protecting the equality of life. Perhaps the term is, like euthanasia, so misused and misunderstood that it should simply be banned from our lexicon. But no matter how one comes out on this question, the issues of normalcy, social worth, and resource allocation are, overtly and covertly, playing an increasing role in court decisions regarding the care and treatment of various categories of patients. The latest, in a series that includes *Saikewicz, Quinlan, Becker,* and *Fox,* is the case of Earle Spring, a senile patient suffering from chronic kidney failure in a nursing home (*In the Matter of Earle Spring,* 405 N.E. 2d 115 Mass. 1980).

The case provides an opportunity to explore how, though courts heroically attempt to avoid using the term, they inevitably have to deal with issues it represents. And it is suggested that their reluctance to speak to such issues directly leads them, at times, to give untenable rationales for some of their decisions. This "journey to fantasyland" may be necessary for courts because their decisions are precedents for other people similarly situated, and they therefore do not have the luxury of making a decision that applies to only one person.

At the time his wife and son sought court approval for removal of Mr. Spring from kidney dialysis, he was seventy-eight years old. After hearing their testimony and that of the kidney specialist, the Probate Court agreed that treatment could be discontinued. Complicated appeals followed for almost a year,

"Quality of Life in the Courts: Earle Spring in Fantasyland" by George J. Annas. Reprinted with permission of George J. Annas and The Hastings Center Report 10(August, 1980): 9–10.

and a final opinion by the Massachusetts Supreme Judicial Court was not issued until May 13, 1980, about a month after Mr. Spring died.

The Court's Opinion

The court's opinion came as a major disappointment to many hospital administrators and their advisors who had hoped for a blueprint describing in detail when they did and did not have to seek court immunity. Instead the court restated its position in *Saikewicz,* although in much clearer language: "Our opinions should not be taken to establish any requirement of prior judicial approval that would not otherwise exist."

The court also added overly generous language on criminal liability which should reassure Massachusetts doctors:

Little need be said about criminal liability: there is precious little precedent, and what there is suggests that the doctor will be protected if he acts on a *good faith judgment* that is *not grievously unreasonable by medical standards* (emphasis supplied).

Since these seem to have been the two issues that most upset and concerned the medical profession, clarification of these points must be viewed as a significant, positive development.

But the most disturbing aspect of the case is the court's loose language on the enormous issue of the "quality of life" of nursing home patients. The court found that the conclusion that Mr. Spring "would, if competent, choose not to receive the life-prolonging treatment" was "not clearly erroneous."

By so doing, it dismissed any reference to quality of life, simply saying, "The problem of impairment of 'quality of life' associated with Saikewicz's mental retardation has no analogue in the present case." But the case seems to have been decided on quality of life considerations.

Mr. Spring himself, for example, had *never* stated any preferences regarding medical treatment he might require after he became incompetent, and the relevant evidence provided by the family members is virtually nonexistent. Most dealt with the fact that, while competent, Mr. Spring had led a vigorous, active life, which he was no longer able to do. But it is almost always true that activity declines as people age, and this alone does not mean that people want to cease living. The only specific opinion rendered came from his wife, who stated that, based on their long years of marriage, she believed "he wouldn't want to live." No evidence was offered as a basis for this conclusion.

Since on this reading, the decision cannot properly rest on Mr. Spring's own preferences, it must rest on some view (his family's or the court's) of what people like Spring want or "deserve." In this regard, the court also took the view that Mr. Spring's kidney condition was "irreversible and incurable." But this is true of all patients who suffer from chronic kidney failure and are not candidates for transplantation. However, the advent of hemodialysis has made this condition controllable. An analogy can be drawn to diabetes, another irreversible and incurable disease, which is also controllable. If Mr. Spring were senile and a diabetic, should we permit the withholding of insulin merely because of the "irreversible and incurable" nature of this disease? If the answer is no, it seems to follow that a distinction between "lifesaving" and "life-prolonging" is also a meaningless one, since both dialysis and insulin could be viewed as either, depending on the perspective.

The Court's Approach to Senility

Even more telling is the court's approach to senility. The Probate Court's conclusion that Mr. Spring need not be continued on dialysis seems to be based largely on its view that senility is an "incurable, permanent, and irreversible illness," and its conclusion that no treatment could restore Mr. Spring to "a normal, cognitive, integrated, functioning existence." Unfortunately, the Massachusetts Supreme Court adopted this language in describing Mr. Spring when it stated, "The treatment did not cause a remission of the disease or restore him even temporarily to a *normal, cognitive, integrated, functioning* existence, but simply kept him alive."

The same statement, rephrased, reads, "If one is not and cannot be returned to a normal, cognitive, integrated, functioning existence, but can simply be kept alive, it is not required that one be kept alive." It is suggested that such a standard, if one can call it that, is so vague and sweeping as not to have any legal pedigree at all. For example, it encompasses almost all severely mentally retarded persons, and certainly all senile persons in nursing homes. It argues that only life which is "normal" (however that is defined) and involves "integrated functioning" (however that is defined) is worthy of legal protection.

Phrased another way, there are some categories of people who are so abnormal or ill-functioning that the state has no interest in seeing to it that their lives are preserved. This is proba-

bly true, but such a class must surely be carefully, rigidly, and narrowly defined.

Quinlan and Saikewicz

A similar approach, but with a much more narrow definition, was enunciated in the *Quinlan* case. There the court said, without ever once using the phrase "quality of life," that there is a certain class of patients who can be treated differently from others. Specifically, if the guardian, family, physician of a patient, and a hospital ethics committee all agree that there is "no reasonable possibility of returning to a cognitive, sapient state," then life-support measures may be withdrawn with legal immunity. This carefully circumscribed test can be viewed simply as a judicial expansion of a "brain-death" criteria, in the sense that if the patient meets the court-defined criteria, there is no legal requirement to continue treatment. *Quinlan* can thus be viewed as either a "brain death" case or the first full-fledged quality of life decision (in the sense that it defined a category of patients who need not be treated).

Saikewicz specifically declined to define the severely mentally retarded as a class that did not have to be treated with cancer chemotherapy directly. On the other hand, by adopting the "substituted judgment test" for a group of patients (that is, the severely retarded) to whom it can never apply, to protect their autonomy (something they never had), the court actually reached the same conclusion: severely mentally retarded patients never have to be provided with cancer chemotherapy as long as the therapy is painful or distressing.

The court forced itself to use a criterion that cannot be applicable to Saikewicz himself because of its fear of explicitly adopting a quality of life standard, which "demeans the value of the life of one who is mentally retarded." The court described the term "quality of life," which had been used by the lower court judge in *Saikewicz*, as "vague and perhaps ill-chosen" and states "to the extent that this formulation equated the value of life with any measure of the quality of life, we firmly reject it." However, the court *did* accept the concept as applied to an *individual*. Specifically, it could be taken into account by Saikewicz himself (read, by the judges) "as a reference to the continuing state of pain and disorientation precipitated by the chemotherapy treatment."

And, while in *Spring* the same court argued that they are not defining the senile patients who live in our nation's nursing homes as a class who do not deserve expensive medical treatment, in fact this seems to be what is at work behind the scenes. While discounted by the court, the physician involved focused his own testimony on the quality of life issue. He said that he himself decides whether or not to discontinue treatment on the basis of "whether a person is a *real person*, whether the person is happy to be alive, *whether other people around him or her are happy to have him alive*" (emphasis supplied).

The quality of life issue was also explicitly stated by the Appeals Court: "To what extent should aggressive medical treatment be administered to preserve life after life itself, for reasons beyond anyone's control, has become irreversibly burdensome?" The question, of course, is "burdensome to whom?" Certainly Mr. Spring's senile condition was troublesome, and perhaps even burdensome, to his family, physician, and the nursing home personnel. But the issue is, does senility alone make a person's life so burdensome that medical treatment can justifiably be withheld from him? The decision in *Spring* can be read as an indication that the answer to this question may be affirmative.

But perhaps this is the best we can do. Perhaps openly acknowledging that we are willing to treat the retarded or the senile differently from the "normal" patient is so offensive to society's view of the equality of citizens that its explicit acknowledgment is impossible. If this is true, and if we still want to be able to make a decision not to treat a senile or retarded person in the same way as a "normal" person, then we do need "make-believe" reasons that we can feel comfortable with. Substituted judgment seems to be one such invention from fantasyland. Whether our fairy tale experience with it will have a happy ending, however, is far from certain. What seems more certain is that, at least on a macro level, society is likely to enter tomorrowland with much more explicit decision-making regarding resource allocation. In the words of a dissenting Justice in a hypothetical case set in the year 2002:

> The energies of the National Health Agency should be directed toward the young and the middle-aged and toward making life more enjoyable and richer. It should not be directed toward prolonging the agony of death and the miseries of old age . . . we should allocate resources toward medical and health measures that make our lives worth living, rather than those that prolong lives that are not worth living. *Minerva v. National Health Agency*, 40 U.S. 2d 345 (2002) (Euterpe, J., dissenting) reprinted in *American Journal of Law and Medicine* 3:59 (1977).

GUIDELINES

28

"Quality of Life"

The Hastings Center

Whether to consider the "quality of life" of patients when deciding about forgoing life-sustaining treatment is one of the major moral dilemmas of modern medicine. Medicine has developed the capacity to delay death, but the lives thus prolonged may not be worth living to some of these patients. Moreover, in making treatment decisions there is often a question of which choice will produce a better "quality of life" for the patient, but it is often not clear how to answer that question.

Some view the term "quality of life" as a euphemism for the judgment that certain individuals, who are in very poor condition, are valueless to society and ought to be allowed to die. That kind of a judgment would be unethical and we reject it; the ethical justification for sustaining a person's life is not determined by his or her worth to society. In contrast we consider "quality of life" to be an ethically essential concept that focuses on the good of the individual, what kind of life is possible given the person's condition, and whether that condition will allow the individual to have a life that he or she views as worth living. In this second sense, the life of an individual is evaluated not according to its worth to others, but according to its worth to the individual himself or herself. Even a person with a serious illness or extremely disabling condition can find satisfaction in life. There is no single "quality of life" experienced by all people with a certain condition. The satisfactions, joy, burdens, and suffering experienced vary tremendously from one person to the next.

When people with decisionmaking capacity make "quality of life" judgments to determine their own medical treatment preferences, that is generally accepted as ethically sound. In fact, patients and health care professionals make judgments about "quality of life" all the time outside of termination of treatment contexts. A common goal of various kinds of medical treatment (for example, rehabilitative care) is

" 'Quality of Life' " by The Hastings Center Staff in Guidelines on the Termination of Life-Sustaining Treatment and the Care of the Dying, 1987, pp. 133–135. Reprinted with permission of Indiana University Press.

the enhancement of the patient's "quality of life." Indeed, health care professionals should always try to enhance the quality of a patient's life, as evaluated from the patient's perspective. When a surrogate or health care professional makes such a "quality of life" judgment instead of a patient, however, discomfort arises. It is all too easy for surrogates and professionals to project their own attitudes about "quality of life" onto the patient, either in applying the patient's own previously stated preferences and values to the treatment choice or in deciding what a reasonable person in the patient's circumstances would want.

Even if the surrogate and professional avoid this kind of projection, the question remains what relevance does "quality of life" have and what should it mean? Some people believe that we should consider the "quality of life" of persons without decisionmaking capacity even when we know nothing of the patient's treatment preferences and the patient's subjective experience of his or her condition. This risks adopting a "quality of life" standard in the sense of worth to society. Others maintain that "quality of life" judgments should simply not

be made for persons who lack decisionmaking capacity; but a failure to do so may condemn some patients to lives of indignity, pain, or burden that no person with decisionmaking capacity would choose.

The best we can do in these circumstances is to allow individuals to choose for themselves before they become incapacitated, or allow their surrogates in consultation with health care professionals to choose as they would have wanted—as best we can know—after they lose decisionmaking capacity. At the same time, we must scrutinize surrogates' decisions and health care professionals' assessments in order to guard against their projecting their own attitudes about "quality of life" onto the patient.

By allowing patients and their surrogates to make choices that consider "quality of life," we diminish the risk of forcing lives of pain, indignity, or overwhelming burden on those who are helpless. By applying the patient's view of "quality of life" we also avoid denigrating the worth of individual human beings, and instead respect their values and beliefs.

29

Guidelines for Legislation on Life-Sustaining Treatment

National Conference of Catholic Bishops Committee for Pro-Life Activities

Introduction: Moral Principles

Our Judeo-Christian heritage celebrates life as the gift of a loving God, and respects the life of each human being because each is made in the image and likeness of God. As Christians we also celebrate the fact that we are redeemed by Christ and called to share eternal life with Him. From these roots the Roman Catholic tradition has developed a distinctive approach to fostering and sustaining human life. Our tradition not only condemns direct attacks on innocent life, but also promotes a general view of life as a sacred trust over which we can claim stewardship but not absolute dominion. As conscientious stewards we see a duty to preserve life while recognizing certain limits to that duty, as was reiterated most recently in the Vatican *Declaration on Euthanasia*. This and other documents have set forth the follow-

ing moral principles defining a "stewardship of life" ethic:

(1) The Second Vatican Council condemned crimes against life, including "euthanasia or wilful suicide" (Gaudium et Spes 27). Grounded as it is in respect for the dignity and fundamental rights of the human person, this teaching cannot be rejected on grounds of political pluralism or religious freedom.

(2) As human life is the basis and necessary condition for all other human goods, it has a special value and significance; both murder and suicide are violations of human life.

(3) "Euthanasia" is "an action or an omission which of itself or by intention causes death, in order that all suffering may in this way be eliminated" (Declara-

"Guidelines for Legislation on Life-Sustaining Treatment" by the National Conference of Catholic Bishops Committee for Pro-Life Activities, 1984. Reprinted with permission of The National Conference of Catholic Bishops.

tion on Euthanasia). It is an attack on human life which no one has a right to make or request. Although individual guilt may be reduced or absent because of suffering or emotional factors which cloud the conscience, this does not change the objective wrong of the act. It should also be recognized that an apparent plea for death may really be a plea for help and love.

(4) Suffering is a fact of human life, and has special significance for the Christian as an opportunity to share in Christ's redemptive suffering. Nevertheless there is nothing wrong in trying to relieve someone's suffering as long as this does not interfere with other moral and religious duties. For example, it is permissible in the case of terminal illness to use pain-killers which carry the risk of shortening life, so long as the intent is to relieve pain effectively rather than to cause death.

(5) Everyone has the duty to care for his or her own health and to seek necessary medical care from others, but this does not mean that all possible remedies must be used in all circumstances. One is not obliged to use "extraordinary" means— that is, means which offer no reasonable hope of benefit or which involve excessive hardship. Such decisions are complex, and should be made by the patient in consultation with his or her family and physician whenever possible.

Although these principles have grown out of a specific religious tradition, they appeal to a common respect for the dignity of the human person rather than to any specific denominational stance. We offer them without hesitation to the consideration of men and women of good will, and commend them to the attention of legislators and other policy-makers. We see them as especially appropriate to a society which, whatever its moral and political pluralism, was founded on the belief that all human beings are created equal as bearers of the inalienable right to life.

Legislative Guidelines

Today the application of these principles to the legislative debate regarding treatment of the terminally ill is both difficult and necessary. The medical treatment of terminally ill patients, including the withdrawal of extraordinary means, has always been subject to legal constraints. Since 1975, however, an increasing number of court decisions and legislative enactments have interpreted and changed these constraints. Some decisions and enactments have been constructive, but others have not. Technological changes in medicine occur so rapidly that it is difficult to keep pace with them. These changes have had a drastic effect on the physician/patient relationship, and make much more difficult the decision process by which a patient determines treatment with the counsel and support of physician and family.

As problems and confusions surrounding the treatment of terminally ill patients continue to multiply, new legislation dealing with this subject is being enacted in some states and proposed in many others. Yet the law relating to the treatment of terminally ill patients still differs from state to state, and does not always adequately reflect the moral principles which we endorse. The Church therefore feels an obligation to provide its guidance through participation in the current debate.

In light of these considerations, we suggest the following as ways of respecting the moral principles listed above as well as related concerns of the Church, whenever there is a debate on whether existing or proposed legislation adequately addresses this subject. Such legislation should:

(a) Presuppose the fundamental right to life of every human being, including the disabled, the elderly and the terminally ill. In general, phrases which seem to romanticize death, such as "right to die" or "death with dignity," should be avoided.

(b) Recognize that the right to refuse medical treatment is not an independent right, but is a corollary to the patient's right and moral responsibility to request reasonable treatment. The law should demonstrate no preference for protecting *only* the right to *refuse* treatment, particularly when *life-sustaining* treatment is under consideration.

(c) Place the patient's right to determine medical care within the context of other factors which limit the exercise of that right—e.g., the state's interest in protecting innocent third parties, preventing homicide and suicide, and maintaining good ethical standards in the health care profession. Policy statements which define the right to refuse treatment in terms of the patient's constitutional rights (e.g., a "right of privacy") tend to inhibit the careful balancing of all the interests that should be considered in such cases.

(d) Promote communication among patient, family and physician. Current "living will" laws tend to have the opposite effect—that of excluding family members and other loved ones from the decision-making process. As a general rule, documents and legal proceedings are no substitute for a physician's personal consultation with the patient and/or family at the time a decision must be made on a particular course of treatment.

(e) Avoid granting unlimited power to a document or proxy decision-maker to make health-care decisions on a patient's behalf. The right to make such decisions on one's own behalf is itself not absolute, and in any event cannot be fully exercised when a patient has had no opportunity to assess the burdens and benefits of treatment in a specific situation. Laws which allow a decision to be made on behalf of a mentally incompetent patient must include safeguards, to insure that the decision adequately represents the patient's wishes or best interests and is in accord with responsible medical practice.

(f) Clarify the rights and responsibilities of physicians without granting blanket immunity from all legal liability. No physician should be protected from liability for acting homicidally or negligently. Nor should new legal penalties be imposed on a physician for failing to obey a patient's or proxy's wishes when such obedience would violate the physician's ethical convictions or professional standards.

(g) Reaffirm public policies against homicide and assisted suicide. Medical treatment legislation may clarify procedures for discontinuing treatment which only secures a precarious and burdensome prolongation of life for the terminally ill patient, but should not condone or authorize any deliberate act or omission designed to cause a patient's death.

(h) Recognize the presumption that certain basic measures such as nursing care, hydration, nourishment, and the like must be maintained out of respect for the human dignity of every patient.

(i) Protect the interests of innocent parties who are not competent to make treatment decisions on their own behalf. Life-sustaining treatment should not be discriminatorily withheld or withdrawn from mentally incompetent or retarded patients.

(j) Provide that life-sustaining treatment should not be withdrawn from a pregnant woman if continued treatment may benefit her unborn child.

These guidelines are not intended to provide an exhaustive description of good legislation, or to endorse the viewpoint that every state requires new legislation on treatment of the terminally ill. They outline a general approach which, we believe, will help clarify rights and responsibilities with regard to such treatment without sacrificing a firm commitment to the sacredness of human life.

Approved for publication by the
NCCB Administrative Committee
November 10, 1984

30

Child Abuse and Neglect: Prevention and Treatment

Department of Health and Human Services

§1340.15 Services and treatment for disabled infants.

(a) *Purpose.* The regulations in this section implement certain provisions of the Child Abuse Amendments of 1984 including section 4(b)(2)(K) of the Child Abuse Prevention and Treatment Act governing the protection and care of disabled infants with life-threatening conditions.

(b) *Definitions.* (1) The term "medical neglect" means the failure to provide adequate medical care in the context of the definitions of "child abuse and neglect" in section 3 of the Act and §1340.2(d) of this part. The term "medical neglect" includes, but is not limited to, the withholding of medically indicated treatment from a disabled infant with a life-threatening condition.

(2) The term "withholding of medically indicated treatment" means the failure to respond to the infant's life-threatening conditions by providing treatment (including appropriate nutrition, hydration, and medication) which, in the treating physician's (or physicians') reasonable medical judgment, will be most likely to be effective in ameliorating or correcting all such conditions, except that the term does not include the failure to provide treatment (other than appropriate nutrition, hydration, or medication) to an infant when, in the treating physician's (or physicians') reasonable medical judgment any of the following circumstances apply:

(i) The infant is chronically and irreversibly comatose:

(ii) The provision of such treatment would merely prolong dying, not be effective in ameliorating or correcting all of the infant's life-threatening conditions, or otherwise be futile in terms of the survival of the infant; or

(iii) The provision of such treatment would

"Child Abuse and Neglect: Prevention and Treatment" by the Department of Health and Human Services. Reprinted from The Federal Register 50 (April 15, 1985), No. 72: Rules and Regulations, part 1340, pp. 14887–14892.

be virtually futile in terms of the survival of the infant and the treatment itself under such circumstances would be inhumane.

(3) Following are definitions of terms used in paragraph (b)(2) of this section:

(i) The term "infant" means an infant less than one year of age. The reference to less than one year of age shall not be construed to imply that treatment should be changed or discontinued when an infant reaches one year of age, or to affect or limit any existing protections available under State laws regarding medical neglect of children over one year of age. In addition to their applicability to infants less than one year of age, the standards set forth in paragraph (b)(2) of this section should be consulted thoroughly in the evaluation of any issue of medical neglect involving an infant older than one year of age who has been continuously hospitalized since birth, who was born extremely prematurely, or who has a long-term disability.

(ii) The term "reasonable medical judgment" means a medical judgment that would be made by a reasonably prudent physician, knowledgeable about the case and the treatment possibilities with respect to the medical conditions involved. . . .

Appendix to Part 1340—Interpretative Guidelines Regarding 45 CFR 1340.15 —Services and Treatment for Disabled Infants

This appendix sets forth the Department's interpretative guidelines regarding several terms that appear in the definition of the term "withholding of medically indicated treatment" in section 3(3) of the Child Abuse Prevention and Treatment Act, as amended by section 121(3) of the Child Abuse Amendments of 1984. This statutory definition is repeated in §1340.15(b)(2) of the final rule.

The Department's proposed rule to implement those provisions of the Child Abuse Amendments of 1984 relating to services and treatment for disabled infants included a number of proposed clarifying definitions of several terms used in the statutory definition. The preamble to the proposed rule explained these proposed clarifying definitions, and in some cases used examples of specific diagnoses to elaborate on meaning.

During the comment period on the proposed rule, many commentors urged deletion of these clarifying definitions and avoidance of examples of specific diagnoses. Many commentors also objected to the specific wording of some of the proposed clarifying definitions, particularly in connection with the proposed use of the word "imminent" to describe the proximity in time at which death is anticipated regardless of treatment in relation to circumstances under which treatment (other than appropriate nutrition, hydration and medication) need not be provided. A letter from the six principal sponsors of the "compromise amendment" which became the pertinent provisions of the Child Abuse Amendments of 1984 urged deletion of "imminent" and careful consideration of the other concerns expressed.

After consideration of these recommendations, the Department decided not to adopt these several proposed clarifying definitions as part of the final rule. It was also decided that effective implementation of the program established by the Child Abuse Amendments would be advanced by the Department stating its interpretations of several key terms in the statutory definition. This is the purpose of this appendix.

The interpretative guidelines that follow have carefully considered comments submitted during the comment period on the proposed rule. These guidelines are set forth and explained without the use of specific diagnostic examples to elaborate on meaning.

Finally, by way of introduction, the Department does not seek to establish these interpretative guidelines as binding rules of law, nor to prejudge the exercise of reasonable medical judgment in responding to specific circumstances. Rather, this guidance is intended to assist in interpreting the statutory definition so that it may be rationally and thoughtfully applied in specific contexts in a manner fully consistent with the legislative intent.

1. *In general: the statutory definition of "withholding of medically indicated treatment."*

Section 1340.15(b)(2) of the final rule defines the term "withholding of medically indicated treatment" with a definition identical to that which appears in section 3(3) of the Act (as amended by section 121(3) of the Child Abuse Amendments of 1984).

This definition has several main features. First, it establishes the basic principle that all disabled infants with life-threatening conditions must be given medically indicated treatment, defined in terms of action to respond to the infant's life-threatening conditions by providing treatment (including appropriate nutrition, hydration or medication) which, in the treating physician's (or physicians') reasonable medical judgment, will be most likely to be effective in ameliorating or correcting all such conditions.

Second, the statutory definition spells out three circumstances under which treatment is not considered "medically indicated." These are when, in the treating physician's (or physicians') reasonable medical judgment:

—The infant is chronically and irreversibly comatose:
—The provision of such treatment would merely prolong dying, not be effective in ameliorating or correcting all of the infant's life-threatening conditions, or otherwise be futile in terms of survival of the infant; or
—The provision of such treatment would be virtually futile in terms of survival of the infant and the treatment itself under such circumstances would be inhumane.

The third key feature of the statutory definition is that even when one of these three circumstances is present, and thus the failure to provide treatment is not a "withholding of medically indicated treatment," the infant must nonetheless be provided with appropriate nutrition, hydration, and medication.

Fourth, the definition's focus on the potential effectiveness of treatment in ameliorating or correcting life-threatening conditions makes clear that it does not sanction decisions based on subjective opinions about the future "quality of life" of a retarded or disabled person.

The fifth main feature of the statutory definition is that its operation turns substantially on the "reasonable medical judgment" of the treating physician or physicians. The term "reasonable medical judgment" is defined in §1340.15(b)(3)(ii) of the final rule, as it was in the Conference Committee Report on the Act, as a medical judgment that would be made by a reasonably prudent physician, knowledgeable about the case and the treatment possibilities with respect to the medical conditions involved.

The Department's interpretations of key terms in the statutory definition are fully consistent with these basic principles reflected in the definition. The discussion that follows is organized under headings that generally correspond to the proposed clarifying definitions that appeared in the proposed rule but were not adopted in the final rule. The discussion also attempts to analyze and respond to significant comments received by the Department.

2. *The term "life-threatening condition."*

Clause (b)(3)(ii) of the proposed rule proposed a definition of the term "life-threatening condition." This term is used in the statutory definition in the following context:

[T]he term "withholding of medically indicated treatment" means the failure to respond to the infant's *life-threatening conditions* by providing treatment (including appropriate nutrition, hydration, and medication) which, in the treating physician's or physicians' reasonable medical judgment, will be most likely to be effective in ameliorating or correcting all such conditions [, except that]***[Emphasis supplied].

It appears to the Department that the applicability of the statutory definition might be uncertain to some people in cases where a condition may not, strictly speaking, by itself be life-threatening, but where the condition significantly increases the risk of the onset of complications that may threaten the life of the infant. If medically indicated treatment is available for such a condition, the failure to provide it may result in the onset of complications that, by the time the condition becomes life-threatening in the strictest sense, will eliminate or reduce the potential effectiveness of any treatment. Such a result cannot, in the Department's view, be squared with the Congressional intent.

Thus, the Department interprets the term "life-threatening condition" to include a condition that, in the treating physician's or physicians' reasonable medical judgment, signifi-

cantly increases the risk of the onset of complications that may threaten the life of the infant.

In response to comments that the proposed rule's definition was potentially overinclusive by covering any condition that one could argue "may" become life-threatening, the Department notes that the statutory standard of "the treating physician's or physicians' reasonable medical judgment" is incorporated in the Department's interpretation, and is fully applicable.

Other commentors suggested that this interpretation would bring under the scope of the definition many irreversible conditions for which no corrective treatment is available. This is certainly not the intent. The Department's interpretation implies nothing about whether, or what, treatment should be provided. It simply makes clear that the criteria set forth in the statutory definition for evaluating whether, or what, treatment should be provided are applicable. That is just the start, not the end, of the analysis. The analysis then takes fully into account the reasonable medical judgment regarding potential effectiveness of possible treatments, and the like.

Other comments were that it is unnecessary to state any interpretation because reasonable medical judgment commonly deems the conditions described as life-threatening and responds accordingly. HHS agrees that this is common practice followed under reasonable medical judgment, just as all the standards incorporated in the statutory definition reflect common practice followed under reasonable medical judgment. For the reasons stated above, however, the Department believes it is useful to say so in these interpretative guidelines.

3. *The term "treatment" in the context of adequate evaluation.*

Clause (b)(3)(ii) of the proposed rule proposed a definition of the term "treatment." Two separate concepts were dealt with in clause (A) and (B), respectively, of the proposed rule. Both of these clauses were designed to ensure that the Congressional intent regarding the issues to be considered under the analysis set forth in the statutory definition is fully effectuated. Like the guidance regarding "life-threatening condition" discussed above, the Department's interpretations go to the applicability of the statutory analysis, not its result.

The Department believes that Congress intended that the standard of following reasonable medical judgment regarding the potential effectiveness of possible courses of action should apply to issues regarding adequate medical evaluation, just as it does to issues regarding adequate medical intervention. This is apparent Congressional intent because Congress adopted, in the Conference Report's definition of "reasonable medical judgment," the standard of adequate knowledge about the case and the treatment possibilities with respect to the medical condition involved.

Having adequate knowledge about the case and the treatment possibilities involved is, in effect, step one of the process, because that is the basis on which "reasonable medical judgment" will operate to make recommendations regarding medical intervention. Thus, part of the process to determine what treatment, if any, "will be most likely to be effective in ameliorating or correcting" all life-threatening conditions is for the treating physician or physicians to make sure they have adequate information about the condition and adequate knowledge about treatment possibilities with respect to the condition involved. The standard for determining the adequacy of the information and knowledge is the same as the basic standard of the statutory definition: reasonable medical judgment. A reasonably prudent physician faced with a particular condition about which he or she needs additional information and knowledge of treatment possibilities would take steps to gain more information and knowledge by, quite simply, seeking further evaluation by, or consultation with, a physician or physicians whose expertise is appropriate to the condition(s) involved or further evaluation at a facility with specialized capabilities regarding the condition(s) involved.

Thus, the Department interprets the term "treatment" to include (but not be limited to) any further evaluation by, or consultation with, a physician or physicians whose expertise is appropriate to the condition(s) involved or further evaluation at a facility with specialized capabilities regarding the condition(s) involved that, in the treating physician's or physicians' reasonable medical judgment, is needed to assure that decisions regarding medical intervention are based on adequate knowledge about the case and the treatment possibilities with respect to the medical conditions involved.

This reflects the Department's interpretation that failure to respond to an infant's life-threatening conditions by obtaining any further evaluations or consultations that, in the treating physician's reasonable medical judgment, are necessary to assure that decisions regarding medical intervention are based on adequate knowledge about the case and the treatment possibilities involved constitutes a "withholding of medically indicated treatment." Thus, if parents refuse to consent to such a recommendation that is based on the treating physician's reasonable medical judgment that, for example, further evaluation by a specialist is necessary to permit reasonable medical judgments to be made regarding medical intervention, this would be a matter for appropriate action by the child protective services system.

In response to comments regarding the related provision in the proposed rule, this interpretative guideline makes quite clear that this interpretation does not deviate from the basic principle of reliance on reasonable medical judgment to determine the extent of the evaluations necessary in the particular case. Commentors expressed concerns that the provision in the proposed rule would intimidate physicians to seek transfer of seriously ill infants to tertiary level facilities much more often than necessary, potentially resulting in diversion of the limited capacities of these facilities away from those with real needs for the specialized care, unnecessary separation of infants from their parents when equally beneficial treatment could have been provided at the community or regional hospital, inappropriate deferral of therapy while time-consuming arrangements can be effected, and other counterproductive ramifications. The Department intended no intimidation, prescription or similar influence on reasonable medical judgment, but rather, intended only to affirm that it is the Department's interpretation that the reasonable medical judgment standard applies to issues of medical evaluation, as well as issues of medical intervention.

4. *The term "treatment" in the context of multiple treatments.*

Clause (b)(3)(iii)(B) of the proposed rule was designed to clarify that, in evaluating the potential effectiveness of a particular medical treatment or surgical procedure that can only be reasonably evaluated in the context of a complete potential treatment plan, the "treatment" to be evaluated under the standards of the statutory definition includes the multiple medical treatments and/or surgical procedures over a period of time that are designed to ameliorate or correct a life-threatening condition or conditions. Some commentors stated that it could be construed to require the carrying out of a long process of medical treatments or surgical procedures regardless of the lack of success of those done first. No such meaning is intended.

The intent is simply to characterize that which must be evaluated under the standards of the statutory definition, not to imply anything about the results of the evaluation. If parents refuse consent for a particular medical treatment or surgical procedure that by itself may not correct or ameliorate all life-threatening conditions, but is recommended as part of a total plan that involves multiple medical treatments and/or surgical procedures over a period of time that, in the treating physician's reasonable medical judgment, will be most likely to be effective in ameliorating or correcting all such conditions, that would be a matter for appropriate action by the child protective services system.

On the other hand, if, in the treating physician's reasonable medical judgment, the total plan will, for example, be virtually futile and inhumane, within the meaning of the statutory term, then there is no "withholding of medically indicated treatment." Similarly, if a treatment plan is commenced on the basis of a reasonable medical judgment that there is a good chance that it will be effective, but due to a lack of success, unfavorable complications, or other factors, it becomes the treating physician's reasonable medical judgment that further treatment in accord with the prospective treatment plan, or alternative treatment, would be futile, then the failure to provide that treatment would not constitute a "withholding of medically indicated treatment."

This analysis does not divert from the reasonable medical judgment standard of the statutory definition; it simply makes clear the Department's interpretation that the failure to evaluate the potential effectiveness of a treatment plan as a whole would be inconsistent with the legislative intent.

Thus, the Department interprets the term "treatment" to include (but not be limited to) multiple medical treatments and/or surgical procedures over a period of time that are designed to ameliorate or correct a life-threatening condition or conditions.

5. The term "merely prolong dying."

Clause (b)(3)(v) of the proposed rule proposed a definition of the term "merely prolong dying," which appears in the statutory definition. The proposed rule's provision stated that this term "refers to situations where death is imminent and treatment will do no more than postpone the act of dying."

Many commentators argued that the incorporation of the word "imminent," and its connotation of immediacy, appeared to deviate from the Congressional intent, as developed in the course of the lengthy legislative negotiations, that reasonable medical judgments can and do result in nontreatment decisions regarding some conditions for which treatment will do no more than temporarily postpone a death that will occur in the near future, but not necessarily within days. The six principal sponsors of the compromise amendment also strongly urged deletion of the word "imminent."

The Department's use of the term "imminent" in the proposed rule was not intended to convey a meaning not fully consonant with the statute. Rather, the Department intended that the word "imminent" would be applied in the context of the condition involved, and in such a context, it would not be understood to specify a particular number of days. As noted in the preamble to the proposed rule, this clarification was proposed to make clear that the "merely prolong dying" clause of the statutory definition would not be applicable to situations where treatment will not totally correct a medical condition but will give a patient many years of life. The Department continues to hold to this view.

To eliminate the type of misunderstanding evidenced in the comments, and to assure consistency with the statutory definition, the word "imminent" is not being adopted for purposes of these interpretative guidelines.

The Department interprets the term "merely prolong dying" as referring to situations where the prognosis is for death and, in the treating physician's (or physicians') reasonable medical judgment, further or alternative treatment would not alter the prognosis in an extension of time that would not render the treatment futile.

Thus, the Department continues to interpret Congressional intent as not permitting the "merely prolong dying" provision to apply where many years of life will result from the provision of treatment, or where the prognosis is not for death in the near future, but rather the more distant future. The Department also wants to make clear it does not intend the connotations many commentors associated with the word "imminent." In addition, contrary to the impression some commentors appeared to have regarding the proposed rule, the Department's interpretation is that reasonable medical judgments will be formed on the basis of knowledge about the condition(s) involved, the degree of inevitability of death, the probable effect of any potential treatments, the projected time period within which death will probably occur, and other pertinent factors.

6. *The term "not be effective in ameliorating or correcting all of the infant's life-threatening conditions" in the context of a future life-threatening condition.*

Clause (b)(3)(vi) of the proposed rule proposed a definition of the term "not be effective in ameliorating or correcting all the infant's life-threatening conditions" used in the statutory definition of "withholding of medically indicated treatment."

The basic point made by the use of this term in the statutory definition was explained in the Conference Committee Report:

Under the definition, if a disabled infant suffers from more than one life-threatening condition and, in the treating physician's or physicians' reasonable medical judgment, there is no effective treatment for one of those conditions, then the infant is not covered by the terms of the amendment (except with respect to appropriate nutrition, hydration, and medication) concerning the withholding of medically indicated treatment. H. Conf. Rep. No. 1038, 98th Cong., 2d Sess. 41 (1980).

This clause of the proposed rule dealt with the application of this concept in two contexts: first, when the nontreatable condition will not become life-threatening in the near future, and second, when humaneness makes palliative treatment medically indicated.

With respect to the context of a future life-threatening condition, it is the Department's interpretation that the term "not be effective in ameliorating or correcting all of the infant's life-threatening conditions" does not permit the withholding of treatment on the grounds that one or more of the infant's life-threatening conditions, although not life-threatening in the near future, will become life-threatening in the more distant future.

This clarification can be restated in the terms of the Conference Committee Report excerpt, quoted just above, with the italicized words indicating the clarification as follows: Under the definition, if a disabled infant suffers from more than one life-threatening condition and, in the treating physician's or physicians' reasonable medical judgment, there is no effective treatment for one of these conditions *that threatens the life of the infant in the near future,* then the infant is not covered by the terms of the amendment (except with respect to appropriate nutrition, hydration, and medication) concerning the withholding of medically indicated treatment; *but if the non-treatable condition will not become life-threatening until the more distant future, the infant is covered by the terms of the amendment.*

Thus, this interpretative guideline is simply a corollary to the Department's interpretation of "merely prolong dying," stated above, and is based on the same understanding of Congressional intent, indicated above, that if a condition will not become life-threatening until the more distant future, it should not be the basis for withholding treatment.

Also for the same reasons explained above, the word "imminent" that appeared in the proposed definition is not adopted for purposes of this interpretative guideline. The Department makes no effort to draw an exact line to separate "near future" from "more distant future." As noted above in connection with the term "merely prolong dying," the statutory definition provides that it is for reasonable medical judgment, applied to the specific condition and circumstances involved, to determine whether the prognosis of death, because of its nearness in time, is such that treatment would not be medically indicated.

7. *The term "not be effective in ameliorating or correcting all life-threatening conditions" in the context of palliative treatment.*

Clause (b)(3)(iv)(B) of the proposed rule proposed to define the term "not be effective in ameliorating or correcting all life-threatening conditions" in the context where the issue is not life-saving treatment, but rather palliative treatment to make a condition more tolerable. An example of this situation is where an infant has more than one life-threatening condition, at least one of which is not treatable and will cause death in the near future. Palliative treatment is available, however, that will, in the treating physician's reasonable medical judgment, relieve severe pain associated with one of the conditions. If it is the treating physician's reasonable medical judgment that this palliative treatment will ameliorate the infant's *overall* condition, taking all individual conditions into account, even though it would not ameliorate or correct *each* condition, then this palliative treatment is medically indicated. Simply put, in the context of ameliorative treatment that will make a condition more tolerable, the term "not be effective in ameliorating or correcting *all* life-threatening conditions" should not be construed as meaning *each and every* condition, but rather as referring to the infant's *overall* condition.

HHS believes Congress did not intend to exclude humane treatment of this kind from the scope of "medically indicated treatment." The Conference Committee Report specifically recognized that "it is appropriate for a physician, in the exercise of reasonable medical judgment, to consider that factor [humaneness] in selecting among effective treatments." H. Conf. Rep. No. 1038, 98th Cong., 2d Sess. 41 (1984). In addition, the articulation in the statutory definition of circumstances in which treatment need not be provided specifically states that "appropriate nutrition, hydration, and medication" must nonetheless be provided. The inclusion in this proviso of medication, one (but not the only) potential palliative

treatment to relieve severe pain, corroborates the Department's interpretation that such palliative treatment that will ameliorate the infant's overall condition, and that in the exercise of reasonable medical judgment is humane and medically indicated, was not intended by Congress to be outside the scope of the statutory definition.

Thus, it is the Department's interpretation that the term "not be effective in ameliorating or correcting all of the infant's life-threatening conditions" does not permit the withholding of ameliorative treatment that, in the treating physician's or physicians' reasonable medical judgment, will make a condition more tolerable, such as providing palliative treatment to relieve severe pain, even if the overall prognosis, taking all conditions into account, is that the infant will not survive.

A number of commentors expressed concerns about some of the examples contained in the preamble of the proposed rule that discussed the proposed definition relating to this point, and stated that, depending on medical complications, exact prognosis, relationships to other conditions, and other factors, the treatment suggested in the examples might not necessarily be the treatment that reasonable medical judgment would decide would be most likely to be effective. In response to these comments, specific diagnostic examples have not been included in this discussion, and this interpretative guideline makes clear that the "reasonable medical judgment" standard applies on this point as well.

Other commentors argued that an interpretative guideline on this point is unnecessary because reasonable medical judgment would commonly provide ameliorative or palliative treatment in the circumstances described. The Department agrees that such treatment is common in the exercise of reasonable medical judgment, but believes it useful, for the reasons stated, to provide this interpretative guidance.

8. *The term "virtually futile."*

Clause (b)(3)(vii) of the proposed rule proposed a definition of the term "virtually futile" contained in the statutory definition. The context of this term in the statutory definition is:

[T]he term "withholding of medically indicated treatment" ∗∗∗ does not include the failure to provide treatment (other than appropriate nutrition, hydration, or medication) to an infant when, in the treating physician's or physicians' reasonable medical judgment, ∗∗∗ the provision of such treatment would be *virtually futile* in terms of the survival of the infant and the treatment itself under such circumstances would be inhumane. Section 3(3)(C) of the Act [emphasis supplied].

The Department interprets the term "virtually futile" to mean that the treatment is highly unlikely to prevent death in the near future.

This interpretation is similar to those offered in connection with "merely prolong dying" and "not be effective in ameliorating or correcting all life-threatening conditions" in the context of a future life-threatening condition, with the addition of a characterization of likelihood that corresponds to the statutory word "virtually." For the reasons explained in the discussion of "merely prolong dying," the word "imminent" that was used in the proposed rule has not been adopted for purposes of this interpretative guideline.

Some commentors expressed concern regarding the words "highly unlikely," on the grounds that such certitude is often medically impossible. Other commentors urged that a distinction should be made between generally utilized treatments and experimental treatments. The Department does not believe any

special clarifications are needed to respond to these comments. The basic standard of reasonable medical judgment applies to the term "virtually futile." The Department's interpretation does not suggest an impossible or unrealistic standard of certitude for any medical judgment. Rather, the standard adopted in the law is that there be a "reasonable medical judgment." Similarly, reasonable medical judgment is the standard for evaluating potential treatment possibilities on the basis of the actual circumstances of the case. HHS does not believe it would be helpful to try to establish distinctions based on characterizations of the degree of general usage, extent of validated efficacy data, or other similar factors. The factors considered in the exercise of reasonable medical judgment, including any factors relating to human subjects experimentation standards, are not disturbed.

9. *The term "the treatment itself under such circumstances would be inhumane."*

Clause (b)(3)(viii) of the proposed rule proposed a definition of the term "the treatment itself under such circumstances would be inhumane," that appears in the statutory definition. The context of this term in the statutory definition is that it is not a "withholding of medically indicated treatment" to withhold treatment (other than appropriate nutrition, hydration, or medication) when, in the treating physician's reasonable medical judgment, "the provision of such treatment would be virtually futile in terms of the survival of the infant and the treatment itself under such circumstances would be inhumane." §3(3)(C) of the Act.

The Department interprets the term "the treatment itself under such circumstances would be inhumane" to mean the treatment itself involves significant medical contraindications and/or significant pain and suffering for the infant that clearly outweigh the very slight potential benefit of the treatment for an infant highly unlikely to survive. (The Department further notes that the use of the term "inhumane" in this context is not intended to suggest that consideration of the humaneness of a particular treatment is not legitimate in any other context; rather, it is recognized that it is appropriate for a physician, in the exercise of reasonable medical judgment, to consider that factor in selecting among effective treatments.)

Other clauses of the statutory definition focus on the expected *result* of the possible treatment. This provision of the statutory definition adds a consideration relating to the *process* of possible treatment. It recognizes that in the exercise of reasonable medical judgment, there are situations where, although there is some slight chance that the treatment will be beneficial to the patient (the potential treatment is considered *virtually* futile, rather than futile), the potential benefit is so outweighed by negative factors relating to the process of the treatment itself that, under the circumstances, it would be inhumane to subject the patient to the treatment.

The Department's interpretation is designed to suggest the factors that should be taken into account in this difficult balance. A number of commentors argued that the interpretation should permit, as part of the evaluation of whether treatment would be inhumane, consideration of the infant's future "quality of life."

The Department strongly believes such an interpretation would be inconsistent with the statute. The statute specifies that the provision applies only where the treatment would be "virtually futile in terms of the survival of the infant," and the "treatment *itself* under such circumstances would be inhumane." (Emphasis supplied.) The balance is clearly to be be-

tween the very slight chance that treatment will allow the infant to survive and the negative factors relating to the process of the treatment. These are the circumstances under which reasonable medical judgment could decide that the treatment itself would be inhumane.

Some commentors expressed concern about the use of terms such as "clearly outweigh" in the description of this balance on the grounds that such precision is impractical. Other commentors argued that this interpretation could be construed to mandate useless and painful treatment. The Department believes there is no basis for these worries because "reasonable medical judgment" is the governing standard. The interpretative guideline suggests nothing other than application of this standard. What the guideline does is set forth the Department's interpretation that the statute directs the reasonable medical judgment to considerations relating to the slight chance of survival and the negative factors regarding the process of treatment and to the balance between them that would support a conclusion that the treatment itself would be inhumane.

Other commentors suggested adoption of a statement contained in the Conference Committee Report that makes clear that the use of the term "inhumane" in the statute was not intended to suggest that consideration of the humaneness of a particular treatment is not legitimate in any other context. The Department has adopted this statement as part of its interpretative guideline.

10. *Other terms.*

Some comments suggested that the Department clarify other terms used in the statutory definition of "withholding of medically-indicated treatment," such as the term "appropriate nutrition, hydration or medication" in the context of treatment that may not be withheld, notwithstanding the existence of one of the circumstances under which the failure to provide treatment is not a "withholding of medically indicated treatment." Some commentors stated, for example, that very potent pharmacologic agents, like other methods of medical intervention, can produce results accurately described as accomplishing no more than to merely prolong dying, or be futile in terms of the survival of the infant, or the like, and that, therefore, the Department should clarify that the proviso regarding "appropriate nutrition, hydration or medication" should not be construed entirely independently of the circumstances under which other treatment need not be provided.

The Department has not adopted an interpretative guideline on this point because it appears none is necessary. As noted above in the discussion of palliative treatment, the Department recognizes that there is no absolutely clear line between medication and treatment other than medication that would justify excluding the latter from the scope of palliative treatment that reasonable medical judgment would find medically indicated, notwithstanding a very poor prognosis.

Similarly, the Department recognizes that in some circumstances, certain pharmacologic agents, not medically indicated for palliative purposes, might, in the exercise of reasonable medical judgment, also not be indicated for the purpose of correcting or ameliorating any particular condition because they will, for example, merely prolong dying. However, the Department believes the word "appropriate" in this proviso of the statutory definition is adequate to permit the exercise of reasonable medical judgment in the scenario referred to by these commentors.

At the same time, it should be clearly recognized that the statute is completely unequivocal in requiring that all infants receive "appropriate nutrition, hydration, and medication," regardless of their condition or prognosis.

Dated: March 29, 1985.
Dorcas R. Hardy,
Assistant Secretary for Human Development Services.

Approved: April 5, 1985.
Margaret M. Heckler,
Secretary.

31

Providing Food and Fluids to Severely Brain Damaged Patients

New Jersey Catholic Conference

This brief is filed on behalf of the amicus curiae New Jersey Catholic Conference (hereinafter "the conference"). The New Jersey Catholic Conference is composed of the Roman Catholic bishops of the Archdiocese of Newark, the Dioceses of Camden, Metuchen, Paterson, Trenton and the Byzantine Catholic Diocese of Passaic. The conference provides a means by which the bishops may speak on matters of public policy.

At issue here is whether a 31-year-old woman, who according to her treating physician is severely brain damaged but not terminally ill, may be denied food and fluids at the request of her spouse. The conference has a keen interest in the case at hand particularly since the disciplines of theology, law and medicine intersect here; hence it hopes that the moral and philosophical insights of Catholic ethical teaching may be helpful to the court as it decides this case. (The conference does not intend to ana-

lyze the decision of the court below in light of prior judicial precedent, believing that more properly to be the function of the parties in this matter.) In addition, the conference has great concern with respect to the effect the decision of this court would have in the 15 hospitals and numerous extended health-care facilities operated under Catholic auspices in this state, because the policies of these institutions are governed by Catholic moral principles. (Our fears have been realized in the ruling in *Matter of Requena,* No. P-326-86E (Ch. Div. Sept. 24, 1986), aff'd.—N.J. *Super.* (App. Div. 1986), which compels a Catholic hospital to violate its moral and ethical principles by allowing a patient to refuse nutrition and hydration. More will be said about this issue *infra.*

The laws society enacts recognize both the need to protect and promote the common good and basic rights of the individual human person resident in or a citizen of the commu-

---

"Providing Food and Fluids to Severely Brain Damaged Patients" by the New Jersey Catholic Conference. Reprinted from Origins 16 *(January 22, 1987):582–584.*

nity governed by the respective legislators. Our case deals with a most fundamental right, that is, the right to life, and the corresponding duty of society to protect that right. The denial of food and fluids, of nutrition and hydration, ultimately results in starvation, dehydration and death. It is direct. It is unnatural, as unnatural as denying one the air needed to breathe, or murder by asphyxiation.

Society and society's laws consider the person who starves himself as suicidal. Society and society's laws should oppose the intervention by other parties which may enable or facilitate suicidal starvation, however willing the victim. See N.J.S.A. 2C:11-3; N.J.S.A. 2C:11-6.

From our Judaeo-Christian heritage, the Catholic Church has developed a distinctive approach to fostering and sustaining human life. Our tradition not only condemns direct attacks on innocent life, but also promotes a general view of life as a sacred trust over which we can claim stewardship but not absolute dominion. A positive duty to preserve life is part of this tradition. Consequently, the conference maintains that nutrition and hydration, which are basic to human life, and as such distinguished from medical treatment, should always be provided to a patient. Withdrawal of nutrition and hydration introduces a new attack upon human life.

This court should carefully avoid any decision which draws its conclusions from an analysis of the "quality of life" of the patient. Moreover, it is equally important that this court not establish guidelines which would allow euthanasia. Society has an obligation not only to protect and promote human life, but also to respect the human life of a person who is seriously ill or dying. Attempts to deal with death within the narrow parameters of a legal

definition generally ignore the far-reaching responsibilities that society has to protect human life and to provide care and compassion for each member of the human family in a manner consistent with human dignity. McHugh (ed.), *Death, Dying and the Law*, at 59 (1976). The court should not overly restrict the judgment of moral and medical decision makers by trying to decide judicially what may be perceived as acceptable public policy.

Although our moral principles have grown out of a specific religious tradition, they appeal to a common respect for the dignity of the human person rather than to any specific denominational stance. They are particularly appropriate to a society which was founded on the belief that all human beings are created equal as bearers of the inalienable right to life.

On Sept. 16, 1986, this amicus filed a motion for leave to file a brief amicus curiae. On Oct. 2, 1986, this court entered an order granting the New Jersey Catholic Conference leave to file a brief amicus curiae. See appendix at 1.

Argument

As moral teachers the bishops of the New Jersey Catholic Conference condemn all offenses against life itself such as murder, genocide, abortion, euthanasia or willful suicide. These crimes damage not only the individual person but also the common good. The entire human race is called to protect human life and every time we fail to do so we injure society at large. The interest of the state embraces "two separate but related concerns: an interest in preserving the life of the particular patient and an interest in preserving the sanctity of all life." *Matter of Conroy*, 98 N.J. 321, 349 (1985).

Our teaching is grounded in respect for the dignity and fundamental rights of the human person and cannot be rejected on grounds of political or religious pluralism.

Our religious principles sharpen our concern for human dignity and our regard for the laws of nature and nature's God, but we join the broad common stream of ethical consciousness when we ask the court not to look favorably on a plea for sanctioning starvation as a means of death for a patient who would not otherwise die immediately. In this we make no ethical judgment of the plaintiff. Indeed we can understand their motivation. Our emphasis, rather, is that the corporate conscience of the nursing home reflects traditional public policy which has brought us our laws against aiding suicide and euthanasia, and has resulted in the type of patient care which balances duty and benefits to society against a spurious "right to die" and relief from burdens sustained regularly by a multitude of suffering but non-terminal patients across the nation.

The conference maintains that nutrition and hydration, being basic to human life, are aspects of normal care, which are not excessively burdensome, that should always be provided to a patient. Nutrition and hydration are clearly distinguished from medical treatment. Medical treatment is aimed at curing a disease. Nutrition and hydration are directed at sustaining life. Medical treatment is therapeutic; nutrition and hydration are not, because they will not cure any disease. For that fundamental reason we insist that nutrition and hydration must always be maintained. As the Pontifical Academy of Sciences noted in its report on "The Artificial Prolongation of Life and the Exact Determination of the Moment of Death": "If the patient is in a permanent coma, irreversible as far as it is possible to predict,

treatment is not required but care, including feeding, must be provided" (emphasis added), Catholic New York, Nov. 7, 1985 at 7. The bishops' Committee for Pro-Life Activities views nutrition and hydration in this way:

"Because human life has inherent value and dignity regardless of its condition, every patient should be provided with measures which can effectively preserve life without involving too grave a burden. Since food and water are necessities of life for all human beings, and can generally be provided without the risks and burdens of more aggressive means for sustaining life, the law should establish a strong presumption in favor of their use." ("Statement on Uniform Rights of the Terminally Ill Act," Committee for Pro-Life Activities, National Conference of Catholic Bishops, (1986); See also "Declaration on Euthanasia," Vatican Congregation for the Doctrine of the Faith, (1980) at 10.).

Indeed, in 1984, amendments to the federal "Child Abuse Prevention and Treatment Act" defined the withholding of life-sustaining treatment from handicapped infants as a form of neglect to be investigated by state child protective agencies. See 42 U.S.C.A. 5103(b)(2)(K). Infants who are "chronically and irreversibly comatose" need not receive most forms of medical treatment, but must be provided with "appropriate nutrition and hydration." See 42 U.S.C.A. 5102(3).

In testifying before Congress on these amendments, U.S. Surgeon General C. Everett Koop observed: "The bottom line in all these cases is that you must nourish the patient (severely handicapped newborn infants). Whether an infant in a hospital is denied food and care, or whether an infant at home is denied food and care, the result is the same; it is child abuse." P.L. 98-457, 1984 U.S. Code

Cong. and Adm. News, 2927. These amendments followed the "Principles of Treatment of Disabled Infants" issued in 1983 by a broad coalition of leading medical associations and advocacy organizations for the disabled. This document provided: "It is ethically and legally justified to withhold medical or surgical procedures which are clearly futile and will only prolong the act of dying. However, supportive care should be provided, including sustenance as medically indicated and relief of pain and suffering. Pediatrics, vol. 73, no. 4, (April 1984), at 559. We cannot understand why failure to provide nutrition and hydration to a handicapped child constitutes actionable child abuse but withdrawal of nutrition and hydration from an incompetent adult would be permissible.

Others have recognized that the provision of nutrition and hydration does not constitute medical treatment. Food and water are the most basic means of caring for human beings and are the most powerful symbols of human care. Callahan, "On Feeding the Dying," 13 Hastings Center Report 22 (October 1983): Derr, "Nutrition and Hydration as Elective Therapy: Brophy and Jobes From an Ethical and Historical Perspective," Issues in Law and Medicine, Vol. 2, no. 1, (July 1986). The withholding or withdrawal of food and fluids is distinguishable from the withholding or withdrawal of medical or surgical therapy by its finality. As Professor Meilaender of Oberlin College has noted, "deprive a person of food and water and she will die as surely as if we had administered a lethal drug, and it is hard to claim that we did not aim at her death." Meilaender, "On Removing Food and Water: Against the Stream," 14 Hastings Center Report, 11, 12 (December 1984). A number of

unwholesome consequences flow from withholding the nourishment that sustains all life. "A social decision to compel or permit physicians to deny food and fluids for patients who are capable of receiving and utilizing them . . . attacks directly the very foundation of medicine as an ethical profession." Derr, *supra* at 31. Modern societies have attempted to get rid of retarded, psychotic, senile, handicapped and racially undesirable citizens by a systematic withholding or withdrawal of foods and fluids. Siegler and Weisbard, "Against the Emerging Stream: Should Fluids and Nutritional Support be Discontinued?," 145 Arch. Internal Med. 129, 130 (January 1985).

Another relevant consideration when nutrition and hydration are withdrawn is the specific effect of that act. A person who withdraws these ordinary means to preserve life is instrumental in bringing about the death of the patient. When the patient dies, death does not come from the original disease. The patient dies of starvation. When this is done with the intention to end or shorten the life of the patient, it is intentional euthanasia.

There is no dispute that nutrition and hydration are beneficial because they would preserve the permanently unconscious patient's life. Nor can it be said that the care involved in feeding is burdensome to the permanently unconscious patient. Meilaender, *supra* at 13. In fact, the court below indicated that Mrs. Jobes "appears to be pain free," Matter of Jobes, No. C-4971-85E (Ch. Div. 1986), S.O. at 13. Meilaender reaches the following conclusion: "For the permanently unconscious person, feeding is neither useless nor excessively burdensome. It is ordinary human care and is not given as treatment for any life-threatening disease. Since this is true, a decision not to offer such care can enact only one intention: to take the life of the unconscious person." Meilaender, *supra* at 13. Seen in this way, it is clear that withdrawal of nutrition and hydration from a permanently unconscious person would be unethical.

What is being placed squarely at issue by the decision of the court below is the usefulness of prolonging the life of a patient who is not dying but is in what is claimed to be a persistent vegetative state. Simply put, the court below made a judgment as to the quality of life of the patient. Earlier this court specifically rejected decision making based on assessments of the personal worth or social utility of another's life, or the value of that life to others. *Matter of Conroy, supra* at 367. To make a decision on the quality of life is in the view of many to practice euthanasia by omission. Euthanasia is understood as any act or omission which either by nature or intention brings on the death of the patient to end suffering. Since bringing on death is directly intended in quality of life decisions, such decisions fulfill the definition of intentional euthanasia by omission. Connery, "Quality of Life," *Linacre Quarterly,* (February 1986) at 33.

The argument that if nutrition and hydration merely prolong biological life there is no obligation to use them is open to serious challenge, as Connery has observed. As long as evidence of human life is present, and it is present until death occurs, a living human person exists. It cannot be said to be mere biological life. The only thing of certainty with severely brain-damaged persons is that the patient cannot communicate with the outside world. It is not known whether the patient can receive communications from the outside. Nor can we rule out some kind of interior life. To posit

that there is only biological life in a human being who is still alive is a judgment which goes beyond scientific evidence.

A major difficulty with a quality of life approach is that it puts "one on a slippery slope with no braking power." Connery, *Linacre Quarterly, supra* at 33. Once the line between quality of treatment and quality of life is crossed, there is no effective way of drawing another line. Today food and nutrition is withdrawn from someone in a persistent comatose state; tomorrow such care is withdrawn from someone suffering from Alzheimer's disease. Siegler, *supra* at 130. Indeed, in a recent article clinicians advocated the withholding of nutrition and hydration from severely and irreversibly demented patients and perhaps at times from elderly patients with permanent mild impairment of competence, a group they referred to as the "pleasantly senile." Wanzer et al. "The Physician's Responsibility Toward Hopelessly Ill Patients," 310 N. Eng. J. Med. 955 (1984). The Catholic bishops of New Jersey, along with the National Conference of Catholic Bishops, have squarely rejected the "quality of life" approach, saying that "life-sustaining treatment should not be discriminatorily withheld or withdrawn from mentally incompetent or retarded patients." "Guidelines for Legislation on Life-Sustaining Treatment," National Conference of Catholic Bishops' Committee for Pro-Life Activities, (Nov. 10, 1984), at 4.

One facet of the decision of the court below with which we agree is its judgment that the nursing home "shall have the right to refuse to participate in the removal of such feeding device and to refuse to permit any feeding device to be removed while Mary Ellen Jobes is a resident of that nursing home." *Matter of Jobes, supra,* S.O. at 17. To the same effect, see *Brophy* v. *New England Sinai Hospital Inc.,* N4152 (Mass. Sup. Jud. Ct., Sept. 11, 1986) S.O. at 31. The court further ruled that the husband of Mrs. Jobes has the right to take her to his home where the feeding tube could be removed under medical supervision. *Matter of Jobes, supra,* at 17. The court quite properly did not compel the nursing home to violate its moral and ethical principles by acceding to the request of the patient's spouse that nutrition and hydration be withdrawn. Further the court correctly did not force the nursing home to find another health facility to accomplish the requested action. We maintain that a private or religiously sponsored hospital or health care facility should not be compelled to violate its moral and ethical principles directly or indirectly. Regrettably that is precisely what occurred in the recent case of *Matter of Requena, supra.* In that case the trial court compelled a hospital run by a Catholic religious order of sisters to accept the decision of a woman who is suffering from amyotrophic lateral sclerosis to refuse artificial feeding. The court further ordered that the patient not be removed from the hospital without her consent, rejecting the hospital's offer to assist her in transferring to another institution. S.O. at 12. We submit this decision is an unwarranted and unjustified judicial interference with the moral and ethical policy of a private or religiously sponsored hospital. Moreover, we believe the court's action impermissibly burdens religious belief, practice or governance in violation of the First Amendment of the U.S. Constitution. Significantly, neither the trial court nor the appellate division in considering the Requena case mentioned the proper standard of review with re-

spect to decisions of governing boards of hospitals, which was set forth by this court in *Guerrero* v. *Burlington County Mem. Hosp.* 70 N.J. 345 (1976). In that case the court held that courts have consistently "evinced a sensitivity to the need of hospital administrators to be able reasonably to exercise their discretion without judicial interference, at the same time remaining alert to strike down action that is discriminatory or unfair." A fair reading of the opinions in Requena discloses no evidence of an unreasonable exercise of discretion on the part of the hospital administrators.

Conclusion

We believe that we have presented good and compelling reasons why this court should recognize that nutrition and hydration are basic to human life and consequently must always be provided to a patient. We acknowledge that our position has not been upheld by those courts which recently have grappled with this issue. See e.g. *Matter of Conroy, supra; Brophy* v. *New England Sinai Hospital Inc., supra.* We submit that these decisions have gone too far. We urge this court to stop the trend toward a public policy which does not advocate the preservation of life. In deciding this case, we respectfully request this court to keep in mind its words in Conroy that "it is best to err, if at all, in favor of preserving life." *Matter of Conroy, supra,* at 368. A society which will not sanction death by starvation in Ethiopia should not tolerate it when it is accomplished under medical supervision in a hospital or a nursing home.

32

Georgia Man Asks to Turn Off Life-Supporting Ventilator

Archdiocese of Atlanta

At the court's request, the Most Reverend Eugene A. Marino, on behalf of the Roman Catholic Archdiocese of Atlanta (hereinafter the "archdiocese"), hereby submits this amicus brief relating to petitioner's request for declaratory relief. This brief will address both the legal and ecclesiastical positions relevant to the petitioner's request.

Background

In his petition, Larry James McAfee informed the court that he is a quadriplegic patient being sustained on a ventilator who, as a result, has "no control over his person and receives no enjoyment out of life" (Petition, Para. 2). He suffered a motorcycle accident on May 5, 1985, and has since been paralyzed from the neck down. His lungs no longer function on their own, and he cannot care for himself. He has petitioned the court for an order allowing him to "turn off his own ventilator by means of a mechanical device operated on a timer, that he be provided with a sedative before turning off said ventilator and, thereafter, that said ventilator not be restarted even though such is a life-sustaining medical treatment" (Petition, Para. 3).

Mr. McAfee contends that he is competent to decide as to his medical treatment, that his living relatives all consent to his request for relief, that he has no dependents, that his condition is irreversible and that "the continued treatment by ventilator merely prolongs petitioner's emotional pain and suffering" (Petition, Para. 9).

On Aug. 16, 1989, the court conducted a bedside hearing with Mr. McAfee, along with attorneys for the Fulton-DeKalb Authority and Grady Hospital, and therein received testimony that confirmed the allegations contained in the petition. Thus, the material facts of this case appear not to be contested.

The sole question before the court appears to be whether Mr. McAfee, a competent

"Georgia Man Asks to Turn Off Life-Supporting Ventilator" by the Archdiocese of Atlanta. Reprinted from Origins 19 *(September 28, 1989): 273–279.*

adult, has the right to refuse extraordinary medical treatment, without interference from third parties, even though such refusal will likely result in his immediate death. Recognizing the unsettling nature of this question, the archdiocese neither opposes nor advocates Mr. McAfee's petition, but is of the opinion that granting his request would not be assisting in suicide or undermining the state's and the Roman Catholic Church's interest in preserving life. This amicus brief will present and discuss both legal and ecclesiastical authorities on the issue.

I. Legal Authorities

It has been said that "(t)he law always lags behind the most advanced thinking in every area. It must wait until the theologians and the moral leaders and events have created some common ground, some consensus" (Burger, "The Law and Medical Advances," 67 Annals Internal Med. Supp. 7, 15, 17 (1967), quoted in *Superintendent of Belchertown State School vs. Saikewicz*, 373 Mass. 728, 370 N.E. 2d 417, 423 (Mass. 1977). This case represents a morally troubling issue for this court and for society in general. As to this situation, however, the law, the theologians, moral leaders and events have apparently arrived at "some common ground, some consensus."

A. The Constitutional Right to Privacy

As pointed out in Mr. McAfee's brief, virtually every court that has addressed this issue in recent years has found that competent adult patients have the right, both under common law and constitutional bases, to choose to receive either active, aggressive medical treatment, something less than that or no treatment at all. This right includes the right to choose an early death rather than a later one, but does not include taking direct steps to terminate life. *Griswold vs. State of Connecticut*, 381 U.S. 479, 85 S. Ct. 1678 (1965); *Zant vs. Prevatte*, 248 Ga. 832, 286 S.E. 2d 715 (1982); *Kirby vs. Spivey*, 167 Ga. App. 751, 307 S.E.2d 538 (1983); *Bartling vs. Superior Court*, 163 Cal. App. 3d 186, 209 Cal. Rptr. 220 (1984); *Lane vs. Candura*, 6 Mass. App. 377, 376 N.E.2d 1232 (1978); *In re: Gardner*, 534 A.2d 947 (Me. 1987); *Satz vs. Perlmutter*, 379 So. 2d 359 (Fla. 1980); *Tune vs. Walter Reed Hospital*, 602 F. Supp. 1452 (D.C. 1985); *In re Farrell*, 108 N.J. 335, 529 A. 2d 404 (1987).

In the landmark case of *Griswold vs. State of Connecticut*, 381 U.S. 479, 85 S. Ct. 1678 (1965), the U.S. Supreme Court expressly recognized a constitutional "penumbral" guarantee of privacy inherent within the Bill of Rights. Specifically, in holding that a Connecticut law forbidding the use of contraceptives unconstitutionally intruded upon the right of marital privacy, the court recognized that the various guarantees inherent in the First, Third, Fourth and Fifth Amendments to the U.S. Constitution created "zones of privacy" (*id.* at 1681), and that this inherent right of privacy and repose is "no less important than any other right carefully and particularly reserved to the people." *Id.* at 1682.

B. Georgia Authorities

Relying on this constitutional right of privacy, Georgia courts have consistently upheld the right of competent individuals to refuse medical care or food, even if such refusal resulted in death. For example, in *Zant vs. Prevatte*, 248 Ga. 832, 286 S.E.2d 715 (1982), the superintendent of the Georgia Diagnostic and Classification Center in Butts County petitioned the court for an order authorizing him to impose medical examinations upon a prison inmate against his will "and, if necessary, to force-feed Prevatte to prevent his death." *Id.* at 832. The court found that Mr. Prevatte was sane and rational and that "without food, Prevatte would die within three weeks, sooner if no liquid is taken." *Id.* at 833. It nevertheless concluded that "the state has no right to monitor this man's physical condition against his will; neither does it have the right to feed him to prevent his death from starvation if that is his wish." *Id.* at 834.

Later, in *Kirby vs. Spivey,* 167 Ga. App. 751, 307 S.E. 2d 538 (1983), the heirs of a decedent, Mr. Echols, sued a nursing home and the attending physician, Dr. Spivey, claiming that Mr. Echols' death resulted from Dr. Spivey's malpractice in failing "to diagnose and treat Mr. Echols for renal failure and cancer of the prostate, the conditions alleged to have ultimately led to his death." *Id.* at 751. Prior to his death, Mr. Echols was lucid and, in Dr. Spivey's opinion, "entirely capable of making a rational decision to decline treatment." *Id.* He had no wife or children, and his other relatives never visited him. According to Dr. Spivey, Mr. Echols, upon learning of his illness, refused to authorize further diagnostic testing and treatment and eventually died. The court first turned to the language of O.C.G.A., Sec. 31-9-7, which provides that a person 18 years of age or over has a right "to refuse to consent to medical and surgical treatment as to his own person." It then concluded as a matter of law that "a lucid adult has the right to withhold his consent to suggested and recommended medical procedures" and that "a patient, by virtue of his right of privacy, can refuse to allow intrusion on his person, even though calculated to preserve his life." *Id.* at 753.

The case of *In re L.H.R.,* 253 Ga. 439, 321 S.E.2d 716 (1984), involved a petition for declaratory relief as to whether life-support systems could be removed from a terminally ill infant. In again upholding an individual's right to decline treatment, the court first noted that "in Georgia, as elsewhere, a competent adult patient has the right to refuse medical treatment in the absence of conflicting state interest." *Id.* at 722. It then went on to address the "narrow question" as to "who may exercise this right on behalf of a terminally ill infant who is in a chronic vegetative state with no reasonable possibility of attaining cognitive function." *Id.* The court concluded that "the decision whether to end the dying process is a personal decision for family members or those who bear a legal responsibility for the patient." *Id.* at 723.

Effective July 1, 1984, the Georgia General Assembly enacted the Living Wills Act, O.C.G.A. Sec. 31-32-1 *et seq.* in which it expressly recognized "the right of a competent adult person to make a written directive, known as a living will, instructing his physician to withhold or withdraw life-sustaining procedures in the event of a terminal condition." Although confined to patients who are certified by two physicians as having a "terminal condition" (defined as those having "no reasonable expectation for improvement" and facing imminent death), the statute expressly recognizes "the dignity and privacy which patients have a right to expect" O.C.G.A. Sec. 31-32-1(d). Thus, Georgia law and Georgia courts recognize the personal right of a lucid adult to refuse medical treatment, even if he is not terminally ill and even if such refusal will result in his death.

C. *Authorities From Other Jurisdictions*

As pointed out in the petitioner's brief, other jurisdictions have likewise upheld the right of non-terminally ill competent adults to refuse medical treatment. In *Bartling vs. Supe-*

rior Court, 163 Cal. App. 3d 186, 209 Cal. Rptr. 220 (1984), the California Court of Appeals upheld the right of a non-terminally ill patient to disconnect his ventilator, a situation virtually identical to this:

"In short, the law recognizes the individual interest in preserving the inviolability of the person . . . . The constitutional right of privacy guarantees to the individual the freedom to choose to reject, or refuse to consent to, intrusions of his bodily integrity," *Id.* at 225.

Likewise, in *Lane vs. Candura,* 6 Mass. App. 377, 376 N.E.2d 1232 (1978), the court, in upholding the right of a patient to refuse amputation of a gangrenous leg, stated:

"The constitutional right to privacy, as we conceive it, is an expression of the sanctity of individual free choice and self-determination as fundamental constituents of life. The value of life as so perceived is lessened not by a decision to refuse treatment, but by the failure to allow a competent human being the right of choice," *Id.* at 1233.

D. Medical Authorities

Finally, experts on medical ethics appear to have arrived at a consensus as to a competent patient's right to decline medical treatment under virtually all situations. A 1983 report from the President's Commission for the Study of Ethical Problems in Medicine and Biomedical and Behavior Research concluded, in part:

"(T)he voluntary choice of a competent and informed patient should determine whether or not life-sustaining therapy will be undertaken, just as such choices provide the bases for other decisions about medical treatment. . . . Health-care professionals serve patients best by maintaining a presumption in favor of sustaining life, while recognizing that competent patients are entitled to chose to forgo any treatments, including those that sustain life." *Deciding to Forgo Life-Sustaining Treatment,* at pp. 3, 5 (U.S. Govt. Printing Office, 1983).

Likewise, the American Hospital Association policy and statement of patients' choices of treatment options, approved by the AHA in 1985, provided in pertinent part: "Whenever possible, however, the authority to determine the course of treatment, if any, should rest with the patient," and "the right to choose treatment includes the right to refuse a specific treatment or all treatment."

Finally, the Council on Ethical and Judicial Affairs of the American Medical Association adopted a statement on March 15, 1986, titled "Withholding or Withdrawing Life-Prolonging Medical Treatment" that provided in relevant part that "the social commitment of the physician is to sustain life and relieve suffering. Where the performance of one duty conflicts with the other, the choice of the patient, or his family or legal representative, if the patient is incompetent to act on his own behalf, should prevail."

E. Countervailing State Interests

The legal right to refuse medical treatment is not absolute, however, and can in certain circumstances be limited by one of several countervailing state interests. These overriding interests can include: 1) the preservation of life in general (discussed in *Superintendent of Belchertown State School vs. Saikewicz,* 373 Mass. 728, 370 N.E. 2d 417, 423–427 (Mass. 1977); 2) the prevention of suicide [See *Erickson vs. Dilgard,* 44 Misc. 2d. 27, 252 N.Y.S.2d 705 (N.Y. Sup. Ct. 1962)]; 3) the protection of innocent third persons, such as dependent children (See *Holmes vs. Silver Cross Hosp. of Joliet, Ill.,* 340 F. Supp. 125 (N.D. Ill. 1972); and 4) the preservation of the medical profession's integrity. See Ezekiel J. Emanuel, "A Review of the Ethical and Legal Aspects of Terminating Medical Care," 84 Am. J. Med. 291 (1988). In this case, however, none of these countervailing state interests appears to be applicable or overriding.

In *Jefferson vs. Griffin-Spaulding County Hospital Authority*, 247 Ga. 86, 274 S.E. 2d 457 (1981), the Georgia Supreme Court found that "an expectant mother in the last weeks of pregnancy lacks the right to refuse necessary life-saving surgery and medical treatment where the life of the unborn child is at stake." *Id.* at 90. Thus, in that case, the state's interest in the life of the unborn child outweighed the mother's right to refuse life-sustaining medical treatment. Here, however, Mr. McAfee has no dependent children and, as noted by Justice Hill, "a competent adult does have the right to refuse necessary life-saving surgery and medical treatment (i.e., has the right to die) where no state interest other than saving the life of the patient is involved." *Id.* at 89-90.

F. Refusing Treatment vs. Suicide

Neither the U.S. Constitution nor common law provides an individual with the right to commit suicide, and no court, to date, has authorized anyone or any entity to take direct steps to terminate life. As a matter of civil law, however, several states have held that "declining life-sustaining medical treatment may not properly be viewed as an attempt to commit suicide." *Brophy vs. New England Sinai Hospital Inc.*, 398 Mass. 417, 439, 497 N.E. 2d 626, 638 (1986). Rather: "Refusing medical intervention merely allows the disease to take its natural course; if death were eventually to occur, it would be the result, primarily, of the underlying disease and not the result of self-inflicted injury." *Id.*

In *Brophy*, the petitioning patient was not terminally ill, although he was rendered incompetent as a result of a ruptured aneurysm. Acting on Mr. Brophy's behalf, his wife requested that the hospital stop feeding her husband by way of gastronomy tube. *Id.* at 422, 497 N.E.2d at 628. The court found that removing the feeding tube merely allowed the patient's body to follow its natural course, *id.* at 439, 497 N.E.2d at 638, and rejected the state's argument that the discontinuance of medical treatment constituted suicide.

Similarly, in *Bartling vs. Superior Court*, 163 Cal. App. 3d 186, 209 Cal. Rptr. 220 (1984), the California Court of Appeals found that disconnecting a ventilator on a patient did not assist him in committing suicide, but "merely have hastened his inevitable death by natural causes" 163 Cal. App. 3d 196, 209 Cal. Rptr. 225 (1984). Finally, in the case of *In re Gardner*, 534 A.2d 947 (Me. 1987), the court found that in allowing a patient's ventilator to be disconnected, "the cause of his death will not be his refusal of care but rather his accident and his resulting medical condition, including his inability to (breathe on his own)." *Id.* at 956.

Thus, the legal and medical authorities seem to be in agreement that:

1) Competent adult patients have the right to refuse medical treatment or intrusions on their persons, even if such refusal will likely result in death.

2) This right exists whether the patient is terminally ill or not; and

3) If death occurs, it results from the underlying disease or injury and not from the refusal of care.

II. Ecclesiastical Authorities

This brief will focus on the basic principles which underlie Roman Catholic tradition relative to the artificial prolongation of life. On June 26, 1980, the Vatican Congregation for the Doctrine of the Faith issued a declaration on euthanasia which was approved by His Holiness Pope John Paul II and which represents the official position of the church. The declaration, which is a definitive statement, represents a compilation based on writings and opinions from theological ethicists of the Roman Catholic faith over many centuries and therefore effectively presents what might be described as a universal ecclesiastical consensus on the subject.

A. *The Sanctity of Life*

The Roman Catholic Church views life as "a gift of God's love, which (believers) are called upon to preserve and make fruitful." "Declaration on Euthanasia," p. 3. In light of this view, "intentionally causing one's own death or suicide is therefore equally as wrong as murder; such an action on the part of a person is to be considered as a rejection of God's sovereignty and loving plan." *Id.*

Nevertheless, one must clearly distinguish suicide from that sacrifice of one's life whereby for a higher cause, such as God's glory, the salvation of souls or the service of one's brethren, a person offers his or her own life and puts it in danger. *Id.* In this case, it does not appear that Mr. McAfee seeks to commit suicide.

B. *The Physician's Obligation to His Patient*

The obligation to preserve or prolong life ultimately resides with the patient. If a mentally competent patient decides not to prolong his life, however, a conflict may arise between the patient and his physician. In such a case:

"The obligation of the physician, therefore, is to do nothing to the patient without first informing the patient of what he thinks should be done, with the significant alternatives (including doing nothing), and the probable risks and benefits of each . . . . The doctor's right and responsibility extends only to informing the patient truthfully about his or her terminal condition and the possible ways in which this can be handled medically. The choice among these is the patient's, although this choice cannot be made prudently without honest and substantially complete medical information." *Moral Responsibilities in Prolonging Life Decisions,* Pope John Center, St. Louis, 1981, p. 120.

In making his decision, it is essential that the patient be fully informed and understand the consequences of his decision:

"In numerous cases, the complexity of the situation can be such as to cause doubts about the way ethical principles should be applied. In the final analysis, it pertains to the conscience either of the sick person, or those qualified to speak in the sick person's name, or the doctor's to decide in the light of moral obligations and of the various aspects of the case." "Declaration on Euthanasia," Congregation for the Doctrine of the Faith," June 26, 1980, p. 8.

C. *Ordinary vs. Extraordinary Treatment*

From the perspective of moral theology, there are two major categories of treatment: ordinary and extraordinary. A patient is obligated to accept the former, but may decline the latter if he, in his informed capacity, so chooses. The competent patient (mentally, emotionally and psychologically) is the one to decide whether a medical treatment is ordinary or extraordinary, and his informed, subjective decision should not be subject to interference or criticism.

The two categories are not specifically defined in the "Declaration on Euthanasia," but moral theologians have compiled their own definitions which are helpful. Thus, *ordinary* means of preserving life "are those means commonly used in given circumstances, which this individual in his present physical, psychological and economic condition can reasonably employ with definite hope of proportionate benefit." Cronin, Daniel, "The Moral Law in Regard to the Ordinary and Extraordinary Means of Conserving Life" (dissertation, Pontifical Gregorian University), Rome, 1958, p. 127-28. On the other hand, *extraordinary* means of preserving life are "those not commonly used in given circumstances, or those means in common use which this individual in his present physical, psychological and economic condition cannot reasonably employ, or if he can, will not give him hope of proportionate benefit." *Id.* at 128.

Thus, the category in which a particular treatment falls is necessarily judged by subjective criteria on a case-by-case basis. A means of preserving life may be deemed ordinary for one patient, but extraordinary for another, depending on the patient's particular physical, psychological or economic condition at the time or his perception of the "hope of proportionate benefit" resulting from the treatment.

In making his decision, the patient must focus on a number of questions:

1. What sort of treatment is proposed/ongoing?

2. What degree of complexity or risk is involved?

3. What is the cost and availability of the treatment?

4. Taking into account the state of the patient, including his physical, psychological and economic resources, what result can be hoped for by employing the proposed/ongoing treatment?

D. Ecclesiastical Guidelines

The "Declaration on Euthanasia" provides the following clarifications when reviewing these difficult questions:

—"If there are no other sufficient remedies, it is permitted, with the patient's consent, to have recourse to the means provided by the most advanced medical techniques, even if these means are still at the experimental stage and are not without a certain risk. By accepting them, the patient can even show generosity in the service of humanity.

—"It is also permitted, with the patient's consent, to interrupt these means where the results fall short of expectations. But for such a decision to be made, account will have to be taken of the reasonable wishes of the patient's family, as also of the advice of the doctors who are specially competent in the matter. The latter may in particular judge that the investment in instruments and personnel is disproportionate to the results foreseen; they may also judge that the techniques applied impose on the patient strain or suffering out of proportion with the benefits which he or she may gain from such techniques.

—"It is also permissible to make do with the normal means that medicine can offer. Therefore one cannot impose on anyone the obligation to have recourse to a technique which is already in use, but which carries a risk or is burdensome. Such refusal is not the equivalent of suicide; on the contrary, it should be considered as an acceptance of the human condition or a wish to avoid the application of a medical procedure disproportionate to the results that can be expected or a desire not to impose excessive expense on the family or the community.

—"When inevitable death is imminent in spite of the means used, it is permitted in conscience to take the decision to refuse forms of treatment that would only secure a precarious and burdensome prolongation of life, so long as the normal care due to the sick person in similar cases is not interrupted. In such circumstances, the doctor has no reason to reproach himself with failing to help the person in danger." "Declaration on Euthanasia," pp. 9-10.

In its conclusion, the "Declaration on Euthanasia" states that "life is a gift of God, and on the other hand, death is unavoidable; it is necessary therefore that we, without in any way hastening the hour of death, should be able to accept it with full responsibility and dignity." *Id.* at 11.

Here, Mr. McAfee has testified that as a result of his present condition and his treatment he "receives no enjoyment out of life" (Petition, Para. 2), his "continued treatment by ventilator merely prolongs (his) emotional pain and suffering (Petition, Para. 9), he is currently without economic resources and is being maintained by public funds (Transcript, pp. 10-11); he has discussed his wishes with his family, who consent to his request (Transcript pp. 21-23), he is "still in a lot of pain" (Transcript, p. 18), his condition is irreversible (Transcript, p. 29), and "there is nothing to look forward to" (Transcript p. 18). Applying

the subjective criteria presented by (Bishop) Daniel Cronin to Mr. McAfee's situation, the ventilator, as applied to Mr. McAfee to prolong his life, clearly constitutes an "extraordinary means of preserving life."

Based on the facts as set forth above as well as the basic principles which outline Catholic tradition relative to the artificial prolongation of life, it is the position of the Archdiocese of Atlanta that the patient, Mr. McAfee, has the right under ecclesiastical law either to continue his present treatment or to interrupt that treatment even though such interruption will end in death.

E. Use of Painkillers When Refusing Medical Treatment

Mr. McAfee has requested that he be given a sedative before he activates a timer which will turn off his ventilator. In the opinion of the archdiocese, this request is irrelevant to Mr. McAfee's and this court's decision in this case. The Roman Catholic Church recognizes that while physical suffering is an unavoidable element of the human condition, "it often exceeds its own biological usefulness and so can become so severe as to cause the desire to remove it at any cost." "Declaration on Euthanasia," p. 6.

The Roman Catholic Church teaches:

"(I)t would be imprudent to impose a heroic way of acting as a general rule. On the contrary, human and Christian prudence suggest for the majority of sick people the use of medicines capable of alleviating or suppressing pain, even though these may cause as a secondary effect semiconsciousness and reduced lucidity." *Id.* at 7.

Thus, Mr. McAfee's request for sedation is not offensive to the Roman Catholic Church.

Conclusion

The archdiocese is submitting this brief to be used as guidance for addressing a difficult and unsettling issue. The archdiocese takes no official position as to whether the relief requested by Mr. McAfee should or should not be granted. The consensus of legal, theological and moralistic authorities, however, supports Mr. McAfee's right to refuse further treatment by ventilator, and such refusal in this case would not be the equivalent of suicide. Rather, it can be considered as Mr. McAfee's acceptance of his condition, his wish to avoid the application of a medical procedure disproportionate to the expected results and his desire not to impose excessive expense on his family and the community at large.